PRAISE FOR ANN LOUISE GITTLEMAN:

"I deeply respect and honor the work of Ann Louise Gittleman, whom I consider as a teacher, as well as what she has done to bring intelligence to the world of nutrition."

—Mark Hyman, MD, medical director of Cleveland Clinic's Center for Functional Medicine, thirteen-time *New York Times* bestselling author

"Rather than accepting conventional wisdom, Ann Louise is always lightyears ahead of it. Every time I read her books or attend her talks, I discover something new. She never stops researching, never stops learning, and never stops advancing our field."

—Dr. Kellyann Petrucci, *New York Times* bestselling author, *Dr. Kellyann's Cleanse and Reset*

"From *Fat Flush* to detox, Ann Louise Gittleman is a trailblazer whose impeccable, groundbreaking research and knowledge paved the path for nutritionists today. As she has for the past few decades, Gittleman continues to inspire, motivate, and challenge me today."

—JJ Virgin, four-time *New York Times* bestselling author

"When it comes to wellness through nutrition, Ann Louise Gittleman not only pioneered the field, she continues to be ahead of her time and on top of the game. At *First for Women*, we rely on Gittleman to alert us to the newest scientific studies with the most urgent relevance for our readers—and she always delivers."

—Carol Brooks, editor-in-chief of *Woman's World* and *First for Women* magazines

"Most people have been brought up believing that old age and decline are inevitable. And that becomes their experience. But there is another way. A far more pleasurable way to grow older while maintaining strength, vitality, and joy. That is the message of *Radical Longevity*—a book whose time has truly come."

—Christiane Northrup, MD, *New York Times* bestselling author of *Goddesses Never Age*; *Women's Bodies, Women's Wisdom*; and *The Wisdom of Menopause*

"A longtime guiding light in the world of nutritional medicine, Ann Louise continues to be The First Lady of Nutrition and someone I can always count on for the best information for my patients, my readers, and me. Not only is she knowledgeable and a pioneer in the field but she is a truly caring person who is dedicated to changing the world, one body at a time. I'm proud to call her my friend."

—Hyla Cass, MD, author of *8 Weeks to Vibrant Health*

"I always admired her passion for healing for all, her desire to look deeper, and her healing wisdom."

—Raphael Kellman, MD, of the Kellman Center for Integrative and Functional Medicine and author of *The Microbiome Breakthrough*

"Ann Louise Gittleman, PhD, CNS, is a visionary and pioneer in the world of natural healing. Her bestselling books have revolutionized natural medicine and Ann Louise continues to innovate."

—Izabella Wentz, PharmD, FASCP-Functional Pharmacist, #1 *New York Times* bestselling author of *Hashimoto's Protocol* and *Hashimoto's the Root Cause*

"Ann Louise Gittleman has been a leading innovator in the field of integrative medicine for decades. Her books bring cutting-edge research to health consumers in an easy-to-understand form. She was one of the first to warn of the dangers of our infatuation with low-carb diets, and now science has validated her message."

—Ronald Hoffman, MD, founder of the Hoffman Center, host of *The Intelligent Medicine* podcast

"I recall interviewing her on the radio when I was just starting out in the field of nutritional medicine…I was terrified because she was so much more knowledgeable than I…So I read all her books and became even more impressed. She was one of the greats even back then. She continues to learn, explore, and, best of all, get the message out to millions of adoring fans."

—Fred Pescatore, MD, *New York Times* bestselling author of *The Hamptons Diet*

"Ann Louise is ahead of the nutrition curve. She's always been cutting edge in her approach, having been part of the lineage of nutritional mentors and pioneers who ultimately led the charge forward to the rise in the current twenty-first century health and wellness interests."

—Deanna Minich, PhD, nutritionist and author of *Whole Detox*

"I have known and admired Ann Louise for decades. Her books, like *Radical Longevity*, enable readers to learn cutting-edge information before science announces THEIR 'breakthroughs!'"

—Doug Kaufmann, host of the TV show, *Know the Cause*

RADICAL LONGEVITY

ANN LOUISE GITTLEMAN, PhD, CNS

RADICAL LONGEVITY

**The Powerful Plan to Sharpen
Your Brain, Strengthen
Your Body, and Reverse
the Symptoms of Aging**

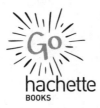

hachette
BOOKS

New York

Copyright © 2021 by Ann Louise Gittleman
Cover design by LeeAnn Falciani
Cover copyright © 2021 by Hachette Book Group, Inc.

Hachette Go, an imprint of Hachette Books
Hachette Book Group
1290 Avenue of the Americas
New York, NY 10104
HachetteGo.com
Facebook.com/HachetteGo
Instagram.com/HachetteGo

First Edition: May 2021

Hachette Books is a division of Hachette Book Group, Inc.
The Hachette Go and Hachette Books names and logos are trademarks of Hachette Book Group, Inc.

The publisher is not responsible for websites (or their content) that are not owned by the publisher.

Print book interior design by Amy Quinn.

Library of Congress Cataloging-in-Publication Data
Names: Gittleman, Ann Louise, author.
Title: Radical longevity : the powerful plan to sharpen your brain,
   strengthen your body, and reverse the symptoms of aging / Ann Louise
   Gittleman.
Description: New York : Hachette Go, [2021] | Includes bibliographical
   references and index.
Identifiers: LCCN 2020044331 | ISBN 9780738286167 (hardcover) | ISBN
   9780306874840 (ebook)
Subjects: LCSH: Longevity—Popular works. | Aging—Prevention—Popular
   works. | Cells—Aging—Popular works.
Classification: LCC RA776.75 .G566 2021 | DDC 612.6/8—dc23
LC record available at https://lccn.loc.gov/2020044331
ISBNs: 978-0-7382-8616-7 (hardcover); 978-0-306-87484-0 (ebook)

Printed in the United States of America

LSC-C

Printing 1, 2021

*To all my fans, friends, and family who
want to live to 120 in the best of health!*

CONTENTS

INTRODUCTION

A New Approach to Aging

I'M NOT A BIG FAN OF "ANTIAGING." IN FACT, I'M PROAGING IN THE SENSE THAT I WANT to continue aging with power, grace, guts, and beauty! I want to be a shining example for radiant longevity by accessing cutting-edge research and combining it with traditional healing wisdom. The exciting news is that it is now possible to live to age one hundred and beyond. It is within our reach and not only possible but plausible with the care, attention, and actions I propose. Yet, for far too many, vibrant longevity is more of a dream than a reality as years of life and happiness dissolve into aches, pains, and an increasing number of age-related degenerative diseases that often progress each advancing year. As my mother used to say, "Getting older ain't for sissies!"

Radical Longevity isn't about "picking your poison" and learning to live longer while tolerating the signs that your body is wearing out. Instead, this book puts to use the many cues your body provides as cries of cellular distress by giving you strategies that answer these distress calls immediately and effectively, *before* you progress into illness and disease. Healthy aging should be a gradual and natural transition, giving our body and our mind time to adjust. Too often, I find that many of us—with each passing year and telltale symptom—feel betrayed by our body. But why should we accept the changes that the body experiences as some sort of extended decline and wind down instead of extending years of youthfulness and pain-free living? All of us are capable of aging while feeling and looking younger than our chronological age. I've spent decades discovering, testing, understanding, and utilizing strategies to turn on longevity genes and turn off disease-promoting genes, opening pathways that boost our longevity and extend years of vigorous living.

Radical longevity is within your reach. You're going to find abundant health strategies throughout the pages of this book, but let's first address mind-set. My personal philosophy about aging is best expressed with the elegant words I love to quote, "I don't regret aging. It is a privilege denied to many." Take that in for just a moment. Why are so many of us giving up valuable years of living because we've accepted some inevitable health fate dictated by outdated ideas and leftover data from times when we knew less and had fewer options? A future full of possibility is what we dreamed about when we were young. Science, medicine, and our understanding of the human body advance every day. Every time we open our eyes in the morning, we're living in a more modern age. Look forward to your future. Embrace and rejoice in your time. I don't regret growing older at all; in fact, I want to make these the best years of my life.

I believe you do too. I know that you wonder whether there could be more waiting for you. You're eager to learn more and you have the will to put some strategies into practice. I know there is more you want to do and that there is so much to enjoy in every day that takes you into your future. That is why I wrote this book . . . for you.

THE SHOULDERS OF GIANTS

My journey to radical longevity started decades ago, and it has been shaped and inspired by four incredibly remarkable women. It all started with my grandmother, Anna, who I actually never met, but for whom I was named. She died at the age of forty-two as the result of a mysterious illness. While on vacation, she had contracted an unidentifiable viral or bacterial infection that could not be successfully treated with the medical knowledge of the time. She developed unrelenting joint pain, brain fog, and neurological symptoms that drove her to the point of seeking to end her life. My grandmother's hopeless struggle underscored my passion to help those suffering and in distress. In fact, I have made it my life's purpose to uncover the underlying root cause of illness.

I unexpectedly discovered the second most important woman in my life while a sophomore at Connecticut College. One very cold winter morning, I walked into the cafeteria and heard two students enthusiastically talking about a book called *Let's Get Well* by Adelle Davis. I immediately ran out and bought all her books. During the late 1960s and early '70s, Davis was a lone voice in the nutrition wilderness. Her teachings made complete sense to me and I practiced what she preached. I ate Tiger's Milk bars for energy, put brewer's yeast into my yogurt, and used safflower oil for my linoleic acid. She was the first to shine a light on the all-encompassing effects of stress on every system of the body and the role stress plays in disease, along with the importance of taking pantothenic acid, the stress vitamin.

Linda Clark was the third woman most helpful along my journey. Her avant-garde books introduced me to topics that expanded my understanding: color therapy, magnetic healing, radiation toxicity, radionics, heavy metals, and essential fatty acids. Clark really sparked my passion for looking outside the box and pushing past accepted limitations.

Hazel Parcells was my last mentor. Dr. Parcells was the capstone of all my experiences and pointed me in the direction of where and how to look for the underlying causes of diseases. She put a magnifying glass on such areas as parasites—which I had never in my wildest dreams considered as a factor in modern diseases. She also expounded on heavy metal toxicity. She discussed the insidious effects of radiation, mold, fungus, and yeast toxicity decades before others began to consider these factors. Dr. Parcells had worked with Los Alamos and the Manhattan Project with the developers of the atomic bomb. She determined ways to neutralize the nuclear radiation from the fallout, which we can still use today.

Most of all, Dr. Parcells taught me by her own longevity that one hundred is the new sixty. She was eighty four years young when I met her—and lived to the incredible age of one hundred six with all her senses and intellect fully intact. On her one hundred sixth birthday, she said, "So many times I'm asked about the secret of my longevity. I can assure you that there are no secrets. There is only the understanding of nature and the everyday practice of nature's laws."

FROM FAT FLUSH TO RADICAL METABOLISM—TO RADICAL LONGEVITY

In my bestselling books *The Fat Flush Plan* and *Radical Metabolism*, I discuss the neglected and overlooked weight-gain factors, beyond just diet and exercise, which are major contributors to our current obesity epidemic. I target liver and gallbladder congestion, sluggish thyroid, excess inflammation, yeast overgrowth, and hormonal imbalance as potent factors "weighing us down" and which also lead to accelerated aging.

Now, I turn my attention to the multiple factors and underlying *Rules* that play a pivotal role in longevity. We live in a wondrous yet still challenging time. Just consider that Alzheimer's is the fastest growing disease in our day and age, more people have cancer now than did in 1971 at the start of the "war on cancer," and the number of individuals with diabetes and prediabetes is more than the entire population of our grandfathers' era.

At the same time, it is exciting to reimagine our future and find new meaning and purpose in our later years in this era of increased longevity. We can fearlessly and boldly embrace lifestyle strategies that address our physical and spiritual needs. We are all yearning to maintain health, create community, and leave a legacy. We're taking salsa lessons. Starting businesses at fifty. Planning our "second act" at sixty-five. Jumping out of airplanes at seventy. Hiking the Himalayas at seventy-five. We're living much longer than our parents and grandparents did. We are "sage-ing," aging wisely and gracefully, growing in all ways as we age. We are driven to retain and regain our vitality. We are on fire with purpose and possibility as we enter the third trimester of our lives. We will not settle for platitudes, and we will not be patronized.

Yet there are several threats to our vitality and overall health. Quite simply, a healthy body depends on a clean body. As we approach our prime-time years, a clean body becomes increasingly unattainable. Toxins are all around us, hiding in the food we eat, surrounding us in the environment, and even created by our body's own metabolic processes. Our immune system weakens from the toxic toll, and we grow old before our time, gaining weight and becoming vulnerable to heart disease, cancer, and a host of autoimmune disorders.

Staying young and healthy in a toxic world can be a daunting task. Although not terribly radical, one of the most reliable, viable, and widely accepted theories today is that aging itself is caused by oxidative stress. Free radicals (also known as reactive oxygen molecules) do their dirty damage to our cells and tissues by weakening and altering cellular membranes, which allow bacteria and viruses to enter the body. Free radical damage destroys genetic coding, resulting in cellular chaos that can led to deteriorating changes in our tissues and organs, including our brain.

Those most fundamental things we do—even breathing and eating—can cause our body to react with an oxidation response. It's perfectly normal. But with a larger toxic burden already present in the body, it's a process that often goes awry. You've likely seen this process in action. When metal becomes oxidized, for example, it develops rust. When you slice open an apple and leave it in the air, you can plainly see that it turns brown. Oxidation turns fats rancid (if you've ever had old olive oil, you know what I'm talking about). You should also know that the same thing happens in your body: Fat becomes rancid—a process that scientists call lipid peroxidation. This process can set your cardiovascular system at risk for the buildup of unwanted lumps of fat and other debris in your arteries. These clogs are often the instigators of heart attacks and strokes.

These free radicals contribute to arthritis by oxidizing joint fluid, making it less lubricating. They can cause DNA damage to your cells, making cell membranes so rigid that nutrients can't get in, and ultimately make the cell so fragile that it breaks, allowing toxins to come in and fluid to drain out before it finally collapses. This is why this process is considered the root cause of aging and disease, from cancer to Alzheimer's.

Most approaches to fighting free radicals focus only on controlling their devastating effects. Yet the root causes of oxidative stress are shockingly ignored: the hidden killer that is iron overload and copper toxicity; the deceptively innocent but potentially harmful substances appropriately known as AGEs (advanced glycation end products) from certain foods and cooking methods; invisible radiation from cell phones and Wi-Fi; and bioincompatible materials in our mouth (dental materials, cavitations, gum infections, and root canals in the oral cavity).

In this book, I identify and expose the top toxic invaders of our time and, most important, I will show you how to eliminate them from your life with a special diet and regeneration program, along with targeted natural prescriptions for wellness. Along the way, you will also be introduced to the magic bullet longevity molecule that can override many lifestyle bad habits—just in case you're not ready to fully clean up your act.

STONE-AGE BODIES

Almost like characters in a science fiction novel, we have left our body behind as we move forward into the technological future. Our body adapted to the natural foods of preindustrial times. It has not evolved in pace with technological change. We're lacking enzymes and metabolic pathways to break down many of today's artificial foods into harmless by-products. Our body was designed with a complex and sophisticated detoxification system. Made up of the skin, lungs, liver, kidneys, blood, bowels, and lymph, the detox system is capable of working with a precision not duplicated in any of humankind's inventions—it truly is a marvel! But the bad news is that, in addition to eliminating the waste products that result from normal metabolic processes, this system has now been forced to rid the body of heavy metals and toxic chemicals, such as drugs, alcohol, pesticides, herbicides, and food additives. And we make it work even harder having to compensate for our sedentary lifestyles, our fast-food diets, and our stressed-out lives.

Our twenty-first-century lifestyle can often overwhelm our biological design. When this happens, we experience any number of devastating symptoms. A toxic body often makes us tense and irritable, and causes us to age prematurely. We may suffer from headaches, insomnia, depression, allergies, poor digestion, bad breath, or skin problems. Long-term toxic overload can lead to immune suppression and chronic illness, such as arthritis, cancer, and Alzheimer's. In response, we may be given artificial drugs—and even artificial organs—to cure the symptoms often caused by artificial food.

DETOXIFY, DON'T RETOXIFY

I know many people are convinced, as I am, that environmental degradation—and the health threats involved—is under way at a pace unimaginable even a decade ago. One difference is that present-day environmental health threats are unlikely to be as straightforward, and therefore not as visible, as threats from cigarette smoke, asbestos, lead, and tanning beds. As our technology grows more complex in leaps and bounds, nature's responses are growing harder even for experts to read with large-scale destruction of natural resources for immediate industrial rewards.

You don't have to have a PhD, or be an ecologist or environmental activist, to protect your family and yourself from what is happening all around you. It's clear that we don't fully understand all the health consequences when we make trade-offs in our lifestyle and in the environment in which we live. But you can take back your power. Radical Longevity begins with becoming aware of hidden dangers where you live and work and play—and then minimizing any negative effects through daily lifestyle changes and nutritional support. The plan includes a comprehensive strategy with clear actions and targeted, customizable strategies for specific concerns.

The Radical Longevity Plan guides you to realistically take control where you can, particularly with the foods you choose to eat and how you prepare them, the water you drink, and the quality of your indoor environment—from your air and light to the company you keep. Organic, properly cleansed food remains the most effective medicine available. Awareness is the first step needed to protect and control your health.

INTRODUCING THE 7 NEW RULES

We will start our work together toward a healthier, more vibrant, ageless body, less prone to disease and premature aging, by looking in detail at your individual symptoms. Are you tired all the time? Do you suffer from persistent GI issues, such as bloating and nausea after eating? Do you have trouble sleeping? Are you bothered by wrinkles, sagging skin, and brown spots? Are you concerned about thinning bones, arthritic joints, and accelerating aches and pains? Are your memory and mental clarity not as sharp as they used to be?

First, you'll take a self-diagnostic quiz to determine the areas you may want to target.

Next, we'll unpack the 7 New Rules for Radical Longevity. When these rules are not adhered to, their mischievous handiwork shows up in practically every degenerative condition known to humans—painful joints, sagging skin, a weakened heart, and a failing memory. Understanding and following the rules can suspend and slow down the aging process, get a jump on preventing the "diseases of aging"—and lead you to look and feel younger than your peers.

The 7 New Rules for Radical Longevity

New Rule #1: Immunity Is Everything
New Rule #2: Take On Toxic Overload
New Rule #3: Stop AGEs (Advanced Glycation End Products)
New Rule #4: Free Up Fascia for Youthful Movement
New Rule #5: Activate Cellular Rejuvenation

New Rule #6: Mind Your Minerals

New Rule #7: Optimize the Gut-Brain Connection

HOW TO GET THE MOST OUT OF THIS BOOK

Attitudes toward aging have evolved into an adoption of "health is the new wealth." We are all becoming increasingly aware of how the efforts we make to set back the clock can serve us for decades to come. We want to upgrade our aging plan and do much more than just the minimum. We want access to new breakthroughs and advanced techniques that keep us well ahead of the detrimental effects of wear and tear on the body accumulated over the years. This plan addresses both the annoying appearances of aging and the damaging internal effects of ongoing bodily demands that determine how we age and at what level of function and overall vitality we operate.

The seven rules that dictate the Radical Longevity Power Plan are detailed in Part 1, followed by a specific set of actions to take in Part 2. The Power Plan includes detailed meal plans featuring specific fortifying foods, delicious and easy-to-prepare recipes, and all that you need to activate the age-busting cooking techniques that will give you bonus years of life. Once you have learned the Rules and have accessed the Power Plan, you'll find targeted strategies that allow every reader to customize their approach in Part 3. These targeted strategies address epigenetics, reversal of developing disease, and actions that change how you experience life on a daily basis. Implementing these comprehensive and leading-edge actions and health strategies can help free you from accepting any limitations that you're placing on yourself and encourages you to take on life through targeted tactics that are game changers where nothing is inevitable and a new era of superaging is within reach. I'm confident that you are going to learn a lot, find things you want to try, and enhance your life and health every day on this healthful journey. You'll be guided through protocols specifically designed to prevent and relieve each lifestyle or environmental issue that is standing in your way.

THE RADICAL LONGEVITY SELF-ASSESSMENT

The best way to point yourself in the right direction is to know your starting point. This questionnaire is both a lifestyle inventory and a detailed personal aging profile. Use this questionnaire as a way to identify areas of your diet, your lifestyle, and your home or office environment that need a tune-up, while also helping you identify the sources of longevity-stealing toxins. This same assessment will also serve as a means to track your progress through the Radical Longevity Program.

RADICAL LONGEVITY QUESTIONNAIRE

IMMUNE SYSTEM	YES	NO
Do you find yourself getting sick more frequently and with longer recovery periods?		
Do you suffer from inadequate sleep and/or chronic stress?		
Do you have an autoimmune illness?		
Are you susceptible to viral illnesses (e.g., colds, flus, and/or Epstein-Barr)?		
TOXINS: HEAVY METALS	YES	NO
Do you use aluminum pots, pans, or foils for cooking?		
Do you eat off unglazed ceramic dishes?		
Do you have MS, ALS, Alzheimer's, or Parkinson's?		
Do you eat fish, seafood, or sea vegetables more than three meals per week?		
Does your jewelry contain nickel or do you wear metal braces on your teeth?		
Are you taking any medications (including over the counter)?		
Do you have possible lead-based paint in your house if it was built before 1978?		
TOXINS: ENDOCRINE-DISRUPTING CHEMICALS	YES	NO
Do you use conventional cleaning products rather than cleaning with natural substances, such as vinegar and baking soda?		
Do you use pesticides on your lawn and garden?		
Do you use synthetic room fresheners or synthetic perfumes rather than essential oils?		
Do you drink out of plastic water bottles?		
Do you use commercial hand sanitizers?		
Do you use commercial arts-and-crafts supplies?		
Do you use personal care products that contain parabens, often found in commercial skin-care products and cosmetics?		
Do you use chemically based nail polish and nail polish removers?		

TOXINS: PARASITES	YES	NO
Have you ever traveled to remote destinations?		
Do you have pets and animals of any kind?		
Do you allow your pets to sleep with you or eat off your plate?		
Do you eat uncooked foods, such as sushi, salad bar fare, or unwashed fruits and vegetables?		
Have you ever suffered from food poisoning?		
Do you have digestive issues, such as diarrhea, constipation, gas, or bloating on a regular basis (3 times per week or more)?		
Do you have food sensitivities, intolerances, or allergies?		

TOXINS: EMFS	YES	NO
Do you sleep with your cell phone or carry it in your pocket?		
Do you have yearly CT scans or X-rays?		
Do you fly more than four times a year?		
Have you ever undergone any type of radiation treatment?		
Do you have a smart meter?		
Do you have Wi-Fi at home or is your neighbor's Wi-Fi signal strong in your home?		
Do you wear a Fitbit or Apple Watch?		

TOXINS: MOLD	YES	NO
Do you use a humidifier?		
Have you ever had a mold issue in your home?		
Do you shampoo indoor carpets frequently (4 times per year) and let them air dry?		
Do you enjoy roasted peanuts, cashews, and pistachios on a regular basis (2–3 times per week)?		
Do you have wall-to-wall carpeting in your home?		

TOXINS: DENTAL INFECTIONS	YES	NO
Do you have dental amalgams (silver fillings) in your mouth?		
Do you have both gold and silver dental amalgams (divergent metals) in your mouth?		
Have you had one or more root canals?		
Are any of your teeth missing?		
Do you have unexplained weakness on one side of your body?		
Have you been told you have a cavitation (hole in your jaw bone where a tooth was removed)—but were not treated (with ozone) for it?		

AGES (ADVANCED GLYCATION END PRODUCTS)	YES	NO
Are you on a higher-fat diet (e.g., keto or Paleo), and/or enjoy cheese, bacon, and butter every day?		
Do you eat meat more than three times per week?		
Do you frequently (more than three times per week) grill, broil, or fry your food?		
Do you use an air fryer?		
Do you indulge in crispy foods, such as crackers, chips, pretzels, cookies, or breakfast cereals, more than five times per week?		

FASCIA	YES	NO
Have you found yourself getting stiffer as you age?		
Have you had one or more surgeries during your life?		
Have you ever been in a car accident?		
Do you use the same repetitive movements on your job (typing, bending, lifting, etc.)?		
Have you been told by a health professional that your posture needs improvement?		
Do you have a sedentary lifestyle or one that involves little or no exercise?		
Are you a shallow breather or someone who does not breathe deeply?		

MINERALS: COPPER	YES	NO
Do you have copper plumbing in your home?		
Do you take a vitamin-mineral supplement with copper?		
Have you ever had a copper IUD?		
Do you use copper cookware?		
Do you avoid red beans, eggs, or pumpkins seeds (high-zinc foods)?		

IRON	YES	NO
Do you have brown "liver" spots on your body?		
Do you cook in cast iron?		
Does your multiple vitamin contain iron?		
Has it been over a year since you donated blood?		
Are you of Northern European descent?		
Do you eat a lot of iron-fortified foods?		
Does heart disease run in your family?		

OPTIMIZE THE GUT-BRAIN CONNECTION: MICROBIOME	YES	NO
Do you take probiotics?		
Do you have a history of frequent antibiotic use?		
Do you avoid fermented foods?		
Do you typically eat your meals alone?		
If you had a crisis, would you have fewer than three friends you could count on?		

	YES	NO
Do find yourself crying easily and overreacting to situations?		
Are you grieving or suffering from a heartbreak?		
Do you have a virtual (or real) community?		

TARGETED STRATEGIES

BRAIN	YES	NO
Does Alzheimer's concern you?		
Have you developed an unexplained tremor in your hand?		
Are you experiencing unrelenting chronic stress?		
Do you take medication for anxiety or depression?		
Have you ever suffered a head injury?		
Do you take any anticholinergic, statin, narcotic, or steroid medications?		
Have you ever had chemotherapy?		

HEART	YES	NO
Does heart disease run in your family?		
Do you have high ferritin, LDL, homocysteine, or CRP levels?		
Are you a smoker?		
Are you a nonexerciser?		
Do you suffer from high trigylcerides?		

BONES	YES	NO
Do you have low vitamin D levels?		
Have you ever fractured a bone as an adult?		
Do you drink fluoridated water or use a fluoridated toothpaste?		
Do you cook with aluminum pans?		
Do you drink a lot of diet sodas?		
Are you a sugar-holic or do you crave sweets?		
Do you drive instead of walk every chance you get?		
Are you unable to balance on one foot for sixty seconds?		
Do you have a job where you sit for most of the day?		
Do you live in a climate that has cold, snowy winters that make it difficult to get outdoors?		

SKIN	YES	NO
Do you reside north of Los Angeles, Phoenix, or Nashville?		
Do you work inside all day?		
Do you expose your eyes and back to the sun?		
Do you have fine lines and wrinkles?		

	YES	NO
Are you vitamin D deficient?		
Have you had more than three sunburns during your lifetime?		
Do you use chemically based sunscreens?		
Have you been diagnosed with skin cancer?		
Do you avoid all fats in your diet?		
HAIR	**YES**	**NO**
Have you noticed your hair thinning as you age?		
Do you skimp on protein in your daily meals and snacks?		
Do you eat a plant-based diet?		
Do you find yourself tired all the time?		
Do you take medications that have coincided with hair loss?		
Do you have low stomach acid?		
Are you hypothyroid?		
HORMONES	**YES**	**NO**
Does any form of hormone replacement therapy frighten you?		
Do you take an unopposed estrogen replacement therapy?		
Is your sex life nonexistent?		
Are you losing muscle strength?		
Do you suffer from depression or anxiety?		
Is sleeplessness or poor-quality sleep an issue in your life?		
DIET	**YES**	**NO**
Do you eat nonorganic fruits, vegetables, meats, grains, and/or dairy products on a daily basis?		
Do you often eat GMO (genetically modified) foods?		
Do you drink unfiltered water?		
Do you cook with herbs, such as rosemary, less than once a week?		
If you own a slow cooker or Instant Pot, do you use it less than four times a month?		
Do you eat out in restaurants more than five times a week?		
Do you eat processed convenience foods more than three times a week?		
Do you have light-colored stools?		
Are you frequently constipated?		
Do you suffer from nausea, heartburn, burping, reflux, gas, or bloating?		
Do you have a history of gallstones or gallbladder surgery?		
Do you often wake up between one and three o'clock in the morning?		

TAKING IT TO THE NEXT LEVEL	YES	NO
Do you believe your biography is your biology?		
Would you like to reprogram your DNA?		
Would you like to replenish your stem cells?		
Would you be willing to try stem cell activators to reboot your body?		
Would you consider using platelet-rich plasma (PRP) therapy for your joints and skin and for wound healing?		

LONGEVITY ASSESSMENT

If you've answered yes to only one or two questions in any category, you rock! You are already doing a great job in your healthy aging regimen. Continue with all the suggestions in this book to maximize and enjoy your vitality and longevity. On the other hand, if you've answered yes to three or more questions in a category, then this book and its protocols are a top priority for you. The material in the following pages may be just the ticket to help you rewind your biological clock and reduce your total toxic load from environmental challenges. You'll feel younger, more energetic, with glowing skin and a sharper brain, in no time at all. The good news is that the keys to reversing your condition, and reclaiming your health, start on the next page.

PART ONE

7 NEW RULES FOR RADICAL LONGEVITY

CHAPTER 1

NEW RULE #1: IMMUNITY IS EVERYTHING

In this chapter, you'll learn . . .

- Which hormone, vitamin, and mineral are each #1 in creating strong immunity
- How one device in your home can help ensure respiratory health
- Why hand washing with soap is so critical and more effective than hand sanitizer

---

OUR IMMUNE SYSTEM IS OUR FIRST RESPONDER DEFENDING AND PROTECTING US from potentially disruptive, harmful invaders. Our overall immunity determines how we will weather any onslaught of bacteria, mold, fungus, virus, parasites, heavy metals, and chemicals. Additionally, our immunity is subject to highly inflammatory lifestyle factors, such as a diet high in processed and refined carbohydrates, a high intake of sugar and grains, stress, lack of sleep, reduced exercise, unexpected trauma, and physical challenge and change as we advance through life. While we are meant to be strong and resilient throughout life, we are more at risk for autoimmune conditions and infections when our toxic burden "runneth over" and the immune system is unable to function in the way it was designed to optimally perform.

The reason the Rules work together, much as the systems in your body, is that every day your DNA is being damaged in some way. A *healthy* person replaces or repairs their damaged DNA at about the same rate that it was damaged. This is why it is so critical to address our overall health as we age, so that we are advancing our healing, repair, and restoration, not relaxing into "normal" decline over the years. When your hair starts to gray, skin starts to sag, or memory starts to fade, these are signs your body is not able to do all the DNA repair it needs, and oxidative damage is accumulating. Think of these as calls to action rather than an inevitable trajectory of your life and health. Because your immune system is a full-body defense system, the information throughout *Radical Longevity* can have either a direct or indirect impact on your immunity. For that reason, I suggest that you begin your approach in the following way:

Invest. Your immunity fortifies you and is an important assurance in vibrant living. You'll see suggestions and recommendations throughout this book, some dealing directly with immunity and others that affect the immune system as a result of your overall health. It is important to begin thinking about your life holistically—body, mind, spirit, and environment. All are intricately and elegantly connected, and each affects the others. Your time, money, and energy are your resources to use and rely on as you make decisions about how you will invest in your present and future well-being.

Be vigilant and take action. Don't wait to start taking corrective steps, believing "It will get better." That is outdated thinking—we now know that repair is our best defense and early action can greatly reduce recovery time from any challenge or injury.

Every effort counts. Be they small or large, inexpensive or more costly, your efforts count and either add to, or subtract from, vibrant health. Don't ever think that one simple action a day won't make a difference. Everything counts.

Upgrade and update. New science is emerging all the time that tells us more about how to enhance our health. Don't get stuck on any one remedy; be open to trying something new or at another level.

Be your own laboratory. Notice the results as you make changes and increase effort. Keep a diary or create a checklist of desired and expected outcomes that you want to see and at what level and frequency. If you don't actively take notice of the effects of your efforts, you're missing a great chance to fine-tune what you need. Your health-care practitioner is reliant on your compliance with follow-through and your ability to articulate what is going on as a result. Everybody is different, so you are always going to know more about your own body and experience than anyone else.

Note that before you begin taking any supplements, you should check with your health-care provider for any issues or contraindications.

THE ROCK STAR OF IMMUNITY—VITAMIN D

Let's start with the basics. As most of us are already aware, vitamin D is essential to maintain strong bones and reduce the risk of fractures. It stimulates the absorption of calcium and magnesium and promotes mineralization and strengthening of the collagen matrix in bone, increasing bone density and overall health of bone tissue. This process starts in the intestine, then the signal travels to the bones and bone marrow, and once the bone marrow is involved, so is the immune system. Interestingly, a 2012 Spanish study compared vitamin D levels in blood levels drawn from three age groups. The seniors studied (ages sixty to eighty-six) showed lower vitamin D levels than the other age groups. This versatile vitamin is not just for bone health. It plays an important role in respiratory health. Through its influence in lung development and respiratory muscle strength as well as reduction of inflammation, it triggers a powerful immune response to foreign invaders. In fact, researchers have found that a deficiency in vitamin D is a risk factor for developing respiratory tract infections. It turns out that vitamin D is such a powerful immune factor for the respiratory tract that the lungs actually produce their own active form of vitamin D.

In addition to fortifying the immune system in general, vitamin D contributes to creating a stronger barrier to viruses by increasing the antimicrobial compounds in mucous membranes—our first line of defense. These membranes are found in your nose, mouth, eyes, lungs, and windpipe. Research supports that vitamin D improves viral immunity by strengthening mucous membranes.

The best form of vitamin D is sunshine. Opt for at least fifteen to twenty minutes at midday in direct sunlight. You want as much of your skin exposed to natural sunlight as possible, with particular attention to legs and arms (be mindful not to burn). And no, sitting by a window is not enough. You need to physically be in the sunlight. This becomes increasingly important in the winter months when we stay indoors and typically have less exposure to sunlight. Natural vitamin D becomes even more critical as the cold and flu season takes hold.

Vitamin D is fat-soluble, so it will typically be found in fatty foods. Sources include beef liver, cheese, egg yolks, fatty fish and fish oil, and even mushrooms, which seem to be the only nonfat food source rich in this vitamin. Like magnesium, vitamin D supports calcium absorption, helping to create strong bones.

As it stands, the RDI (Recommended Daily Intake) for vitamin D is 600 IU (international units) per day. However, in 2014, research from the University of Alberta showed that the official RDI of vitamin D from the National Academy of Medicine is significantly lower than needed to maintain a healthy body. According to the researchers' statistical analysis, the RDI should actually sit at 8,895 IU per day to ensure that the vast majority of the population has adequate vitamin D in their system. The researchers do note that this dose is higher than any previously studied dose, and caution should be taken when interpreting this number. I recommend a daily vitamin D intake of 2,000 to 5,000 IU of the D_3 fat-soluble version of the vitamin, which is more bioactive than D_2. Ask your health-care practitioner to ascertain your vitamin D level in a blood test and strive for levels of 50 to 80 ng/ml. Ideally, vitamin D should be taken along with vitamin K_2 to be sure that the increased level of calcium that is being absorbed is directed to your bones and not your arteries.

VITAL VITAMIN C

Of course, most of us know the wonders of vitamin C, yet still, many of us don't think to take it until we begin to feel a little under the weather. Vitamin C is essential to our immunity. It can help prevent respiratory infections as well as help treat and heal infections. Note that our body does not store vitamin C, so you need daily intake. Period. Exclamation point! I recommend a time-release vitamin C, with a recommended daily dosage of 2 to 5 g daily.

ZINC

If vitamin D is the body's #1 immunity vitamin, then zinc is the body's number one immunity mineral (and there's another connection between the two: vitamin D has been linked to improved zinc absorption). Necessary for over three hundred enzyme-dependent processes, zinc's importance to your immune system starts with its ability to control many of the reactions to harmful invaders. In fact, a zinc-dependent enzyme is crucial for daily DNA repair; zinc is also critical to the white blood cell's ability to attack invading bacteria and viruses and eliminate them. Without adequate levels of zinc, the immune system can be erratic, resulting in massive inflammation. Any zinc deficiency can impair immune system function; our immunity often declines as we age in direct relation to declining levels of zinc. Zinc deficiency has been linked to pneumonia and other respiratory infections in seniors.

Good dietary sources of zinc include beets, seafood, eggs, and pumpkin seeds. Although I typically recommend anywhere from 15 to 45 mg of zinc daily, many people over the age of fifty are highly deficient and need to take more. Just keep in mind that the greater your zinc intake, the more likely it is to lower other mineral levels, including copper, manganese, molybdenum, chromium, and the insulin mimic vanadium. Zinc needs to be balanced with copper in an 8:1 ratio of zinc to copper. It is important to test your zinc levels with the most accurate testing, which is RBC Zinc, rather than a plasma or serum blood test. Ideally, your zinc level should be in the upper half of normal. Ask your doctor to order this.

COUNT ON QUERCETIN

Quercetin is an antioxidant-rich anti-inflammatory that inhibits histamine release, making quercetin-rich foods natural antihistamines. Also valued for its antiviral effect, it has been known to diminish the ability of a virus to infect cells and impede replication of infected cells. This powerful ability to block viral activity, along with its antihistamine effects, has made it an ideal contributor to respiratory health.

Foods rich in quercetin include capers, quinoa, asparagus, cranberries, apples, kale, okra, spinach, elderberries, and red grapes.

Quercetin supplementation is recommended at 500 mg, two or three times a day.

MELATONIN: THE IMMUNE WARRIOR HORMONE

The body's number one antioxidant hormone, melatonin bolsters your immune system in an amazing way. It increases the antioxidant activity of two powerful chemicals, superoxide dismutase (SOD) and glutathione perioxidase. SOD is an anti-inflammatory that helps repair cells, specifically the damage they incur from the most common free radical in the body—superoxide. Much like SOD, glutathione is a powerful antioxidant and detoxifier. Like a resident handyman, it can repair free radical damage on the spot as well as clean up any toxins and the injury they cause. Melatonin keeps both of these in the fight. Recommended dosage is 1 to 3 mg, preferably in a time-release form.

QUALITY SLEEPING HELPS YOU GROW NEW STEM CELLS

Getting enough sleep is essential for healthy bone marrow, which is where stem cells are made. These stem cells are essential for repairing everything from your immune system to your brain to your bones, and so much more. Stanford researchers have found that a sleep deficit of just four hours is enough to cut the activity of these stem cells in half. For stem cells to travel to where they're needed in your body, you first need to get a full night's sleep. Your investment in getting more high-quality sleep is one of the best you can make.

SOAK IN THE GOOD STUFF

A nice hot soak can help build immunity by raising your body's pH to an optimal level between 7.30 and 7.45, which makes it a less hospitable "terrain" for bacteria and viruses. Apple cider vinegar is especially good for relieving aches and pains as well as helping to eliminate uric acid deposits and carbon-based pollution through the skin. I recommend the following soak twice per week during the cold and flu season and once per week at other times of the year.

→ Run a tub of the hottest water you can manage. Test the water to prevent any scalding. Pour in 2 cups of organic apple cider vinegar.

→ While immersed, sip a glass of warm water mixed with 1 teaspoon of organic apple cider vinegar.

→ Get out of the bath when the water is cool. Don't shower for at least four hours afterward.

THE AIR YOU BREATHE

A 2019 Harvard University study analyzed hundreds of virus risk factors, including such contributors as age, hand washing, contact with larger numbers of people, adequate sleep, and flu shots. Its findings concluded that the biggest risk factor in determining whether someone developed a respiratory infection was related to the dryness of the air they were breathing. Those studied who were breathing drier air were found to be far more likely to develop an infection. Dry air enables a virus to travel farther and survive longer. Researchers also explained that dry air harms our natural immune barriers—our mucous membranes, whereby they become thinner and less protective.

The answer: a humidifier with an optimal range of humidity from 40 to 60 percent. I suggest prioritizing adding a humidifier in the room where you sleep, since many immune functions and repair are taking place during sleep, as well as having a somewhat controlled environment for a prolonged period of time. However, if possible, you might want to add personal humidifiers to your office, kitchen, and other areas where you spend significant amounts of time.

SOAP, NOT SANITIZER

Much of 2020 was dominated by the mandate to wash our hands. We all know to do it and that it saves lives as well as greatly protects against illness through reducing exposure to bacteria and viruses as well as mold and parasites. What you may not know is that it is the preferred protector because hand washing with soap gives two levels of protection, whereas hand sanitizer provides only one. Since most viruses have a fatty outer layer, soap binds with the fat layer at a molecular level and both kills and eliminates viruses—hand sanitizer simply kills the virus but can leave remnants of it on your hands. Therefore, some virus remnants may not be completely neutralized, leaving you with less protection.

If you wash your hands whenever soap and water are available, using the twenty-second approach and covering all areas of both hands (including tops of your hands, thumbs, and in between your fingers), it is the much better choice. For times when soap and water are not available and hand sanitizer is your best option, be sure it contains at least 60 percent alcohol. Any lower concentration may not kill viruses. I personally use a waterless soap called EssentiaClenz, made with natural plant oils, including thyme, which according to the EPA has been found to contain virus-killing thymol.

Proactively supporting your immune system with key nutrients and lifestyle habits clears a path for your body to be able to age more gracefully. Now, let's turn to minimizing toxins to further reduce the toxic load that weighs so heavily on modern-day immunity.

CHAPTER 2

NEW RULE #2: TAKE ON TOXIC OVERLOAD

In this chapter, you'll learn . . .

- How misbehaving minerals and heavy metal exposure lead to memory loss, osteoporosis, and GI woes
- About everyday products that hijack your estrogen receptors and increase your fat storage while robbing you of precious energy
- Why parasites are the great masqueraders—disguising themselves as more recognizable diseases
- About the newest digital toxin that may be compromising your health by breaking down DNA, creating blood barrier links and systemic inflammation
- How to help your body mop up age-promoting toxic overload

OUR EFFORTS TO HAVE VITALITY AS WELL AS A LONG LIFE, IN LARGE PART, RELY ON our ability to rid ourselves of toxins. We are the first generation to have been exposed to a constant sea of chemicals. As unbelievable as it may sound, we are now more likely to get sick from the indoor air in our home or office than from the air outside. According to the EPA, indoor air pollution is one of the leading health risks. In fact, some chemicals may be nearly one hundred times more concentrated indoors than outdoors.

Estimates suggest that each of us stockpiles about seven hundred different types of pollutants in our body. Researchers are now finding that babies are born with over two hundred chemicals in their bloodstream; there's rocket fuel in breast milk, lead in drinking water, and the list goes on. This early and constant bombardment of toxins takes its toll on our ability to detox and ultimately can cost us our health. Adding insult to injury, many of the very medicines that are supposed to benefit us often come with an alarming number of unwanted additives with detrimental side effects, making them villains in our aging process. While we must make an ongoing effort to rid our body of toxins as we age, we also have to address our toxic overload that has accumulated during our years of living. Detox, repair, and rejuvenate are our primary tasks at this stage of life.

You can live to one hundred—and beyond—in nearly perfect health, as many people around the world are doing. It's not as hard as you may think. However, to do that, you need to understand what's going on inside your body and why you're accumulating toxins faster than you can eliminate them. For the first time in a century, American life spans are getting *shorter* because of the rise in such preventable diseases as heart disease, cancer, diabetes, and Alzheimer's. To recalibrate our biological clock and restore optimal health, we must look at the effects of toxic overload in the body as a major contributor to the underlying causes of premature and accelerated aging.

IDENTIFY YOUR TOXIN OVERLOAD

It's difficult to vanquish the foe you don't know, so identifying the toxins you've been exposed to is the first step to freeing yourself from this unwelcome burden. Once you know who your toxic invaders are, you can take targeted steps to eliminate them from your body and reenergize and restore health to your cells.

HEAVY METALS

Living in today's world has made our body a lifetime stockpile of way too many toxins. Aluminum, lead, mercury, and copper are so pervasive in twenty-first-century life that it is difficult to figure out which metal is to blame for one's ill health; each can be devastatingly damaging. Emerging evidence now suggests that many of these and other metals suppress the immune system by producing free radicals that, in turn, help accelerate the aging process as well as degenerative disease.

The metals discussed in this chapter are all in everyday use. Although some are actually therapeutic and beneficial in small amounts (copper, iron, and manganese, for example), they can be toxic in greater quantities. Others, such as mercury, aluminum, and lead, can be toxic to certain individuals no matter how small the amount.

I consider the removal and avoidance of toxic metals to be as essential to my Radical Longevity Program as breathing is to life. Even though efforts toward prevention are well advised and to be applauded, without a systematic and deliberate effort to rid your body of accumulated toxins, your longevity and quality of life will be compromised. After introducing you to the toxic metal sources all around us, I will explain how to eliminate their toxic effects. Let's first understand why and how they accumulate in the first place.

ELEMENTAL RELATIONSHIPS

Part of the wondrous mystery of the body is the ongoing need to compensate for something it determines as lacking. It turns out that when you are deficient in one element, your body will use another element in that group to fill its place. The only problem is the new element is quite often toxic and can't perform the functions for which the deficient one is meant.

Take, for example, the case of iodine. It is an essential building block of your thyroid hormones, T3 (tri-iodo-thyronine; hyphens added so you can see how important the iodine is) and T4 (thyroxine). Your thyroid takes the iodine from your food and converts it into these hormones. But when iodine is deficient, your body substitutes another element.

Iodine is in the group known as halogens, which also contains fluoride, bromide, and chloride. Chloride is already in such abundant use in the body, it can't be pulled away to perform thyroid functions. This leaves fluoride—found primarily in drinking water, tea, and toothpaste—and bromide—found mainly in processed white flour and flame retardants on furniture and clothing (more on these later in the chapter).

When the body makes thyroid hormones with bromide or fluoride, they aren't as biologically active as hormones made properly with iodine—but they still show up on a blood test in the same way. This means you'll feel all the symptoms of hypothyroidism, an underactive thyroid, but you will appear to have normal thyroid hormone levels on blood tests.

This is similar to how your body uses mercury or cadmium when zinc is deficient. And once these impostors bind to the target receptor sites, they stick like glue and are very challenging to unseat. First, you have to supplement to restore your zinc or iodine stores; then you have to keep supplementing to flood these receptor sites, so you can outcompete the attached toxic metals. Keep in mind that part of the attack plan underlying each of these toxic accumulations of heavy metals is to address the deficiency first. Otherwise, the undesirable metal will keep being substituted, making your efforts that much harder and prolonged.

ALUMINUM

Aluminum is able to cross the blood-brain barrier, and its toxicity is believed to be associated with neurodegenerative diseases, including Parkinson's, dementia, and Alzheimer's. It is also commonly found in vaccines.

Symptoms of aluminum toxicity include mental confusion and memory loss, muscle weakness, heartburn, colic, flatulence, ulcers, spasms of the esophagus, appendicitis, dry skin and mucous membranes, constipation, and immune problems, among others. Due to its astringent quality, aluminum can irritate the mucous membranes in your gastrointestinal tract and destroy the protein-digestive enzyme pepsin in your stomach. Aluminum also hampers your body's utilization of calcium, magnesium, phosphorus, and vitamin A, increasing your risk for osteoporosis.

Aluminum is present in a wide variety of kitchenware, from aluminum foil to pots and pans. If it's in your kitchen and made of metal, it potentially contains aluminum. The problem is, when your food encounters aluminum, small particles can make their way into and accumulate over time in your body.

CADMIUM

We are most likely to be exposed to cadmium from cigarette smoking or secondhand smoke, as well as many e-cigarettes and vaping products. Surprisingly, it can be found in chocolate of all varieties and also in some seaweeds, including nori (which is used in sushi and as a dried snack). Other common sources include metal containers, cookware with a cadmium-containing glaze, electroplated ice cube trays, and antiseptics.

Cadmium has been linked to lung and prostate cancer, chromosome damage, and reduced birth weight. Loss of smell, runny nose, shortness of breath, coughing, weight loss, irritability, and fatigue result from long-term exposure to cadmium fumes, accompanied by yellow rings on the teeth, bone pain, and kidney damage.

FLUORIDE

Fluoride, the substance said to strengthen tooth enamel, is another savior-turned-disabler that is added to our water as a dental aid. It is also becoming prevalent in our food supply due, for example, to such pesticides as cryolite, commonly used as a filler in commercially prepared animal feed. Fluoride is a potent factor in aging. It is a primary culprit in the calcification of the pineal gland, and along with aluminum is known to weaken the immune system and cause heart disease, birth defects, and genetic damage. More than 150 studies now show fluoride's neurotoxicity and links to bone and brain diseases, diabetes, cancer, and digestive disorders.

LEAD

As you've undoubtedly heard in the news, lead in drinking water from corroded lead pipes is a huge concern today. Besides being a common contaminant in chocolate and in many imported products (including glazed pottery), vintage dishware, and glass-ware, recent testing identified lead as a contaminant in a host of dietary supplements, particularly those with inferior manufacturing standards. Purchasing your supplements from a reputable company with strict sourcing and production standards is money well spent.

No level of lead exposure is considered safe. Lead is distributed to your brain, liver, and kidneys and accumulates in your teeth and bones over time. Once stored in the bone, lead will remain there for twenty-five to thirty years. Even low levels of lead may cause osteoporosis, cognitive problems, and hearing loss. Chronic exposure to low levels of lead has also been shown to cause hypertension and cardiovascular disease.

Most lead dust we inhale gets absorbed into the lower respiratory tract. The liver can't metabolize inorganic lead, so it must be bound by bile in the intestines and excreted or it will be absorbed into our tissues.

MERCURY

Mercury, a potent neurotoxin, is at the root of a wide variety of disorders. There is no known "safe" level of mercury exposure. We are exposed to mercury mainly through dental amalgams, fish and seafood (especially larger fish, such as tuna, swordfish, mackerel, and sea bass), medications, personal care products, agricultural chemical residues, and high-fructose corn syrup.

Mercury causes demyelination of nerve fibers (damage to the nerves' protective myelin sheath) and slowing of the nerve conduction velocity. Mercury can also cause tinnitus and hearing loss, among other commonly recognized age-related illnesses.

Although many (not all) dentists now use safer composites, those of us who received a mouthful of silver amalgam mercury fillings during our younger years often still have them. And these fillings have slowly been leaking one of the most poisonous substances on the planet—mercury—into our body ever since, representing 50 percent or more of an adult's mercury exposure. If you still have amalgam fillings, it's imperative that you seek the advice of a biological dentist trained in safe mercury removal.

Hidden Dental Infections from Root Canals, Cavitations, and Implants

Teeth are a living tissue. Although they seem solid, they are porous, with fluid constantly flowing through them to cleanse all the layers of the tooth. This creates an environment for the microbiome to live in, the community of microorganisms that contribute to both the health and disease of your mouth. When the infection from tooth decay reaches the root of the tooth, the choices are to do a root canal or have the tooth extracted. Both of these choices can lead to hidden infections near the bone, which can lead to systemic disease in your body.

A tooth with a root canal no longer has fluid flowing through it, which allows unhealthy bacteria to grow deep inside, near the bone. The tooth is essentially dead with no oxygen flowing through it, providing the perfect environment for a long-term, low-grade infection to exist. These infections also travel to other parts of the body, such as the heart, and are a known cause of heart disease.

A cavitation is an infection of unhealed bone where a tooth has been extracted. If the tooth cavity is not cleaned thoroughly and the periodontal ligament isn't removed when the tooth is removed, the infection that caused the tooth decay moves into unhealed bone and can even form a cyst that is a potent source of infection. These hidden infections are hard to find; they occasionally show up on an X-ray, but more commonly they're found by a biological dentist who knows what to look for.

Dentists who practice biological dentistry believe that each tooth is connected to an organ. This means your digestive woes, irritable bowel syndrome, or even liver dysfunction may be linked to the anaerobic bacteria leaking into your system from root canals, cavitations, and/or implants affecting these teeth. Have a thorough examination by a biological dentist and take on these toxins (see Resources).

NICKEL

If you suffer from lactose intolerance or "leaky gut," nickel may be to blame. Remember the problem with mineral deficiencies and poor substitutes? Nickel is so similar to zinc that when you have a zinc deficiency, your body will use nickel instead. Nickel is mutagenic, causing chromosome damage by binding DNA and other cellular proteins. So, when nickel tries to play a role in the more than three hundred enzyme reactions that zinc catalyzes, metabolic mayhem is the result. Nickel exposure is also a known instigator of lung irritation, asthma, and even lung and nasal cancers.

The Dirty Dozen

The Environmental Working Group (EWG) has identified the following chemicals as the "Dirty Dozen Endocrine Disruptors." You will see some of our heavy metal invaders on this list since heavy metals are multitasking toxins.

1. BPA (canned foods, plastics)
2. Dioxin (processed foods, especially commercial animal products)
3. Atrazine (herbicide often found in tap water)
4. Phthalates (plastics, PVC, fragrances, personal care products)
5. Perchlorate (rocket fuel, also shows up in tap water)
6. Fire retardants (clothing, carpet, upholstery, bedding)
7. Lead
8. Arsenic
9. Mercury
10. Perfluorinated chemicals (PFCs) (nonstick cookware; stain- and water-resistant coatings on clothing, furniture, and carpets)
11. Organophosphate pesticides (nonorganic foods)
12. Glycol ethers (cleaning products)

GLYPHOSATE

Many of us grew up enjoying bread and pasta, and the incidences of gluten sensitivity were practically unheard of. All of a sudden, there seems to be an explosion of gluten-sensitive individuals here in the US. According to detox expert Linda Lancaster, "Glyphosate is a powerful metal binder that binds with mercury and aluminum, making them more toxic. It not only disturbs the detoxification process of the liver, but also helps the metals make their way into the bloodstream." It's interesting to note that when American vacationers eat pasta or bread in other countries, such as Italy, for example, they are often able to tolerate the foods. What is going on? The answer just might lie with the method of wheat harvesting.

Here in the US, the practice since the 1990s has been to spray wheat fields with a chemical, such as Roundup, several days before the combine harvesters work through the fields. The end result is designed to be an earlier and more robust harvest. Sounds great, right? In addition, glyphosate can migrate through water from the chemically treated field into organic fields, and we now know that glyphosate is being used to treat other grain and legume products after harvesting. Unfortunately, glyphosate, the active ingredient in Roundup, has been linked to damaged gut flora, cancer, leaky gut, and autoimmune illnesses such as rheumatoid arthritis, and combines with both mercury and aluminum. When these pollutants are addressed, the pain of many age-related diseases, such as brain and memory conditions, as well as Lyme disease and fibromyalgia, can improve remarkably.

TARGETED SOLUTIONS

Our strategic plan against the unrelenting assault of everyday toxins, combined with the toxic overload that we've acquired through years of living, requires us to be proactive. Addressing toxins is important at every stage of life, but your actions today determine the toxic toll on your body for decades to come. You can outsmart and reverse any potential health crisis in the making.

> Note that before you begin taking any supplements, you should check with your health-care provider for any issues or contraindications.

Consider chelation therapy. This procedure consists of the administration of chelators (or binders), such as the intravenously given EDTA (ethylene diamine tetra-acetic acid) and dimercaprol/DMPS (usually administered as a shot or a pill). These substances bind with toxic metals in the tissues for excretion in the blood and urine. Urine is then collected in a special container for twenty-four hours, after which a portion is sent to a lab for analysis. For the name of a physician in your area who practices chelation therapy, call the American College for Advancement in Medicine (see Resources).

ALUMINUM SOLUTIONS

Remove aluminum sources. Check such products as deodorants and antiperspirants, medications (including antacids, antidiarrheals, and over-the-counter painkillers), dental work, and soy-based infant formula, which commonly contain aluminum. Remove as many aluminum sources from the kitchen as possible and find suitable substitutes.

Supplement with silica. Consider drinking silica-rich water, such as Fiji. You'll find detailed information on aluminum-proofing your kitchen in Chapter 9.

CADMIUM SOLUTIONS

Avoid smoking, secondhand smoke, e-cigarettes, and all forms of vaping. One single cigarette may contain approximately 1 to 3 mg of cadmium. Vaping also has cadmium and nickel inside the vapor.

Avoid exposure to cadmium-laden products. Make sure your cookware does not contain a cadmium glaze, nor should any other metal container coming in contact with food or water. Jewelers, potters, welders, painters, sculptors, and photographers need to be especially careful with the products they use.

Avoid eating cadmium-laden foods. Seafood, such as mussels and nori, are typically high in cadmium.

Supplement with zinc. Low levels of zinc are associated with a two- to threefold increase in the risk of cadmium-induced renal damage.

MERCURY SOLUTIONS

Avoid foods and products that contain high levels of mercury. These include large fish as well as such medications as Preparation H, certain contact lens solutions, and diuretics.

Supplement with selenium. A lack of selenium and/or lipoic acid has been connected to mercury toxicity. Consider taking selenium (no more than 200 mcg daily).

Mind your dental health. Check out www.Iabdm.org/location for a dentist who is trained in correct removal protocols and procedures.

LEAD SOLUTIONS

Avoid as many sources of lead as possible. You (and especially children) should keep away from lead-based paint chips. Use a good-quality water filter to remove lead in the home (see Resources).

Test for contamination. If you want to test your vintage china pattern for possible lead contamination, you can order a lead-testing kit (see Resources).

Consider adding extra calcium. Calcium is the mineral antagonist to lead (at least 500 mg daily of calcium hydroxyapatite).

NICKEL SOLUTIONS

Remove as many nickel sources as possible. Avoid cheaply made jewelry, which is a common allergen. Cookware (some stainless steel is composed of 14 percent nickel) and hydrogenated fats (including vegetable oil), which use nickel in the processing, are major sources of nickel. Other sources include tobacco, e-cigarettes or vapes, piercings, and vehicle exhaust. DO NOTE: e-cigarette vapors are often four times higher in nickel than is tobacco smoke.

FLUORIDE SOLUTIONS

Find substitutes for products that contain fluoride. Look for toothpaste that doesn't contain fluoride and avoid kombucha at all costs because it is a highly concentrated source of fluoride-rich tea. Remember that the common tea plant is a bioaccumulator of fluoride, so find young tea leaves and limit all black, white, and green teas to no more than two cups daily.

Invest in a good water filter. Fluoride should and can be removed through reverse osmosis or ceramic purification home water filtration (see Resources).

Balance with boron. Supplement at least 3 mg of boron daily to help detox fluoride from your thyroid and your pineal gland.

GLYPHOSATE SOLUTIONS

Substitute other grains for wheat. Baking with unhybridized flour, such as einkorn, which has an entirely different genetic makeup than modern wheat, can be a great alternative for many with gluten sensitivity. The gluten in einkorn lacks the high-molecular-weight proteins that many people can't digest. Because einkorn does contain gluten, it is *not* recommended for those with celiac disease.

Sourdough bread is known to help break down gluten in wheat. Be advised, however, that the sourdough bread must be baked using select *Lactobacilli* and nontoxic flour. It's best to get it from a qualified baker who makes it from scratch. Many individuals who are grain intolerant can also use tigernut flour or chestnut flour.

Supplement with fulvic and humic acid minerals. They can help offset glyphosate toxicity and are found in the products Restore and Biome Medic (see Resources). Use as directed.

Go for glycine. Since glyphosate can displace glycine, a key amino acid in many metabolic reactions, it is best to supplement with at least 3,000 mg of glycine per day if you are eating glyphosate-rich foods.

HIDDEN HITCHHIKERS

The metals and minerals that overwhelm our body and become toxic are just one part of ridding our body of toxins. We continue with digging deeper into the effects of toxic overload from parasites, mold, radiation, and electropollution, which wipe out our health at the cellular level.

PARASITES

This section is purposely designed to open up a can of worms. Typically, we think of parasites as a problem in developing countries. More than thirty years ago, the chief of pathobiology at Walter Reed Army Institute of Research, Peter Weina, PhD, FACP, told me, "We have a tremendous parasite problem right here in the United States—it's just not being identified." The truth is that one in three of us in the US, and likely many more, is harboring these unwanted invaders, and it's time this epidemic is finally brought into focus. A study in the *American Journal of Tropical Medicine and Hygiene* found that approximately 32 percent of the 2,896 Americans tested were positive for parasitic infections, and at least forty-eight states have fought measurable outbreaks. Increased international travel; improperly washed fruits and vegetables; undercooked/raw fish, meat, and poultry (think sushi bars, carpaccio); polluted soil and water; and inadequate hygiene (particularly in daycare and senior centers) all contribute to the spread of parasites.

I believe these statistics would soar if we included the tick-borne parasites that are becoming increasingly more common. According to the Centers for Disease Control and Prevention (CDC), the number of reported cases of Lyme disease in the US alone has tripled in the past twenty years, and even they note that the reported cases are only a fraction of the total number of people afflicted.

Parasites, ranging from the microscopic amoeba to yards-long tapeworms, can zap your vitality and steal the nutrients from your body. They also have the habit of disguising themselves as other diseases. Basically, parasites create damage to the host body (meaning *you*) in six ways:

→ They destroy cells in the body faster than cells can be regenerated, thereby creating an imbalance that results in ulceration, perforation, or anemia.

→ They produce harmful toxins. In cases of chronic infection, parasites can cause an increase in the numbers of eosinophils, the white cells that normally fight off pathogens. When the level of eosinophils is elevated, they can actually cause tissue damage, resulting in pain and inflammation.

→ The presence of parasites irritates the tissues of the body, inducing an inflammatory reaction.

→ Contact dermatitis is a condition in which some parasites invade the body by penetrating the skin. Other parasites may even perforate and damage the intestinal lining.

→ The size and/or weight of the parasitic cysts, especially if they are located in the brain, spinal cord, eye, heart, or bones, produces pressure effects on these body parts. Obstruction, particularly of the intestine and pancreatic and bile ducts, can also occur.

→ The presence of parasites depresses immune system functioning while activating the immune response. This can eventually lead to immune system exhaustion.

The five most common parasites found in the human body are

→ Toxoplasmosis
→ Giardia
→ *Blastocystis hominis*
→ Roundworms
→ Tapeworms

PARASITES: THE GREAT MASQUERADERS

Over 130 different "hidden invaders" can account for over 385 diseases and disorders. Their symptoms go way beyond the gastrointestinal tract. Parasites may be the underlying cause of some of the most prevalent insidious and mysterious disorders of our time. The list can include constipation, diarrhea, gas and bloating, persistent flu-like symptoms, teeth grinding, anemia, secondary gluten intolerance, casein intolerance, lactose intolerance, Crohn's disease, bile duct congestion, enlarged liver or spleen, or sleep disturbances. Just remember one thing, above all else: as my revered mentor, Dr. Hazel Parcells, taught me so many decades ago, *parasites are the most immunosuppressive agent known to humans.*

Here are some of the most common warning signs:

→ **Sugar cravings.** A diet high in simple carbs, such as sugar, white flour, and milk, can fuel your uninvited guests, even so-called natural sweets—honey, rice syrup, fruit juice sweeteners—provide instant nourishment for your internal hitchhikers.

→ **Anxiety.** Toxoplasmosis infection has been dramatically and significantly linked to general anxiety disorder (GAD).

→ **Secondary dairy and gluten intolerance.** Many parasites, such as roundworm and giardia, can trigger secondary lactose and casein intolerance, so avoiding milk and cheese is a must. Because of the damaged intestinal villi, giardia can also precipitate a type of gluten intolerance. With any protozoan infection that can damage the intestinal villi, it is always a good idea to reduce the intake of grains.

→ **Food and environmental allergies.** Parasites irritate and sometimes perforate the intestinal lining, increasing bowel permeability to large undigested molecules and activating the body's immune response, causing allergic reactions.

→ **Anemia.** If enough parasites are present, you can lose enough blood to cause iron deficiency or anemia.

→ **Constipation.** Some worms, because of their shape and size, can block the bile duct and intestinal tract, making elimination difficult and infrequent.

→ **Gas and bloating.** Some parasites live in the upper small intestine, making persistent abdominal distention a frequent sign of uninvited guests.

→ **Irritable bowel syndrome.** Parasites can inflame the intestinal cell wall, leading to various GI symptoms and malabsorption of vital nutrients.

→ **Joint and muscle aches/pains.** Some parasites can migrate and encyst in joint fluids and muscles, leading to chronic inflammation.

→ **Skin conditions.** Parasites can cause allergic skin reactions, such as eczema, hives, rashes, and sores.

→ **Overall fatigue.** You may also experience dark circles under the eyes, and bruxism (grinding of the teeth).

TARGETED PARASITE SOLUTIONS

If you suspect you have a parasite, try the following solutions. Even if you don't know if have a parasite, these strategies will be helpful.

Always wash your hands after handling your pet. Use a brush to scrub under your fingernails, where parasitic cysts can hide.

Wear light-colored clothing when walking outdoors. Frequently check yourself and your fellow travelers for ticks on your skin and clothing. If you take off the tick soon after its attaches, you lower your risk of infection.

Use lemongrass essential oil as a natural tick repellent. Combine
the oil with a carrier oil, such as almond or jojoba, and apply to ankles and
legs before walking outdoors.

Up your digestive enzymes and probiotics. These make your stomach
and gut acidic—an inhospitable environment for the critters to take root.

Try antiparasitic supplements. For microscopic parasites, consider an
herbal formula consisting of cranberry concentrate, grapefruit seed extract,
Artemisia annua, pomegranate, peppermint, slippery elm, and bromelain.
Cranberry is especially important because its organic acids kill parasites by
breaking down their protein structure and stimulating the release of parasitic
waste. Para-Key, which is part of My Colon Cleansing Kit (see Resources), is
a great parasitic remedy.

For larger worms and flukes, try an herbal tincture. Those containing black walnut, wormwood, centaury, male fern, orange peel, cloves, and
butternut squash can be especially helpful in triggering release of the parasites' hooks and suckers from the intestinal tract. Tinctures containing these
ingredients are often especially effective against the newly uncovered human
rope worm. Try Verma-Plus (see Resources).

Try deep colon cleansing. Home enemas and colonic irrigation can play
an important role in cleansing the colon of parasites. Garlic enemas are especially helpful in eliminating pinworms.

As always, check with your health-care provider before starting any supplement
regimen.

For a More Definite Diagnosis

If you or anyone in your family shows signs of parasites (and your health-
care practitioner lacks experience with these kinds of infections), you
may want to consider an Expanded GI Panel (see Resources), which allows
you to collect saliva and stool samples in the privacy of your own home.
The panel tests for the following:

- Pathogenic bacteria, including *H. pylori* and *C. difficile*, *Candida albicans*, and fungus

(continues)

(continued)

- Protozoa and worms, including giardia, *Blastocystis hominis*, round-worm, *Toxoplasma gondii*, *Trichinella spiralis*, and tapeworm
- Allergies to gluten, cow's milk, eggs, and soy
- Intestinal function markers, including GI immunity

After the lab analyzes your samples, my office can review your results, and recommend personalized diet, lifestyle, and supplementation changes.

MOLD

In many sensitive or immunosuppressed individuals, mold alone is a leading cause of environmental illness. But, to be clear, this is *not* a mold allergy—the mycotoxins from mold are *poison*, and to react to long-term exposure is to experience the symptoms of low-grade poisoning. Immunosuppression magnifies the effects of the poisonous mycotoxin exposure and being more sensitive than others does not mean you're the only one being affected—it just makes you the proverbial canary in the coal mine.

Mold exposure can cause many of the symptoms we associate with unhealthy aging, including difficulty finding words, forgetfulness, weakness, balance and coordination issues, achy joints, and other signs of neurotoxicity. Bronchial and sinus disorders as well as depression and chronic fatigue have also been linked to mold exposure.

The most insidious source of environmental mold takes place inside walls and other hidden areas where you may live and work, from plumbing leaks, roof or vent leaks, and HVAC condensation and drainage issues. Forty percent of the air in your home comes from the basement or crawl space, so these areas are another primary source of mold-producing spores that can spread throughout the house. The other predominant mold-producing areas are the kitchen and bathroom, as well as overwatered houseplants, damp carpets, and memory foam mattresses.

Such mycotoxins as *Alternaria, Aspergillus, Chaetomium, Cladosporium, Penicillium,* and *Stachybotrys* (toxic blood mold) can lead to diverse symptoms, including environmental or food allergies, anxiety, and phobias, especially agoraphobia. Other symptoms may include

| asthma | change in appetite | chronic fatigue |
| cancer | chronic bronchitis | confusion |

depression	hoarseness	rheumatoid arthritis
difficulty concentrating	inflammation of the ear	shortness of breath
digestive issues	learning disabilities	skin problems
eye irritation	lupus (SLE)	vertigo
fatigue	memory loss	wheezing
fibromyalgia	multiple chemical	
headaches	sensitivity	
histamine intolerance	nosebleeds	

If you have at least five of these symptoms, then you've most likely been exposed to mold.

> **Track down hidden mold.** If you're experiencing symptoms of mold toxicity, even if you don't see visible mold, it's a good idea to test your environment for it. I suggest that you get the EPA-approved test called the ERMI (Environmental Relative Moldiness Index) Analysis (EPA-licensed MSQPCR) from www.mycometrics.com (see Resources). This test can identify the molds, bacteria, toxins, and viruses that may be negatively affecting your health. The kits you can buy at the hardware store don't differentiate between outdoor and indoor molds in your home, so don't waste your money. If you think you'll need to get your insurance company involved, consider hiring a building biologist to do the detective work for you.

For personal mold sensitivity or toxicity indication, Dr. Ritchie Shoemaker developed the Visual Contrast Sensitivity (VCS) test, which you can find on his website. This is a simple, inexpensive visual test you can do on your computer. A positive result may suggest a neurotoxin exposure, such as mold. You'll want to follow up with your health-care practitioner for additional testing. For more information, please see Resources.

Another test I've found valuable is the mycotoxin urine test from RealTime Labs (see Resources). This test measures mycotoxins in your urine but can't tell you when you were exposed. If your ability to detox is impaired, you may have mycotoxins in your tissues but aren't able to excrete them, so your urine test is negative even though your tissues have high levels. The best way to use this test is to measure your detox progress by taking the test before you start the five-day detox in the Radical Longevity Plan, then again after you've completed your detox to see if there's still more work to do.

TARGETED MOLD SOLUTIONS

It's important to understand that recovery doesn't happen overnight; persistence pays off when it comes to mold sickness and toxic mold exposure. While available testing will give you some clue about your mold exposure, there is no one test that definitively tells you that you are currently being exposed to mold. Getting a complete physical exam done will rule out other dangerous causes of these symptoms that you don't want to overlook and gives you a good starting place to evaluate your overall health. First up, **mold-proof your body**:

> **Address candida.** People who already have other fungal issues, such as candida, are more susceptible to mold illness because the environment inside the body is already set up for fungus to thrive.
>
> **Keep your diet clean and full of sulfur-rich foods, to encourage glutathione production.** Cut out the sugars, processed foods, and foods known to have mold toxins in them, such as peanuts, grains, and cheese.
>
> **Use gentle binders to tie up mold.** Consider making a cocktail out of cilantro (Nutramedix), chlorella powder (BioPure), takesumi activated charcoal (made from bamboo), and food-grade clay, such as Living Clay's Detox Clay. Combine several drops of the cilantro tincture with about 1 teaspoon of the powders in a small glass with about 4 ounces of water. Take this binder cocktail daily about thirty minutes before eating any food.

I've also had a lot of success with oil of oregano (not the essential oil) at one to two gelcaps twice daily, Y-C Cleanse, and high dose vitamin C (to bowel tolerance), along with a binder (e.g., charcoal, citrus pectin, or zeolite or bentonite clay), and good liver detoxification support. Magnesium (to bowel tolerance) is a safe choice to help get things moving along.

Next, you'll want to **mold-proof your space**:

> **Create an open space.** This helps provide adequate ventilation.
>
> **Maintain bare floors.** Get rid of carpets, especially wall-to-wall carpets. If you do want to have rugs, use throw rugs that you can launder. Vacuuming can't eliminate all contaminants, but if you do, use vacuum cleaners with rotating heads and HEPA filters. Do not use wet-method carpet shampoos, as this allows mold growth beneath the surface of the carpet and padding.
>
> **Maintain clean surfaces.** Regularly disinfect surfaces that people frequently touch—including door handles, phones, remote controls, and

computer keyboards—with a disinfectant, or straight 60 percent (or greater) alcohol.

Prevent dishwashing mold. After cleaning dishes, dry them with a clean dishcloth or let them air dry in the dish rack. Don't stack dishes wet, as that can foster the growth of bacteria.

Change and wash your dishcloths daily. Wet dishcloths are welcoming homes to bacteria and mold. And above all, please don't use sponges—the holes harbor bacteria and mold that you can't get out, even if you boil them.

Keep the outdoors outdoors. Remove your shoes when entering your home, to avoid tracking in mycotoxins and mold spores from outdoors.

Use dehumidifiers. Dehumidifiers lower indoor humidity of damp air that would otherwise encourage the growth of mold, mildew, and bacteria. Please note that dehumidifiers are just for a dampness issue, such as in a basement.

Repair leaks. Leaky roofs and walls lead to accumulated dampness that allows the growth of fungus and mold. Leaky faucets add to the humidity of your house.

Get out of a moldy environment. You must leave—at least temporarily—as soon as you find out you have a mold problem. Anything porous—such as paper, books, photographs, or clothing—carries mold spores in it, so mold experts say it's best to get rid of these things.

Remediate for mold. If your home (or office) tests positive for mold spores, you must find the source and get a certified specialist to properly remediate the space. It's not enough to spray bleach on the problem areas; this causes the mold to sporify and become airborne.

Invest in a good air cleaner. After remediation, you'll need high-quality air cleaners throughout your home to filter the mold spores and mycotoxins that are still circulating. Even though the source of the mold is gone, the spores and mycotoxins linger and can cause an exacerbation of symptoms.

ENERGY ZAPPERS: RADIATION AND ELECTROPOLLUTION

Radiation damages living tissue by removing electrons from other atoms or molecules with which it comes into contact. These radioactive particles get into our body via air, water, or food, destroying tissues, organs, cells, and genes.

According to Dr. Parcells, natural low-level radiation has been around in the environment for decades. And for years, we lived harmoniously with it. Starting in the 1930s, low-level radiation from X-rays, microwaves, electronic equipment, and nuclear power has pumped tremendous amounts of radioactivity into the environment. And it doesn't just stay in one place. Because radioactivity is airborne, it can be transported for hundreds of miles beyond its origin.

Radiation shortens our life span. Its cumulative effect can cause premature aging, cancer, leukemia, genetic mutations, abnormal blood clotting, thyroid dysfunction, and numerous other health problems. It can create mental impairment. It zaps our immune system, leaving us vulnerable to a host of nonspecific ailments.

Radiation does its damage by entering the body and attaching to the cells where it stays for a very long time, absorbing large amounts of minerals and trace elements, leaving the body with little reserves to carry on its normal functions of digestion, absorption, elimination, and reproduction.

EMF: THE DIGITAL TOXIN THAT MAY BE RUINING YOUR HEALTH

The most underreported toxin of our time is a digital toxin: electromagnetic fields (EMFs) and the rollout of 5G is making this an even more urgent problem that we can no longer ignore. EMFs are an insidious form of nonionizing radiation that can cause fatigue, sleep problems, migraines, back pain, depression, cognitive issues (impaired reaction time, brain fog, memory loss), heart problems, digestive disturbances, cataracts, chronic inflammation, even brain tumors and cancer.

I know because I had a rare (thankfully benign) tumor of the parotid gland (a salivary gland) a number of years ago. I realized that my being tethered to my cell phone for hours every day—to the point of even sleeping with it—had brought about my body's attempt to protect me by isolating the toxins inside a tumor, which was located on the left side of my neck where I routinely held my cell phone while talking. My parotid tumor turned out to be one of several kinds of tumors linked to cell phone use.

As I brought to light in my book *Zapped*, over a decade ago, the most common sources of this twenty-first-century toxin are cell phones, cordless phones, Wi-Fi, and smart meters. The explosion in sales of smartphones, iPads, smart thermostats, and smart doorbells is a good indicator that there is no end in sight.

WHY EMFS ARE HARMFUL

Medical experts around the world are sounding the alarm, but the advent of 5G for the sake of faster internet capability is happening despite the health concerns not being addressed by the majority of governmental agencies. The American Academy of Pediatrics, for example, has repeatedly called for federal action to protect children from EMF exposures. They cite research showing that just living near mobile phone base stations is associated with an increased risk for sleep disturbances, dizziness, headaches, depression, and memory problems.

The International Association of Firefighters has officially opposed cell towers on fire stations since 2004, when research demonstrated the serious neurological damage—including memory problems, intermittent confusion, and feelings of weakness—firefighters suffered from the EMF they radiate.

And in 2015, more than 230 scientists in forty-one countries studied the biological and health effects of nonionizing EMFs due to the evidence of negative health effects even at low levels and sent an urgent international appeal to the United Nations. To date, there are more than 1,800 studies summarizing the cognitive, neurological, and immune system effects (*BioInitiative Report*, 2007, 2012). Research by Martin Pall, PhD, demonstrates the connection between microwave exposure and oxidative stress and the serious link to the increasing number of neurological disorders. EMF comprises frequencies, modulation patterns, and other characteristics that constantly disrupt sympathetic nervous system activity and raise cortisol. Changes in this stress hormone level have been linked to everything from accelerated aging and erratic sleep patterns to lower immunity and autoimmune problems, cardiovascular disease, and blood sugar imbalance. EMFs can damage every system in the body—from major organs, such as the brain and heart, down to individual cells and even DNA.

SCRAMBLED CELLULAR COMMUNICATION

Studies have found that even low-level EMFs may rupture delicate cell membranes, releasing calcium from cells as well as changing the way calcium ions bind to the surface of the membrane. Since calcium ions are the glue that holds together cell membranes, which are only two molecules thick, the membranes are likely to weaken and tear, allowing toxins to enter and contents to spill out. They literally become unglued.

CALCIUM DYSREGULATION

No fewer than twenty-three studies have shown that voltage-gated calcium channels (VGCCs) play an enormous role in EMF effects. When calcium ions pour into one or more of your one hundred billion brain cells, which use calcium in small doses to make neurotransmitters, they may release those chemical messengers too soon, too often, or at the wrong time, creating false messages that tell you that you're in pain or bring on neurological symptoms, such as headaches, an altered sense of taste or smell, tingling, numbness, or mental fog.

There are good reasons why your body reacts to EMFs as though they were public enemy number one:

- Using your cell phone just thirty minutes a day can increase brain tumor risks by 40 percent.
- Holding a cell phone to your ear allows between 10 and 80 percent of the EMFs to penetrate 2 inches into your brain.

THE 5G HEALTH HAZARD—COMING TO YOUR TOWN SOON

Hundreds of scientists and doctors from forty different countries have studied the adverse biological and health effects from the involuntary exposure to 5G EMF and microwave radiation—and the news is not good. They have reached out to the FCC, European Union, and even the United Nations, requesting further research into the health risks and environmental impact of 5G as it is being rolled out.

Here in the US, according to Harvard reports, the Federal Communications Commission (FCC) is owned by the wireless industry leaders it regulates, and these leaders, during a US Senate hearing, were so bold as to say they haven't done any 5G safety studies—and don't plan to. However, independent research done through the $30 million US National Toxicology Program (NTP) Study on Cell Phone Radiation found that the heart and brain cancers detected in their study are the same as those found to be increased in people who have used cell phones for more than ten years. With major studies like these, why is there not more concern over 5G safety issues?

THE CORE OF THE SAFETY CONTROVERSY

There are currently hundreds of studies showing harm to both human health and the environment from radiofrequency electromagnetic fields (RF-EMF) radiation that cellular towers and phones emit:

→ A review of 113 studies showed that 70 percent found a significant effect on wildlife, with reproduction, development, and navigation affected most.

→ RF-EMF damages trees around cell towers and affects their growth.

→ 5G frequencies used in weapons are proven to cause damage to humans. This research review has found that millimeter waves can increase oxidative stress and inflammation, affect metabolic processes, alter gene expression, and promote rapid cell growth.

Very high levels of RF-EMF radiation can rapidly heat biological tissue and cause harm. This is how microwave ovens cook food—and how we may get our concerns over 5G heard.

WHAT 5G AND YOUR MICROWAVE HAVE IN COMMON

Can you imagine turning on your microwave oven and opening the door and then being exposed to that level of radiation for the rest of your life? This is comparable to what we could be exposed to with 5G. Until now, the wavelengths of all the generations of wireless telecommunications technology, including 4G, have traveled along the surface of the skin. 5G is different, and those wavelengths will automatically be absorbed by our skin, which results in a rise in temperature of the skin that we can easily measure.

The shorter-millimeter waves of 5G require more towers and cell stations than we've ever seen before—potentially even one mini cell tower per every two to eight houses. So, your RF-EMF exposure could increase exponentially within a matter of months, effectively creating a global microwave oven.

When food is cooked in a microwave oven, the amino acids change shape, rendering them unusable by the human body. Microwave exposure to humans shows the same amino acid changes, rendering your body's own DNA building blocks unusable and leading to circulatory disturbances and DNA changes that may lead to cancer.

The bottom line is that until lawmakers hear the concerned scientists—as they had to with cigarette smoke and DDT—it's up to us to protect ourselves and teach the most vulnerable among us how to protect themselves as well.

TARGETED RADIATION SOLUTIONS

Plants, herbs, and other foods. Rosemary, hemp seeds, and hemp seed oil are all known to absorb radiation and mitigate its effects in the body. Bee pollen and propolis, dried primary-grown nutritional yeast, lecithin, thymus glandular extract, cysteine, pectin, charcoal, and germanium all help the body fight off the ravages of radiation. Miso soup is also a known radiation protector.

Sweating. Detox radiation through exercise, sauna, or sweating outside in a hot climate.

Homeopathic cell salts. Twelve cell salts, of which kali phosphoricum is the most effective, can be taken under the tongue several times a day.

Herbal aids. Ginseng, and shiitake and maitake mushrooms fight radiation.

Heavy-duty antioxidants. Glutathione, catalase, lipoic acid, grape seed extract, pine bark, and vitamins A, C, and E can mop up free radical damage.

TARGETED RF-EMF AND 5G SOLUTIONS

The foundation of your EMF defense plan should be minimizing your exposure while supporting your body's innate ability to protect and heal itself.

Support your body's natural calcium channel blockers by increasing your magnesium intake. Magnesium acts as a natural calcium channel blocker to offset the calcium dysregulation that is impacted by EMF exposure. Studies show that calcium channel blockers significantly reduce the effects of EMF, making this an effective natural solution. I recommend 5 mg of magnesium per pound of body weight (see Resources).

Use home, car, and cell phone protectors. The whole house protection, whole car protection, and cell phone neutralizer from Aulterra (see Resources) are all I need to protect myself.

Avoid buying 5G-enabled devices.

Use a battery-powered alarm clock. Use a clock that does not have a light, if possible. Never use your cell phone as an alarm clock!

Make it a habit to turn off the electricity to your bedroom at night. This may seem strange at first, but it can be very helpful especially if you suffer from insomnia.

Hardwire your home. You can have a safer connection by opting for Ethernet connections and eliminating Wi-Fi altogether. If you DO have Wi-Fi, always turn it off at night while you're sleeping.

Trade in your microwave oven for a steam convection oven. It's a much safer alternative that will heat your food just as quickly!

Smart is not always better. Those new smart appliances, TVs, and thermostats depend entirely on wireless signals.

Shield your smart meter or refuse it if you can. If you must have a smart meter on your home, consider adding a shield. Some Faraday shields have been shown to reduce radiation by 98 to 99 percent! (See Resources.)

Avoid wireless baby monitors. Hardwired monitors are much safer. If that is not an option, consider moving your baby's bed nearer to your own bedroom.

Replace fluorescent lights with incandescent bulbs. Just being in close range of fluorescent bulbs can result in the transfer of unwanted current to your body.

Decorate your home with plants that help eliminate and absorb electromagnetic radiation. Particularly helpful varieties include cactus, snake plant, spider plant, betel leaf plant, stone lotus flower, aloe vera, ivy, asparagus fern, mustard greens, and rubber plant.

Surround yourself with shungite. This black, lustrous, noncrystalline stone absorbs and neutralizes unnatural frequencies due to its unique molecular structure of hollow carbon cages known as fullerenes. Wear it in jewelry or keychains or purify drinking water with 100 g of shungite per liter of water.

CELL PHONE SAFETY SOLUTIONS

Your cell phone is likely your greatest exposure to EMF radiation, yet the adverse effects of cell phones and other wireless technologies may take years—even decades—to develop. EMF exposure, just like other toxins, is cumulative.

Carry your phone in an EMF-blocking bag. A good choice is the Faraday bag (see Resources).

Reduce overall exposure. Keep your cell phone on airplane mode or off when not in use. Reconnect with nature, eat well, and support your body's detoxification efforts.

Keep your cell phone away from your head. When talking on your cell phone, use the speakerphone option and hold the phone a minimum of 3 feet away from you. A healthy alternate is an air tube headset (see Resources).

Limit cell phone use to areas with excellent reception, and use only briefly. Phones use more power (and therefore emit more radiation) in areas of poor reception. Use a cell phone only for very short periods of time and only when necessary.

Consider using an old-fashioned landline in your home.

CALCIUM DYSREGULATION SOLUTIONS

Supplement with 5 mg per pound of body weight to balance ratio of magnesium to calcium. Optimum calcium dose: maximum of 500 to 1,000 mg per day for all ages, provided there is sufficient magnesium and vitamin D intake via foods and/or supplements. If taking supplements, this is best taken in 400 to 500 mg dosages. My personal favorite is Osteo-Key (see Resources). Good food sources include dairy foods, dark leafy greens, almonds, pecans, sunflower seeds, parsley, kelp, and burdock.

There's no doubt that taking on toxins can be an overwhelming and daunting task. But rest assured that the Radical Longevity Program is specifically designed to enable you to detox daily, thereby filtering out and eliminating age promoting pollutants. In the next chapter, it's time to explore one of the most pervasive toxic substances of all, hiding right in plain sight. Many so-called health foods and popular cooking techniques contain this substance, which not only accelerates aging but is responsible for many chronic diseases.

CHAPTER 3

NEW RULE #3: STOP AGES (ADVANCED GLYCATION END PRODUCTS)

In this chapter, you'll learn . . .

- What AGEs are and how you can slow the aging process
- About the missing link between inflammation, oxidative stress, and age-related chronic diseases
- The #1 reason HOW you cook is just as important as WHAT you cook
- How to prevent AGE-ing with simple kitchen substitutes

AS WE EXAMINE EACH CONTRIBUTOR TO AGING, THE BIGGEST CULPRIT IS HIDING IN plain sight. AGEs, or glycotoxins, are toxic "sticky" molecules that show their effects throughout your body, from the surface of your skin to the deepest of your cells. They act much like glue in a process known as cross-linking, in which proteins are bound together, overbinding these proteins and making them stiff. They live in your high-fat and protein foods and are produced by how you're cooking these foods.

Glycotoxins are oxidants. Excess glycotoxins cause oxidative stress that plays a huge role in the premature aging process by damaging cells, tissues, and even our DNA. Our body interprets AGEs as irritants and, as with any other irritants, reacts with its built-in defense mechanism: inflammation. As glycotoxins accumulate in tissues, the inflammation becomes pervasive and chronic. The consequences of chronic inflammation, left unchecked, can eventually lead to tissue damage and organ malfunction. AGEs are the likely culprit behind your stiff joints and muscles. Once formed, they clump together and accumulate in the liver and other tissues, causing inflammation and oxidative damage throughout your body. This process is also the link to the common "hardening of the arteries" that many older people experience.

More evidence of AGE damage? Wrinkles, creases, hyperpigmentation, lines, sagging skin, pain, and lethargy—yet we are told that these are "normal" signs of aging. Make no mistake—these are signs of cellular stress from AGEs to iron overload and so much more.

What's most crucial and jaw-dropping to remember about AGEs is that they can compromise the host defense longevity molecule known as SIRT1, which is part of a powerful family of proteins called sirtuins. Sirtuins control major bodily functions, including metabolic and immune mechanisms, fat metabolism, brain function, and insulin resistance.

As Dr. Helen Vlassara, Professor Emeritus of the Mount Sinai School of Medicine, who has devoted over thirty years to studying the effects of AGEs, states so eloquently in her book *Dr. Vlassara's A.G.E.-Less Diet*:

> SIRT1 all but disappears in older adults and in people with chronic diseases such as diabetes. . . . [W]e discovered that SIRT1 was depleted only in those people (or animals) who consistently consumed food with high levels of AGEs, which bring with them high oxidant stress and a high inflammatory state. It would seem, then, that low levels of SIRT1 are not simply a random event caused by getting older or having a chronic disease. Rather, these levels may be due to long exposure to AGE-laden foods. In fact, SIRT1 is low even in young people if they consume a high-AGE diet.

DISCOVERING AGES

AGEs were initially discovered by researchers studying diabetes. When blood sugar rises after a meal, that sugar can travel and attach itself to many different proteins. *Glycation* is the name of the process that binds sugars, such as fructose and glucose, to fats and proteins in the bloodstream. These toxic, sticky, sugar-bound complex proteins are AGEs, and not only do they accumulate faster as you age, but they age you faster as they accumulate. These large molecules stick together and form the flabby, sagging skin on your upper arms, your double chin, the extra breast tissue pillowing underneath your arms, the potbelly below your waist, the dowager's hump on the back of your neck, and the mysterious lumps and bumps that pop up anywhere but seem to come out of nowhere.

AGEs are much more than just a vanity problem. They are a sign that your liver is bogged down and accumulating toxins, and in addition to accelerated and premature aging, they're associated with such chronic diseases as diabetes, Alzheimer's, heart disease, kidney failure, and liver cirrhosis.

The reason AGEs are linked to such a variety of diseases is that they are very versatile in their destruction. Once formed, they clump together and accumulate in your tissues. Your body is smart and reads these as invaders and agitators, so it tries to mount an immune response, which backfires in the form of an overactive, hypersensitive immune system.

MEASURING AGES

It's difficult to measure AGE levels in the body. Currently, the only blood test, for hemoglobin A1c, looks at one protein that gives us a clue. This test tells us what percentage of the hemoglobin in your blood has been glycated (coated with sugar). Because it was initially used for diabetics, the laboratory reference range (around 6 percent) is really only valuable for those with the disease. For optimal longevity in nondiabetics, set your goal of an A1c result of 5 percent or less. Your health-care practitioner can guide you in determining if this test is for you.

Since this is currently the only test that even begins to hint at the extent of AGE damage, it's important to look to your body for the answers. When you look in the mirror, is there anywhere you can pinch an inch or more of rolling, sagging, or lumpy tissue? Do you have cellulite? These are all signs that you are accumulating AGEs.

If you do have signs of AGEs, snap an honest picture of yourself and save it as your "before" photo for comparison. Once you make the changes to what you eat and how you cook your food, you just may find that over time, renewing the health of your cells is renewing the youth of your skin, physique, and overall appearance.

OBESITY AND AGES

It's estimated by the World Health Organization that more than 1.9 billon adults are overweight, and of these, 650 million are obese. Worldwide obesity has tripled just since 1975—and the culprit is our food. The transformation of our food industry began during World War II, which introduced new ways of processing and preserving foods. These convenient, longer shelf-life foods quickly became a part of the everyday American diet.

Processed foods are not just found at the supermarket but also make up foods handed out through drive-thru windows—and our waistline is reflecting this style of eating. The average consumer has developed a taste for highly processed foods, which contain, as we now know, staggering levels of glycotoxins. These glycotoxins are likely affecting our increasing weight as reflected on the bathroom scale even more than the actual calories we consume. Remember, it's not only the foods we eat that can hurt us, but *the way they are cooked* that matters just as much.

You'll want to keep your AGE limit under 8,000 kU per day. Given that a typical double burger with cheese serves up a whopping 6,283 AGE kU/100 g and the French fries that accompany it contain upwards of 1,500 AGE kU/100 g, you can see that it adds up fast *(see the charts on pages 54–56 for AGE contents of common foods).*

YOUR LIVER'S SIGNS OF AGES

Even if you start as the picture of perfect health, if you eat a diet high in AGEs, you increase your risk of insulin resistance, diabetes, and fatty liver disease. The accumulation of AGEs is a sure sign of a liver that is unable to process fats or toxins and is congested and overloaded.

AGEs modify the insulin molecule so it can't function as efficiently, which leads to rising blood sugars. When we have high blood sugar levels, we have the fuel to make more AGEs. Chronically high blood sugar levels make us more prone to insulin resistance, and AGEs encourage this process by changing how our fat cells, muscles, and liver all respond to insulin. Insulin resistance is a hallmark of not only prediabetes and metabolic syndrome but also nonalcoholic fatty liver disease (NAFLD).

NAFLD is caused by the accumulation of fat depositing in the liver, combined with insulin resistance and oxidation. AGEs exacerbate the progression of the disease. The more fat that accumulates in your liver, the less your liver is able to do its jobs of breaking down fats and detoxification, which leads to toxic accumulation of fat and waste products. The end result is a tired, fatty, congested liver. Once your liver is on toxic overload, you feel fatigued and your body loses its hormone balance and its ability to fully detoxify. The following factors all contribute to the vicious cycle of AGE formation:

→ **Toxic metals** from drinking water, dental amalgams, antiperspirants, antacids, swimming pools, and more. The process of glycation can involve toxic metals, especially fluoride, chlorine, and bromine.

→ **Yeast and fungal infections** create the inflammatory conditions that form AGEs. Their very presence is a sign that excess sugar is available for the process of glycation.

→ **Blood sugar imbalances** allow more AGEs to form in the blood.

→ **Antioxidant deficiency** decreases our defenses against AGE formation and makes it difficult for us to break them down.

→ **Dehydration** encourages the formation of AGEs, even if it's at a low level.

The Epigenetics of AGEs

The science of *epigenetics* was born out of research that showed our genes change their expression based on the environment they're in. So, it wasn't our genetics that were to blame for the sudden surge in expanding waistlines and type 2 diabetes, it was what we were feeding our cells that turned on body mechanisms that resulted in type 2 diabetes. When we feed our cells toxins and deplete their necessary nutrients, gene mutations express themselves, which is why one person with a gene defect will become ill from the associated disease, whereas another remains completely healthy. In a nutshell, this means the foods we eat, the water we drink, and the air we breathe are the environmental factors that drive our gene expression—and whether we are healthy or headed for disease.

THE FOODS THAT AGE YOU

It doesn't matter how many miles you run, how much muscle you build, or how much you starve yourself—if your cooking methods are adding to your toxic load, your skin will sag, your tissues will clump together, and your cells will age prematurely. And if your body is already on toxic overload, there's no route for those AGEs to get out, so they go into your tissues and lead to chronic disease.

Fats. Fats and oils are a critical part of our diet, but certain fats are also naturally high in AGEs, so you must take care to choose the proper ones.

Animal-based fats (think: butter) are high in AGEs; processed vegetable oils, even cold-pressed oils, form AGEs the longer they sit on the shelf. Such foods as avocados, extra-virgin olive oil, and raw nuts and seeds are lower in AGEs. You'll want to be mindful that the nuts and seeds you do consume should be refrigerated and they are best eaten raw or very lightly toasted, as roasting can double their AGE content. Raw nuts and seeds should be soaked in water for at least six hours or overnight, for better absorption of nutrients and to neutralize enzyme inhibitors.

A note about keto: While I personally do not recommend the ketogenic diet long term for a variety of health reasons, many have found weight-loss success by using this diet. Keto calls for 75 percent fats, 20 percent proteins, and 5 percent carbohydrates.

With fats composing three-fourths of daily intake, it only makes sense to be sure the type and quality of fats consumed are not causing you to age prematurely.

TABLE 4.1. AGE CONTENT OF SELECTED FATS AND FAT SOURCES

A kilo unit (kU) is one thousand units. You'll want to limit your AGEs to 8,000 kU daily.

FOOD	AGES PER SERVING
Almonds, raw (1 ounce)	1,600 kU
Avocado (1 ounce)	470 kU
Butter (1 tablespoon)	1,890 kU
Olive oil (1 tablespoon)	450 kU
Pumpkin seeds, raw (1 ounce)	560 kU
Sunflower seeds, raw (1 ounce)	750 kU
Sunflower seeds, roasted (1 ounce)	1,400 kU

Proteins. In a recent article published by AARP, it is recommended that men and women aged sixty-five and older eat up to 100 g of protein daily, which is about double the RDA (Recommended Daily Allowance) for adults under sixty-five years of age. It's important to realize that meats are typically higher in AGEs than all other food groups. Although cheeses tend to be high in AGEs, such dairy foods as yogurt are low. No matter what protein source you choose, you can *reduce* the AGE levels of these proteins significantly by choosing the right cooking method.

Animal foods and cheese are far more susceptible to AGE buildup than are plant-based proteins. Just like you, animals are exposed to toxins through their environment and accumulate AGEs. This means they are naturally present in the high-protein animal products you consume.

Think about that breakfast you might have on your way out the door or served at a drive-thru window on your way to work. Bacon, fried for five minutes, has a staggering 11,905 AGEs kU/serving, one large fried egg has approximately 1,237 AGEs kU/serving, and one refrigerator biscuit has 247 AGEs kU/serving. Your day hasn't even really started, and yet you've already put your body in harm's way. Do you really want to follow that up with a cheeseburger and fries for lunch? Can you afford to, nutritionally speaking? I think you'll agree that the answer is a resounding *no*.

TABLE 4.2. AGE CONTENT OF SELECTED PROTEINS

A kilo unit (kU) is one thousand units. You'll want to limit your AGEs to 8,000 kU daily.

FOOD	AGES PER SERVING
Beef steak, grilled (3 ounces)	6,700 kU
Beef steak, stewed (3 ounces)	2,200 kU
Chicken, skinless, grilled (3 ounces)	4,400 kU
Chicken, skinless, poached (3 ounces)	800 kU
Egg, fried (1 large)	1,200 kU
Egg, poached (1 large)	30 kU
Kidney beans, cooked (3 ounces)	190 kU
Pork ribs, roasted (3 ounces)	3,985 kU
Pork tenderloin, braised (3 ounces)	1,000 kU
Salmon, broiled (3 ounces)	3,400 kU
Salmon, poached (3 ounces)	1,550 kU
Soy burger (2 ounces)	60 kU

TABLE 4.3. AGE CONTENT OF SELECTED CHEESES

A kilo unit (kU) is one thousand units. You'll want to limit your AGEs to 8,000 kU daily.

FOOD	AGES PER SERVING
Cheddar cheese (2% milk) (1 ounce)	740 kU
Cheddar cheese (whole milk) (1 ounce)	1,660 kU
Cottage cheese (whole milk) (½ cup)	1,600 kU
Parmesan cheese (2 tablespoons)	2,500 kU
Processed American cheese (1 ounce)	2,600 kU

Vegetables and fruits. When it comes to choosing foods low in AGEs, plants are your best friends, primarily due to their high-water content and naturally low levels of fat and protein. Vegetables contain detoxifying enzymes, fiber, vitamins, minerals, and chlorophyll for radiant good health, and are a rich source of phytochemicals (biologically active compounds) and antioxidants that will stave off the aging process. In Chapter 9, you'll see a list of suggested vegetables and fruits. You'll want to pay special attention to those "bitter foods" noted with an asterisk as I highly recommend these foods.

Cranberries and blueberries contain a phytonutrient that is also particularly helpful in lowering AGE levels.

Fresh is best when it comes to vegetables and fruits, though preserving by canning or freezing does not affect AGE formation significantly. As with meats, the cooking methods used when preparing fruits or vegetables makes a difference. Grilling, roasting, and deep-frying vegetables increases their AGE levels. At this point, it probably won't surprise you that French fried potatoes are significantly higher in AGEs than boiled or steamed potatoes.

TABLE 4.4. AGE CONTENT OF SELECTED VEGETABLES AND FRUITS

A kilo unit (kU) is one thousand units. You'll want to limit your AGEs to 8,000 kU daily.

FOOD	AGES PER SERVING
Apple, baked (3½ ounces)	45 kU
Apple, raw (3½ ounces)	15 kU
French-fried potatoes (3 ounces)	1,000 kU
Peppers and mushrooms, grilled (3 ounces)	261 kU
Plums, dried (1 ounces)	50 kU
Sweet potato, baked (3½ ounces)	70 kU
Tomatoes, raw (3½ ounces)	20 kU

Any food combined with sugar and cooked—such as the grains used in baking—will also form high levels of AGEs. Even honey, maple syrup, fruits, fruit juices, coconut water, milk, and commercial, sweetened nut milks can. Be sure to check the food labels to check how many grams of sugar the foods contain. But you can't simply eliminate animal foods and sugars and resolve your AGE issues because (as we've previously mentioned) *how* you cook your food is just as important as *what* you cook. If you roast, broil, grill, barbecue, fry, sauté, sear, bake, toast, brown, or use high heat in any manner to cook your food, you are creating very high levels of AGEs—regardless of *what* you're cooking. And surprisingly, the dry heat that has been touted as the healthier alternative to frying, known to many as air frying, causes AGEs to form at high levels due to the requisite dry, high heat.

COOKING SOLUTIONS

When it comes to cooking methods that do not raise AGEs, there are a number of delicious options at your disposal. Low heat is the way to go, and wetter is better when cooking your foods.

Slow cooking. This is a great time to use your slow cooker, such as my favorite, the VitaClay cooker. This cooking method retains moisture and enhances an array of flavors. A splash of red wine, broth, juice, or some other liquid added to the combination of meats and vegetables results in not only a tasty meal, but an AGE-less one. Tougher cuts of meats become tender when slow cooked slightly below the boiling point, at or around 200°F.

Simmering. This technique helps lock in key nutrients that might otherwise be lost during high-temperature boiling.

Braising. This cooking method uses a combination of liquid and steam. I suggest that you first lightly brown meat with a high-heat oil, such as ghee (clarified butter), red palm oil, or avocado oil. Acidic foods—especially Mediterranean staples, such as tomatoes, citrus, or vinegar—add flavor and reduce AGEs, as they break down proteins.

Steaming. Asian-style dishes are often prepared using this method, which allows for maximum nutrient absorption and preservation of the food's unique natural texture and taste. Lighter foods, such as vegetables, chicken breast, and shellfish, also benefit from this technique.

Poaching. The idea is to cook more delicate foods (such as fish and duck) at a lower temperature than one would if braising or steaming. The liquid base is best cooked at or around 160° to 185°F.

Marinating. Marinating meats (or fish) in an acidic medium for even just one hour can prevent AGE formation by as much as 50 percent. Use lemon or lime juice, dry organic wine, organic grass-fed broth, olive oil, or apple cider vinegar; and add herbs and spices, such as garlic, mustard, rosemary, thyme, sage, and tarragon for amazing flavor and added health benefits. Per pound of meat, use 4 to 6 tablespoons lemon juice, lime juice, or vinegar plus enough water or other ingredients to cover the food.

TIP: In addition to proper cooking methods, when serving meat or cheese, it helps to add plenty of colorful phytonutrient-rich foods, such as leafy greens, beets, and squash, to your plate, as the antioxidants they contain help defray the AGE-related damaging effects.

TARGETED AGE NUTRITIONAL
AND DETOX SOLUTIONS

Avoid fried foods. They are high in AGEs. Anything fried is not your
friend.

Avoid processed foods. Processed foods, such as chips, cookies, dried milk,
and hot chocolate mixes, are typically prepared using high- and dry heat
methods, increasing their AGE content.

Fill up on phytonutrient-rich vegetables. Naturally low in AGEs, vegetables are a great way to mitigate the damage done by improperly cooked
foods. But vegetables should also be cooked properly to avoid increasing their
AGE content.

Up your antioxidants. Your body needs antioxidants to remove excess
AGEs and to balance your oxidation process so they stop accumulating in
the first place. Vitamins A, C, and E, along with such minerals as selenium
and zinc, should be plentiful in the diet and supplemented through a daily
multivitamin/multimineral.

Bet on benfotiamine. New research suggests that supplementing with
benfotiamine—which is fat-soluble vitamin B_1—can help reverse or greatly
counteract meals high in AGEs better than any other antioxidant. So, if you
can't refrain from broiling, roasting, grilling or air frying, I suggest that you
supplement with benfotiamine-rich Ultra H-3 Plus, which is discussed in the
brain chapter (Chapter 11). In this way, you can hit two birds with one stone
as the benfotiamine in the Ultra H-3 Plus is also helpful in cognitive function
(see Resources).

Love your liver. I recommend gentle herbal cleansing and nourishing support. N-acetylcysteine, alpha-lipoic acid, chlorophyll, choline, and taurine are
all excellent supplemental aids for a tired, toxic liver, as well as coffee enemas.

Prevent AGEs when Dining Out

When eating out, there are three styles of cuisine that tend to use AGE-
less cooking methods:

- **Middle Eastern.** Olive oil, yogurt, chickpeas, and parsley are low in
AGEs and high in antioxidants and vitamins. Bean dips and spreads

such as hummus, stews and soups made with fava beans or split peas, and stuffed cabbage rolls are all excellent choices.

- **Chinese.** These restaurants offer many AGE-less choices, due in large part to their traditional method of steaming. Avoid deep-fried dishes, such as breaded chicken or crispy noodles, and instead opt for soups, steamed dumplings, or marinated beef or chicken stir-fries with vegetables. Skip any heavy, sweet sauces.
- **Mexican.** Skip the fried tortilla chips and choose healthier dishes, such as soups, fresh fish tacos (not fried) made with soft non-GMO corn tortillas, served with guacamole and pico de gallo.

Of all the underlying toxins potentially impacting a long and healthy life, AGEs are likely the most easily controllable. These compounds do not have to be totally eliminated, but they do need to be markedly reduced to a level the body can safely manage. This is exactly where the Radical Longevity 7-Day Menu Plan and recipes found in Chapter 10 come into play. But for right now, let's turn our attention to the physical body and the important topic of fascia for radical health.

CHAPTER 4

NEW RULE #4: FREE UP FASCIA FOR YOUTHFUL MOVEMENT

In this chapter, you'll learn . . .

- What fascia is and why it is so critical to your longevity
- How your arthritis may actually be symptoms of "frozen fascia" and how to restore movement to stiff joints
- Why adhesions form and how they contribute to unexplained pain
- Radically simple solutions for pain-free movement

FAR TOO MANY PEOPLE ACCEPT JOINT PAIN, LIMITED MOBILITY, AND LOSS OF FLEXIBIL-ity as inevitable aging, but it doesn't have to be this way. There is a key player in the tight muscles, painful joints, dimpled thighs, scars, adhesions, and many of the unexplained mystery symptoms plaguing us: fascia.

Fascia, also known as connective tissue, isn't like other tissues in the body. It's complicated and can't be neatly dissected and studied as easily as anatomy. Rich in collagen, fascia is a sheet or band of tissue that provides structure and acts as a divider and support between muscles and other internal organs. This tissue is more than just a layer of packaging, though; it protects every part of you, helps hold the shape of your body, takes part in every movement you make, and is involved in every injury and scar you've ever had.

Your fascia is all connected. It weaves its webs around your six hundred muscles, diving deep and forming pockets difficult to reach from the surface of your skin. In a normal, healthy state, fascia is smooth and relaxed and moves without any restriction. The problems come when you haven't been active or moving much, when you're under stress for prolonged periods of time, or when you lack flexibility or have poor posture.

All of these conditions restrict the movement and flow of fascia, thickening the fibers, clumping it into adhesions (bands of scarlike tissue that form inside your body), and cementing the once freely mobile fibers into one place. This is how fascia can be a factor at the root of your arthritis symptoms.

THE BODY REMEMBERS—THE LEGACY OF TRAUMA

Every type of physical and emotional trauma is recorded in your body long after you may have forgotten all about it. Whenever you experience any kind of surgery (even dental surgery), an accident, an injury, infection, or inflammation, your body gets to work on healing—and this "work" creates internal scars in your fascia, called adhesions, as the first step. These adhesions are made up of tiny strands of collagen—similar to the strands of a nylon rope.

Like any good-quality rope, these adhesions are strong, having been measured with a tensile strength at close to 2,000 pounds per square inch. Unless treated, these adhesions remain in the body after healing. Before you know it, they act much like a straitjacket in the areas of the body where formed, and we confuse them as by-products of aging instead of an accumulation of adjustments made by living.

Later in life, if we experience chronic pain, we may not recognize its source. If we accept that it is just a form of pain, we can overlook repairs that are well within our reach. I experienced this firsthand. Through my own subsequent research, I came to realize that because adhesions are composed of collagen fibers, they do not appear on any diagnostic test. That explains why X-rays, MRIs, ultrasounds, or CT scans do not pick them up.

REVERSING THE DAMAGE

Fascial adhesions that formed years or decades ago from earlier surgeries or traumas are not really necessary anymore, but your body has no way to dissolve them, and we don't even know to look for them until symptoms show up. The good news is you can reverse the damage. Just as muscles stretch and can be massaged into relaxation, fascia can be worked to regain its fluidity and flexibility. The first key to fascia rejuvenation is found in your lymphatic system.

Your lymph is like a liquid tissue that traverses the entire network of your fascia and, in fact, is often referred to as "liquid fascia." Just like blood moves through vessels (which are also a type of fascia), lymph fluid travels from node to node in its network of vessels through the layers of your fascia. While blood is busy delivering nutrients and oxygen to your cells, lymph is busy removing cellular wastes (including unwelcome invaders, such as viruses and bacteria) and maintaining your overall fluid balance. Lymph vessels are surrounded by a network of nerves, so the movement of lymph fluid alone is soothing and healing. When you get your lymph moving and flowing, you also help free up your restricted fascia.

The structure of your fascia comes from collagen, known as "solid fascia." Collagen is the most abundant protein in our body, holding together our tendons, muscles, bones, cartilage, joints, skin, and more. Beginning at age twenty-one, our collagen production slows down at a rate of up to 1 percent a year, causing thinning and weakening of the cartilage in the joints, which later in life often leads to arthritis. There are many types of collagen, and the type made depends on the cell making it. The cells that are primarily responsible for making the collagen of fascia are called fibroblasts. They communicate with one another to adapt to the tension and compression that results from the stretching and movement of fascia and maintain the flexibility of fascia, even under strain. When fascia is dehydrated or pushed beyond its limits, fibroblasts stimulate inflammation as a protective mechanism, but when inflammation persists, fibroblasts can no longer clean, repair, and replace damaged fascia. This is when the trauma leads to adhesion formation.

As mentioned, there currently is no imaging technology available to find adhesions and other fascial traumas when symptoms arise. It's important to listen to your body and trust what it is telling you, so as to find the healing you need. Symptoms of internal adhesions may include bloating and abdominal pain. Scars that are fixed and immobile are also sure to have adhesions beneath the skin.

Cupping Therapy

Cupping is an ancient, drugless way to relieve pain and spasms, and digestive and respiratory woes, to promote relaxation, and to improve the health of your skin, assisting in detoxification. Cups, applied by a qualified practitioner, are placed to provide suction to the skin to stimulate blood and energy flow as a way to relieve pain and inflammation.

While this practice of cupping for deep tissue therapy and lymphatic drainage is well known throughout most of the world, it's relatively undervalued as a newcomer to the United States. However, more than six hundred studies have been done showing its safety and effectiveness for a variety of maladies, from shingles to low back and neck pain, facial paralysis, and asthma, with the most common side effect being bruising at the suction site.

Skillful cupping creates suction when attaching a cup to the surface of the skin, and techniques may include leaving the cup in place or moving it around on oiled skin. Here are five of its amazing health benefits.

1. **Revitalize your skin.** Cupping for deep tissue therapy increases blood and lymph circulation to the skin. The suction opens up capillaries and permits the exchange of gases to your skin cells, releasing congested and stagnant lymph and blood, and also helps remove any toxins from the skin's surface. The cupping procedure focuses mainly on the back of your midsection, but the effects extend throughout the body.

2. **Relieve pain.** There are two basic ways people use cupping for pain. The first is to apply the cups where it hurts—sore muscles (or spasms) and achy joints are the most common sites. The suction from cupping relaxes muscles and releases spasms. The second is to cup along the meridian channels of the body. In a nutshell, meridians are the "highways" by which energy flows through the body.

3. **Respiratory relief.** Relief from asthma, congestion from the common cold, or other respiratory infection is among the most common uses for cupping worldwide.

4. **Revive your digestion.** Cupping stimulates stronger digestion, clears constipation, and improves appetite regulation.

5. **Boost your immunity.** Cupping has been shown to modulate the immune system at the cellular level.

HOW TO FREE UP FASCIA

Fascia can be categorized into liquid or solid, so it's important to know how to deal with both. Liquid fascia solutions can be as simple as stretching or low-impact exercise, as well as

Move your lymph. Since the lymph system doesn't have a pump the way your bloodstream does, it's up to you to get it moving mechanically. Thirty minutes of walking a day is a great way to start.

Go on the rebound. Even five minutes each day on the mini trampoline or rebounder, bouncing lightly, or walking on the balls of your feet, is enough to get your lymph moving.

Hydrate. Lymph fluid is just like any other fluid in your body—you need water to keep the supply up. Stay hydrated all day long so waste products are flushed out of the lymph and it stays free flowing.

Try dry brushing. Lymph is most concentrated in the fascia that's only millimeters below the skin. You don't need anything more intense or invasive than dry brushing to get lymph moving and free up fascia.

Stretch yourself. Tight muscles restrict and tighten fascia over time. This creates a vicious cycle, where the muscles become compressed and tighten even more, which leads to nerve compression and pain. Relax in a warm Epsom salts bath or detox bath, stretch your muscles, and follow it up with rebounding or other light activity to really get your lymph flowing.

Try Yin for the win. When it comes to fascia, gentle yoga is more effective than more intense pressure and exercise. Yin Yoga not only helps you stretch your muscles and get lymph flowing, but holding the poses can facilitate the breaking up of scar tissue and fascial adhesions.

Let yourself go with myofascial release massage. In this technique, the therapist uses gentle pressure to find the areas of restricted movement, and this is not always located right where your pain is. They then apply gentle pressure until the tension releases and move on to the next area to repeat the process. I personally recommend active release technique (ART) practitioners, Barnes practitioners, and those who follow Louis Stecco's work (see Resources).

Solid fascia solutions include eating a proper diet, making sure you get plenty of restorative nutrients, and taking therapeutic treatments, such as myofascial massages.

THE COLLAGEN CONNECTION

Homemade bone broths cooked low and slow for several hours are a superfood for collagen production. The least desirable cuts of meat and bones for soup are some of the most collagen-rich foods available. Although collagen-boosting protein powders are all the rage right now, there is growing concern over what's actually in these powders and whether they're doing more harm than good. Grass-fed meat is best, since animals raised in confined feeding operations contribute to antibiotic resistance and contain antibiotic residues in their meat. Their bones have been found to contain heavy metals, including lead, pesticides, fluoride, and even radiation. Basically, whatever these animals have been fed and exposed to in their environment gets stored in their tissues, especially bone.

When you buy bone broth, unless it's organic, it's likely been sourced from animals raised on factory farms. Remember, bone broths are cooked for extended periods of time, so the bones break down and release their nutrients into the broth—along with their contaminants. Bone broth powders and gelatins are bone broths that are cooked even longer, then dehydrated, which concentrates their toxins even more.

There's no need to expose ourselves to these toxic products to build healthy collagen, which can increase our toxic load over time. Using homemade bone broths or trusted brands, such as Kettle & Fire (see Resources), supplementing with collagen-building nutrients, and avoiding collagen antinutrients, we can provide the optimal conditions for the collagen our body needs to keep connective tissues healthy and strong.

Additionally, daily weight-bearing exercise, such as resistance or weight training or walking, enables cartilage to repair more easily and keeps collagen strong. This type of exercise is essential to rebuilding and repairing our joints as we age.

Note that before you begin taking any supplements, you should check with your health-care provider for any issues or contraindications.

TARGETED LIFESTYLE AND NUTRITIONAL SOLUTIONS

Quit smoking. Nicotine constricts the blood vessels in the skin, causing reduced blood flow and delivery of nutrients and oxygen, which damages delicate tissue. Even the chemicals present in secondhand smoke damage both the collagen and elastin proteins in the skin and fascia, causing skin to thin, wrinkle, and age, while fascia becomes more stiff, weak, and inflexible.

Fortify with vitamin C. Vitamin C in combination with lysine, proline, and EGCG (green tea extract) makes your cells like an impenetrable fortress and strengthens the collagen matrix so no intruders—such as free radicals—can get through and cause damage. Linus Pauling and Matthias Rath, MD, found this combination to be effective even in stopping the spread of cancer. Dr. Rath's Healthy Collagen formula contains 900 mg of vitamin C, 900 mg of L-lysine, and 450 mg of L-proline. The suggested dosage is 1 to 7 g daily.

Rejuvenate with L-arginine. This amino acid is one of the building blocks of collagen; it can also increase nitric oxide production to promote healthy cardiovascular function. The recommended dosage is 1 to 3 g daily with equal amounts of lysine.

Build up with TMG. Trimethylglycine (TMG), an amino acid derivative, is a rich source of glycine, one of the main building blocks of collagen. It's best known for its energy-boosting effects but also promotes healthy brain balance and good digestion, and is commonly recommended for those with an MTHFR genetic defect. The recommended dosage is 2,500 to 6,000 mg taken in two divided doses daily.

Protect yourself with niacin (vitamin B$_3$). Not only does niacin promote healthy collagen production, it also decreases protein glycation, which is the process that forms AGEs. Niacin protects the skin from harmful sunlight radiation and promotes cardiovascular health. Start slowly at 250 mg at bedtime, then increase gradually to 1 to 2 g daily in divided doses. The form best tolerated is inositol hexanicotinate. Endur-acin, a slow-acting, time-released niacin, is typically available in three strengths—250 mg, 500 mg, and 750 mg—for easy compliance with doctor recommendations.

TARGETED SCAR AND ADHESIONS SOLUTIONS

Scars and superficial fascia pain respond well to topical herbs and innovative solutions, breaking up the adhesions underneath and allowing fascia to move more freely.

Erase scars with gotu kola. Gotu kola is an herbal scar remedy that works well topically and internally, fading existing scars, preventing new ones, and encouraging the growth of new skin. Enjoy it as an herbal tea (two cups per day); as a topical paste (combine 2 teaspoons of the dried herb powder with enough water to form a paste, apply directly to healed scar, and cover loosely with a gauze pad; as a tincture (2 teaspoons [10 ml] twice daily in water); or as a supplement (Gotu Kola Complex by MediHerb, one tablet three times daily).

Break up painful adhesions with wheat germ oil. Wheat germ oil, massaged into an existing scar, can help relieve pain and break up adhesions. David L. Hartz, DC, CFMP, also recommends cold laser treatment once the oil is applied, for maximum relief. Consult your local chiropractor or massage therapist for this particular treatment.

Cupping therapy. The International Cupping Therapy Association can assist you in finding a qualified cupping therapist in your area. Visit www .cuppingtherapy.org (see Resources).

The topic of fascia, adhesions, and scars is an underserved area in the longevity world. Freeing up fascia in the form of adhesions and scar tissue may be the missing link to pain-free movement and the ability to release stuck emotions. In the next chapter, we'll take a deeper dive into an emerging topic of great interest on the longevity scene—cellular rejuvenation.

CHAPTER 5

NEW RULE #5: ACTIVATE CELLULAR REJUVENATION

> **In this chapter, you'll learn . . .**
>
> - How to tap into your body's natural healing at the cellular level with omega-6 fats
> - Why membrane medicine is your pathway to cellular performance
> - How to replicate your body's innate cellular communication
> - How to activate your body's own stem cells

REJUVENATION AND REPAIR TRULY START AT THE CELL LEVEL. THE INTELLIGENCE of a cell lies in its membrane, even more than its nucleus. The nucleus houses DNA, but that's about all. It has all the data but initiates none of the activity—functioning more like a library. On the other hand, the cell membrane uses the DNA for reference and then tells it what to do, directing all cellular activities. Biologist and epigenetics scientist Bruce Lipton, PhD, cleverly dubbed these amazing cellular structures "mem-Brains."

Those little mem-Brains are embedded with thousands of hormone receptors. Hormones direct cellular function, but the cell's receptors are responsible for "hearing" those hormone messages. Most of today's rampant endocrine problems are the result of damaged hormone receptors—therefore, the promise of rejuvenation lies in repairing these receptors. Instead, what is typically done is to throw more hormones at the system, which does nothing to fix the problem and actually makes receptors tune out even more. This is called hormone resistance.

One type of hormone resistance involving the metabolism is insulin resistance, which if not addressed may lead to type 2 diabetes. Insulin, made in the pancreas, is the hormone that controls blood glucose levels and storage. Type 2 diabetics have plenty of insulin, but their insulin receptors have gone deaf. The way to reverse hormone resistance is to mend the cell membranes—fixing the problem at its source.

The right dietary fats make membranes more fluid and efficient—especially the omega-6 fatty acids. In fact, omega-6 linoleic acid is a key player in cellular health. It maintains the cell membrane structure and enhances permeability of the membranes—including those in the skin, digestive tract, and blood-brain barrier, preventing toxins from entering the cell.

THE "FORBIDDEN FAT," OMEGA-6

I'm sure you've heard or read that omega-6 fatty acids aren't good for us and we need to focus on omega-3 fats. The reality is more complex and there is a good deal of debate around omega-3 and omega-6 fatty acids in terms of their biological roles and how much we should be eating. Omega-3s and omega-6s are essential fatty acids (EFAs), meaning they are just that—essential. Our body cannot make them, so we must get them from the foods we eat. Omega-3s and omega-6s are both integral parts of the structure and function of cell membranes.

When the scientific community began recognizing inflammation as a major driver of chronic disease, they began to search for the cause. Blood levels revealed most of our diets are extremely top heavy in omega-6 fatty acids, and light on omega-3s—so the omega-6s, as a category, were blamed for inflammation, especially arachidonic acid (AA). Omega-6 fats were labeled "pro-inflammatory" and omega-3s as "anti-inflammatory," and the misguided mantra to simply reduce your dietary omega-6s and increase your omega-3s (e.g., supplement with fish oil) spread like wildfire.

The problem is this is oversimplified. Not all omega-6 fats are equal. It's true that many of us are overloaded in omega-6, but the type of omega-6 we're overloaded with is the toxic kind, mainly oils destroyed by overprocessing. We're talking about those found in French fries, packaged cookies (made with shortening), and junk food loaded with sugar and hydrogenated vegetable oils—all of which are indeed pro-inflammatory. The increased consumption of hydrogenated vegetable oils represents the single largest increase in any type of food over the last century. One estimate is that Americans now consume 100,000 times more vegetable oils than they did in the year 1900.

The pervasive recommendation to avoid omega-6 fats is actually counterproductive to rejuvenation and healthy aging as well as weight loss. It turns out, functional omega-6s are some of the most powerful fats for activating your fat-burning engines. They have positive benefits for the checks and balances of your body's inflammation system. They prevent toxins from entering cells by maintaining cellular membrane structure and enhance permeability in membranes. Omega-6s also help synthesize eicosanoids (tissue-like hormones) involved in day-to-day cellular activities and are involved in the synthesis and transport of cholesterol. The bottom line is that omega-6s are extremely restorative to cell membranes, and strong cell membranes are key to optimal cellular repair and performance.

THE RIGHT RATIO

Thanks to an overabundance of refined vegetable oils, processed foods, grains, and grain-fed meats, our natural essential fatty acid ratio is out of balance. For optimal cellular repair and function, it's important to routinely consume omega-6 and omega-3 fatty acids *in the right balance:* There seems to be a golden ratio of about 4:1. Hemp seed oil comes the closest to meeting this ratio of all omega-6-rich oils.

Historically, traditional diets have provided omega-6–to–omega-3 ratios in the range of 1:1 to 5:1, but the standard American diet has now put it at ratios of up to 20:1. If you have twenty times as many omega-6s as omega-3s, then they are coming from junk—meaning they're damaged and provide no nutritional benefit.

Adding to the problem is that all those junk omega-6s shut down the omega-3s through a mechanism called competitive inhibition. The omega-3s cannot compete with all those omega-6s, and so the junk omega-6s become incorporated into your cell membranes, weakening them and generating all sorts of problems, hence the cell receptor's inability to "hear" the messaging of the cell nucleus.

It may be a challenge to wrap your head around, but it's important to understand that you can be omega-6 dominant and have an omega-6 deficiency, at the same time—the difference is in having *healthy, functional* omega-6s, not just plentiful omega-6.

Surprisingly, most of our cells prefer the omega-6s over the omega-3s—especially our mitochondria, which use omega-6s almost exclusively. One of the reasons for this is the tendency for the omega-3 fatty acids to oxidize. Oxidized fatty acids are as toxic to your cells as rancid fish oil is objectionable to your nose, causing inflammation and accelerated aging.

Believe it or not, health abnormalities appear more quickly when people are omega-6 deficient. And when animals are deprived of both omega-3 and omega-6 fatty acids, abnormalities can be corrected with the omega-6s alone, whereas efforts to correct with only omega-3s make many conditions worse. Omega-3s represent about 14 percent of the total lipids in your brain and nervous system (in the form of EPA and DHA), but the omega-6s make up about 10 percent (in the form of arachidonic acid). It follows that both must be replenished on a regular basis and in the ideal ratio with healthy omega-6 choices, specifically hemp seed oil, at least 1 tablespoon per day or hemp seeds at 3 tablespoons per day.

PROTECT YOUR NATURAL DEFENSES

The radical master gene SIRT1, mentioned earlier, is often dubbed the governing anti-aging controller. It has been credited with not just slowing aging but even reversing it. And, it also has been noted as a "survival factor" in that your body has a collection of natural protective mechanisms known as *host defenses*, of which SIRT1 is the leading player. This team of defenders works to protect our cells and our membranes day in and day out. But today's unprecedented burden of environmental toxins from air, water, and food, especially in the form of AGEs, can compromise and overwhelm these defenders, as discussed in Rule #3.

Simply put, the protection of SIRT1 goes a long way in mitigating many of the ill effects of aging. Beyond decreasing AGE-rich food and AGE-rich cooking practices, another significant way to protect and increase SIRT1 is through the well-researched practice of calorie restriction, sometimes to the tune of 20 percent or more of total calories. Although the reduction of calorie consumption results in a markedly longer life span and fewer age-related diseases, it is impractical to maintain a long-term calorie restricted diet due to severe hunger. It may also be challenging to obtain enough critical nutrients on a severely low-calorie diet. So, it is no wonder that there has been a relentless search for cutting-edge nutraceuticals and technologies. The most promising is resveratrol, a well-researched compound contained in large amounts in red wine and in small amounts in tea, vegetables, fruits, and in the polyphenols found in spices. Resveratrol has been found to effectively mimic the anti-inflammatory activities of SIRT1 by decreasing free radical production, inflammation, and harmful DNA changes. In addition, it activates nitric oxide to dilate blood vessels and improves blood flow, crossing the blood-brain and blood-ocular barriers, and it regenerates mitochondria.

CELLULAR HYDRATION

Proper hydration extends beyond just making sure you drink plenty of water. True hydration involves getting the water inside your cells. Properly hydrated cells are critical to the process of removing toxins and cellular repair and reproduction. A good amount of the water we drink passes through the body and is urinated out. The predominant characteristic of aging is a loss of fuel production by mitochondria. Mitochondrial production is absolutely critical for activities that stave off aging—most important, cellular repair and replacement. Water, having basically two hydrogen molecules for every oxygen molecule along with their electrons, feeds the electrical charge necessary for fuel production. Drinking electrolyte-rich water enhances this electrical charge needed for hydration within the cells. A good approach is to drink free water intermittently infused with electrolytes and watch your stools carefully. If you begin to have loose stools, it is a sign that your body may be sensitive to electrolytes. If this occurs, cut back your intake and build more gradually.

Here are five foods and beverages you can use to increase your cellular hydration:

1. Start your day with a Live Longer Cocktail (page 132). Vegetables and fruits, such as cranberries, are full of electrolytes and rich in fiber, which helps your body absorb water within the cells.
2. Incorporate mucilaginous foods, such as chia seeds, flaxseeds, and such herbs as marshmallow root and slippery elm into your smoothies, salads, and baked goods. The slippery substance that is formed when these items are crushed and mixed with water is what you need for complete hydration.
3. Just add salt. Mineral-rich salts that have some color to them, such as Celtic, Himalayan, and Real Salt, all contain trace minerals and electrolytes that can help hydrate your cells. It's more hydrating to salt your food than it is to add salt to your water, so sprinkle a pinch of your favorite salt over every meal.
4. Drink highly diluted coconut water or cranberry water (for recipe, see page 133), or add a slice of lime, lemon, or cucumber to your water to give your body all the raw materials it needs (electrolytes and water) to support cellular hydration.
5. Add bone broth (I like Kettle & Fire brand) to your soups and stews. When your grandma made you chicken soup to get well, she knew what she was doing! The collagen in these broths is full of electrolytes as well as other nutrients that contribute to cellular hydration.

SLEEP SUPPORTS BODY REPAIR

When you don't get enough sleep, you put your body under stress, depriving it of its critical time to repair tissue, reset hormones, and consolidate memories. The following are ways that you can maximize the rejuvenating gifts of sleep.

Turn off electronics at least one hour before bedtime. Our beloved devices that we can't live without emit a type of light called blue light, which mimics daylight. Your body cannot tell the difference between the kind of blue light you see outside at noon and the kind you see from your device at midnight—and it reacts to both in the same way, reducing the sleep hormone melatonin.

Create a sleep-promoting environment. Sleep in a quiet, dark, cool room—ideally between 62° and 65°F. A warm temperature impedes sleep and causes restlessness.

Additionally, electronics emit electromagnetic radiation (electropollution) that can stress the adrenals, creating intermittent awakenings and fluctuating cortisol levels. Disable all wireless devices within 300 feet of the bedroom, if possible.

Sleep on a schedule. Try going to bed at the same time every night and waking up with the sunrise. I recommend going to bed around ten p.m. This will mimic your natural cortisol rhythm as closely as possible. Getting an hour of morning sunlight, or using extremely bright lights in the morning, could help with falling asleep at night.

Take a warm bath. Researchers suggest that taking a fifteen-minute bath at 105°F approximately ninety minutes before going to bed is helpful. The rise in body temperature, followed by the decline in core temperature, signals the body that it's bedtime. Add some lavender or chamomile essential oil to the bath to enhance relaxation.

Avoid eating or exercising in the two hours before bedtime. Both of these can cause hormonal disruptions, namely with cortisol and insulin, that interfere with sleep.

Create a nighttime routine. Practicing a specific bedtime ritual will establish a set behavior pattern that cues your brain to relax and go to sleep. I strongly encourage you to incorporate relaxation techniques into this routine. Take a warm bath, meditate, or journal to reduce sleep-sabotaging anxiety and quiet your mind and body. You might also try ¼ teaspoon of baking soda before bed to reduce overstimulating acidity that can impede your ability to fall asleep or cause multiple awakenings during sleep.

Be mindful of naps. Try not to nap after four p.m. If you do need a quick reenergizer, try a twenty- to thirty-minute nap in the middle of the day.

SIGNALING MOLECULES ARE KEY TO CELLULAR COMMUNICATION

Redox signaling molecules are created within every cell in the body. In fact, your body is one big redox signaling program. Signaling molecules are believed to be reduced as we age at the rate of about 10 percent per decade. These molecules serve as cellular messengers, helping to keep cells functioning at optimal levels and boosting the body's natural cellular renewal. These amazing molecules act as a communication system, signaling the activation of genetic pathways, supporting total body health, and facilitating improved function for every system of the body. Due to age, environmental toxins, and stress, they are used up and cell signaling is reduced and weakened and cellular communication breaks down, along with restricted gene expression. Most important, these signaling molecules can provide support where your body needs it most, as reflected in cellular meltdown.

Cell signaling in your body is directly involved in regulating gene expression. Genes provide critical data that gives life-sustaining instructions to cells, which then are tasked with carrying out those instructions to keep you alive and healthy. When cell communication breaks down, the signal weakens, and gene expression can be disrupted.

THE PROMISE OF YOUR OWN ADULT STEM CELLS

Twenty-four hours a day, seven days a week, your body is using adult stem cells to repair and renew damaged cells. Adult stem cells are strategically located throughout your body from the time you're an embryo. They continue to be produced throughout your entire lifetime, but the production slows as we age. Not only that, but they become harder to activate as we age too.

These stem cells have far reaching potential—they can be used to build whatever tissue your body is in need of at the time they're called into service. Scientists have found stem cells in brain, liver, skin, muscles, bone marrow, blood, and blood vessels.

Adult stem cell therapy includes everything that stimulates the production and activation of your body's own stem cells to divide and regenerate to stimulate healing of a cell, tissue, or organ. This can be as simple as intermittent fasting, or as complicated as harvesting bone marrow for a stem cell transplant. The type of therapy you need depends on the illness or body repair you're facing.

PHOTOTHERAPY EFFECTS ON YOUR NATURAL STEM CELLS

Now there is promise using phototherapy technology in a wearable patch. Known as X39, this noninvasive, easily applicable patch can be worn daily to help mobilize and reset stem cells to a younger and more vitalized state. Using the power of light it helps to activate the copper-binding tripeptide GHK-Cu, which has the ability to stimulate four thousand genes. When placed on the body, these nano-patches stimulate nerves and acupuncture points to produce myriad age-reducing benefits, including decreased inflammation and wound healing, better sleep, pain reduction, and increased mental clarity.

TARGETED CELLULAR SOLUTIONS

Feed your cell walls with membrane medicine. Since toxins tend to attach to cell membranes, the membrane-stabilizing diet that is present in the Radical Longevity Program helps remove them. A forgotten key to most cellular rejuvenation problems is the rebalancing and revamping of the fats in your diet. Adding biologically potent omega-6s, such as hemp, sesame, safflower, sunflower, or pine nut oil is a surefire way to fuel membrane medicine. The Radical Longevity Plan addresses this gap head-on. It closes and adds a dimensional level of repair to cellular function with its unique omega-6 fats. If your cells are not getting what they need, they will not function properly. Fix the cell and rejuvenation at your very core begins.

Reprogram your DNA with resveratrol. There is now a resveratrol product on the market that was found to "activate nine-fold more longevity genes than plain resveratrol." Called Longevinex, it contains a group of synergistic molecules in addition to resveratrol that reinvigorates cellular repair. Longevinex, 100 mg per day, is recommended (see Resources).

Replicate your body's innate signaling molecules. As the world's only verified supplement containing redox signaling molecules, ASEA Redox Supplement can help reset health on a cellular level and aid in the repair of the body's natural processes. The signaling molecules are suspended in a patented process pristine saline solution composed of the same life-sustaining molecules that natively exist in the human body. This *revolutionary* product has been scientifically tested and has been found to positively impact five genetic pathways. It aids a healthy inflammatory response, helps maintain cardiovascular health and support arterial elasticity, improves overall gut health and digestive enzyme production, and modulates hormone balance to support vitality and wellness (see Resources).

STEM CELL SOLUTIONS

Introduce intermittent fasting. Even during a short-term fast, your body turns to fats for fuel, which boost your intestinal stem cell function. Because of the strong connection between your intestines and your immune system, the positive effects are felt not only with digestion but also immunity.

According to MIT researchers, this one dietary change is enough to reverse age-related stem cell decline.

Lower your blood sugar. Most stem cell therapies require you to have a hemoglobin A1c test done beforehand to measure your blood sugars because elevated blood sugar decreases the life span and number of adult stem cells in the body. The optimal A1c for your stem cells is 5.1 or less. You can effectively lower your blood sugar on the Radical Longevity Plan with the right kind of fats, moderate protein, and low carbohydrates. You can also add chromium at 200 mcg three times a day plus the core mineral zinc. Many people find that blood sugar regulation is even more effective with a product called berberine at 500 to 1,000 mg three times a day.

Add organ meats and bone marrow to your diet. Organ meats are rich in vitamin K_2, which has been shown in studies to activate the stem cells in your blood and bone marrow. Start with grass-fed goose liver, which tops the list of stem cell–boosting foods. Or, if roasting bones with marrow appeals to you more, use the bone marrow like butter and spread it over your favorite savory foods. It's not only anti-inflammatory, rich in collagen, and high in vitamin B_{12}, but it's also loaded with natural stem cell activators.

Avoid drugs that sabotage stem cells. One of the most common treatments for painful joints is steroid injections, but steroids in any form should be avoided for healthy stem cells. This group of medications reduces the adult stem cells' ability to transform into the tissue they're needed for. Also harmful are the quinolone antibiotics, including Cipro and Levaquin. These drugs are harmful to the stem cells of the ligaments and tendons.

Supplement with special cell activators. As we age, even when our body sends the signals for repairs that are needed, fewer cells are able to respond and activate. Three main nutrients can help: (1) vitamin C may increase the number of stem cells in bone marrow, (2) vitamin D_3 can help reverse the stem cell aging process while helping them to activate when needed, and (3) Longevinex resveratrol can help stem cells multiply and differentiate into different types of tissue.

Let there be light. A targeted form of phototherapy found in LifeWave X39 Patches is now available on the market to stimulate cell activation providing support at a cellular level. In turn, these patches regulate thousands of genes, which provides support at the cellular level. It harnesses the power of light to provide real hope in the quest for age reversal and life extension (see Resources).

Today, we are better equipped to care for our health by taking full advantage of the latest cell regenerating daily practices, preventative medicine, and technology advances. The next chapter takes on the topic of misbehaving minerals. Since minerals are the true catalyst of life, imbalances have wide ranging negative impact on every cell, tissue, and organ of the body.

CHAPTER 6

NEW RULE #6: MIND YOUR MINERALS

> ## In this chapter, you'll learn . . .
>
> - About the number one brain-aging trigger hiding in your home
> - How copper is linked to Alzheimer's disease
> - How too much iron impacts aging
> - The critical balance between copper and iron levels
> - How you can "reverse the rust" and fix your fatigue

THERE'S NO DOUBT THAT THE MOST DREADED DISEASE ASSOCIATED WITH GROWING older is . . . Alzheimer's. So, as we look at minerals and why both copper and iron are critical to any discussion about aging, my focus, right from the start, is to make you acutely aware of an ignored but potent Alzheimer's trigger hiding in your own home and what you can do about it NOW.

The reality is, I don't think it is coincidental that the rise of Alzheimer's disease (AD) mirrors the use of copper plumbing in the twentieth century. And neither does Dr. George Brewer, a professor at the University of Michigan Medical School, who is considered one of the country's leading experts on copper toxicity. Dr. Brewer explains that "when I educated myself about the history and current status of AD, two facts made a huge impression on me. These facts were that while we had an epidemic of AD in developed countries, this epidemic wasn't occurring in undeveloped countries. Second, the epidemic was new, starting during the 1900s. These facts gave me what I like to call my first epiphany about AD—namely, some environmental cause of the disease had occurred in developed countries during the 1900s."

So, let's get right into it. Here, in brief, is Dr. Brewer's data summary from the science communication publication *Scientia Global*. This verbatim synthesis of data lends credibility to the assertion that excess inorganic (divalent) copper (or copper-2) has a direct link to Alzheimer's:

→ The addition of 0.12 ppm divalent copper to the drinking water of AD animal models greatly enhanced AD. The US allowance for copper in drinking water is 1.3 parts per million, ten times as high.

→ From one-third to two-thirds of North American drinking water samples contain unsafe levels of divalent copper, according to the animal model studies.

→ The development of the AD epidemic closely parallels in time the increasing use of copper plumbing, beginning in the early 1900s. It is still found in 90 percent of homes in the United States.

→ Japan has shunned the use of copper plumbing and is a developed country with a low prevalence of AD. But when Japanese people migrate to Hawaii, where copper plumbing is used, their AD prevalence matches other developed countries.

→ Ingestion of divalent copper in the form of copper-containing supplement pills has been shown to decrease cognition at six times the normal rate.

→ Monovalent copper is the prevalent form of copper in food and we evolved a safe mechanism for absorbing and handling monovalent copper, but not divalent copper.

→ Unlike organic (monovalent) copper, some divalent copper is absorbed directly into the blood and slowly damages cognition.

THE DIFFERENCE BETWEEN ORGANIC AND INORGANIC COPPER

Simply put, copper comes in two forms, organic and inorganic. *Organic copper* (monovalent) is found in such foods as avocado, asparagus, liver, mushrooms, nuts, and chocolate. Organic copper, considered an essential micronutrient, is, by and large, safely bound to proteins and utilized to help form red blood cells, and for healthy bones, connective tissue, and the immune system. The copper is bioavailable and is critical for your body to build collagen—you can't have radiant, wrinkle-free skin without it. When in balance with zinc (its mineral antagonist), copper is responsible for activating more than thirty enzymes. A number of metabolic functions are dependent upon balanced copper metabolism. These include the formation of the myelin nerve sheaths, the synthesis of neurotransmitters, the production of keratin and melanin, fertility, and the building of the body's connective tissue. So far, so good!

However, *inorganic copper* (divalent) or biounavailable copper is found mainly from environmental sources, like drinking water coming from copper pipes and multivitamin/ mineral supplements. Other common sources of inorganic copper include copper-lined cookware, copper intrauterine devices, dental amalgams, fungicides for swimming pools, and copper wiring often found in homes and offices. This divalent copper accumulates silently and stealthily over a period of many years, causing serious neurological damage by switching on an inflammatory response in the brain that begins to fuse beta-amyloid to plaque, eventually leading to the destruction of brain cells and to Alzheimer's.

Copper toxicity alters our brain and changes the way we age, taking us from healthy, productive, independent individuals to a state of continual dependence and sickness. This process doesn't happen overnight, but its long assault on our brain cells ultimately leads to destruction.

TELLTALE SIGNS OF COPPER TOXICITY

Interestingly, decades before Dr. Brewer made the connection between copper toxicity and Alzheimer's, I was made aware of neurological and other issues associated with the overabundance of copper. Many years ago, Dr. Paul Eck, who was not only my teacher but also my friend and health-care provider, described "copperhead" personality types that are distinguished by their highly charged nervous system, which causes compulsive and sometimes addictive behaviors. These individuals are highly creative and intensely hyperactive.

Other common symptoms associated with copper toxicity include depression, insomnia, anorexia nervosa, anxiety, various skin disorders, hair loss, and allergies.

So, copper has been on my radar for a very long time. In the early 1970s, I worked with a nutritionally oriented psychiatrist at Deepbrook Associates in Newtown, Connecticut, who systematically took hair samples from every new patient. Unbelievably, he would find that many of the children he was treating who were suffering from learning disabilities and hyperactivity were also suffering from a copper imbalance. Once the copper was in check, the hyperactive symptoms disappeared.

As I have discussed, the problematic potential of excess copper is the corresponding *decrease of zinc*. A copper-zinc imbalance also affects the liver's ability to detoxify, as both are needed to activate key liver enzymes. A nutritionally oriented psychiatrist, Carl Pfeiffer, MD, PhD, was instrumental in teaching a whole generation of psychiatrists how a copper excess was at the bottom of many depression, anxiety, and bipolar issues. For his breakthrough work in researching the connection between biochemical imbalances in the body and mental illness, he was inducted into the Orthomolecular Hall of Fame in 2004.

Copper levels also rise and fall in tandem with estrogen levels. If you are deficient in zinc, the balancing mineral to copper, copper levels tend to rise. Weight gain as well as food cravings, mood swings, fatigue, depression, and yeast infections are all common symptoms of copper overload. In fact, migraine headaches are often triggered by an improper copper-to-zinc imbalance, which can influence the restriction of blood vessels.

TARGETED COPPER SOLUTIONS

By implementing these suggested solutions, you can kick copper to the curb and greatly reduce your chances of developing dementia and other debilitating health problems.

- **Avoid taking supplements that contain copper.** Avoid copper-enriched multivitamin/mineral supplements as they most likely contain the inorganic form of copper.
- **Test your drinking water levels.** Many companies offer this service (see Resources). If the level registers 0.01 ppm (0.01 ug/l or less), it is considered safe. Do note that if it is over 0.01 ppm, it is not necessary to change out copper plumbing, which can be very expensive. Simply install a filter that removes copper (such as a reverse osmosis filter) and place on the tap used for drinking and cooking.
- **Remove as many copper sources as possible.** These include copper-lined pots and pans, copper IUDs, and copper dental components.
- **Balance intake of copper-rich foods.** Copper-rich foods include avocado, soy, shellfish, tea, chocolate, nuts, and seeds. Balance with zinc-rich meat, pumpkin, and eggs.
- **Supplement with zinc.** This immune-boosting mineral plays a key role in the healthy function of neurons. Zinc is the "good guy" in brain health. Alzheimer's patients are typically zinc deficient.
- **Bind copper with resveratrol.** Resveratrol is a copper chelator. Check out Longevinex 100 mg of micronized, microencapsulated trans-resveratrol per capsule (see Resources).

WHY WE NEED TO DUMP THE IRON

For most of our young lives, we were told to be sure to get enough iron in our diet and our multivitamins. I knew this all too well as a public health nutritionist. Iron deficiency, with its classic symptoms of debilitating fatigue and shortness of breath, is such a great public health concern that we start screening for it as young as twelve months of age. Lack of iron can stunt a child's development and growth. Processed foods, such as refined rice, flour, and cornmeal, are fortified with iron, and multivitamins are chock-full of it, to ensure that children and women of childbearing age receive adequate amounts.

Once you are around eighteen years old, excess iron starts to accumulate in your blood at the rate of about 1 mg per day. Because of blood loss during monthly menstruation, women of childbearing age have roughly half the circulating iron that men have. Women in this age group also have roughly half the rates of heart disease, cancer, and diabetes.

But what are the effects of all this accumulating iron on men? And women who have gone through menopause? As you age, you need less than you're probably getting. And even though it doesn't get the attention it deserves, too much iron is *not* a good thing. Iron overload as we age is at least as much a concern as iron deficiency is when we are younger—and is just as dangerous. Accumulating iron is not naturally removed by our system except through the blood, via menstruation or blood donation.

IRON: THE NUTS AND BOLTS

It's been estimated that for every 1 percent increase in ferritin (stored iron) levels, your risk for cardiovascular disease shoots up by 4 percent! And the risks don't end at heart disease. Too much iron also accelerates aging, by creating oxidative stress that causes cell damage and unwanted DNA changes. Plus, iron overload has been linked to arthritis, fatty liver disease, metabolic syndrome, type 2 diabetes, and even cancer.

To know the true state of your iron levels, at your next blood test or annual checkup, have your physician order a ferritin test—first and foremost. Once you have your results in hand, you need to know what your numbers mean. There's a normal range for ferritin and then there's an *optimal* range, backed by science and years of research. Normal ranges only let you know you aren't in immediate danger, whereas optimal ranges tell you when you are truly in good health. Ferritin, in both men and postmenopausal women, is optimally between 50 and 70 ng/ml. Ferritin levels below this warrant further blood testing to rule out iron deficiency anemia. These lower, more optimal rates also apply to annual blood donors, in part because blood removal helps keep circulating iron levels lower. Levels above the normal ranges are a sign you are accumulating excess iron.

You'll want to repeat your ferritin test at least every two years, and more often if your ferritin levels are above the optimal range.

YOU'RE NOT WHAT YOU EAT—
YOU'RE WHAT YOU DIGEST

I'm sure you're familiar with the phrase, "You are what you eat," but the truth is that you are what you *absorb*—and what you *accumulate*. This is especially true when it comes to iron. Iron is a critical micronutrient that is essential for human life, primarily because of its role in the formation of hemoglobin. The average adult's body has a total of 2 to 4 g of iron, and over 80 percent of that is contained in the hemoglobin of red blood cells, which help transport oxygen to the rest of our body, along with other critical processes.

Once we accumulate more iron than we need, the protein ferritin stores the excess—until it can't. The excess iron builds up, and this unbound renegade accelerates oxidation, essentially "rusting" your body tissues and organs, aging you prematurely. The result is a dramatic increase in your risk of heart disease, cancer, arthritis, cataracts, diabetes, osteoporosis, liver disorders, diseases of the retina, and brain disorders, such as Alzheimer's disease.

But who is at risk? No one is immune to progressive iron buildup. Although some people have hemochromatosis—the genetic form of iron overload—this disease is rare, affecting less than 1 percent of Americans. The truth is iron overload is a universal threat as you age, regardless of your genetics.

The Mediterranean Diet and the Blue Zone Longevity

When we look for examples of people who are aging well, we need look no further than the Blue Zones, which are areas of the world where people live longer and healthier-than-average lives. Their optimal iron levels are commonly overlooked factors in their healthy aging. According to a study published in *Experimental Gerontology*, the blood tests of those over age ninety living in the Mediterranean Blue Zone (Sardinia) showed almost 40 percent lower levels of ferritin (stored iron) than did middle-aged controls.

Their longevity and optimal iron levels are due in no small part to their traditional Mediterranean-style diet, which is well known among cardiologists for its heart-protective effects. What's their secret? Their diet is perfectly balanced between bioavailable iron sources, iron inhibitors, and absorption enhancers. Their low levels of ferritin are a direct measure of the low level of free iron available to do oxidative or inflammatory damage. In other words, there's nothing "rusting" them from the inside out—and it shows in their long, healthy lives.

(continues)

(continued)

In addition to the healthy fruits and vegetables that are a mainstay of Mediterranean cuisine, it's the healthy fats that truly set the diet apart. Olive oil, omega-6-rich nuts and seeds, and fatty fish, such as sardines, salmon, mackerel, herring, and lake trout, are rich in omega-3s and are a large part of the Mediterranean diet, which also includes limited dairy and red wine in moderation.

YOUR GUT HEALTH AFFECTS YOUR IRON LEVELS

If you have read any of my other books, then you know just how important your digestion is to your overall health—and iron metabolism is no exception. Not only do your pancreatic enzymes dwindle as you age, but your stomach also becomes more alkaline, which causes a whole host of problems with nutrient absorption. If your stomach is too alkaline, it cannot absorb iron, along with other vitamins and minerals.

Iron and your heart. Plain and simple, iron can be a hidden killer that adversely affects the heart. A landmark five-year study conducted in Finland followed 1,900 men with no clinical evidence of coronary disease at the start of the study. Measuring the amount of ferritin in the blood of the participants, the researchers found that for each 1 percent increase in ferritin, the risk of heart attack increased by more than 4 percent. A ferritin level of 200 ng/ml more than doubled the relative risk of heart attack.

Your brain on iron. Accumulating free iron in your brain is the number one risk factor for advancing age. Everyone's need for iron decreases in their fifties and sixties, in large part because the production of myelin slows. Myelin is an important protein-rich, fatty tissue in the brain and nervous system that acts as insulation for every nerve cell you have. Iron helps signal the growth of myelin, so once it stops growing, excess iron begins to accumulate in the brain. Recent advances in MRI technology allow us to see both iron and myelin in the brain. Iron has long been suspected in the development of Alzheimer's disease, and a recent study at the University of California in Los Angeles found higher than normal iron levels in the brains of people with Alzheimer's. Although this disease is still a puzzle to the medical community, with no known cause or cure, this new research shows that the buildup of iron in the brain may be causing free radical reactions that mark the start of this devastating disease. And once iron accumulates, so does copper. Iron and copper are double-edged swords. Even though they are necessary for your health, even a modest excess is enough to age your brain prematurely. The hallmark of Alzheimer's disease is the presence of beta-amyloid plaque; and an excess of iron, followed by an excess of copper, not only leads the brain to hold on to too much beta-amyloid, but will also cause it to produce even more beta-amyloid. A vicious cycle, to be sure.

Alzheimer's disease is not the only danger of excess iron in the brain. When iron deposits in the hippocampus of the brain, which is responsible for short-term memory, memory decline results. When iron accumulates in the temporal and frontal lobes of the brain, which are associated with language and higher functions, language issues arise. Basically, the area of the brain where excess iron deposits form determines the type of damage you will sustain. And brains with the most excess iron deteriorate first and fastest. That's one race you don't want to win, especially as you age.

THE EYES HAVE IT

The Iron Disorder Institute names iron as a contributor to the leading cause of blindness in people over fifty years old: age-related macular degeneration (AMD). Your body's normal systems of checks and balances keep iron out of your well-protected retina, but when iron levels are high and export from your cells is unregulated, iron can accumulate in the retina and damage the macula, leading to AMD. When there are already low oxygen levels or inflammation in the eye from preexisting disease, then iron can accumulate to even higher levels, causing greater damage and leading to blindness.

A LIVER RICH IN IRON MAY BE POOR IN HEALTH

When it comes to iron, your liver is your knight in shining armor; it rallies the troops to conserve and recycle iron when it's low and shields you from harm by storing iron when it's in excess. The liver increases its iron storage to protect your other tissues, namely your heart and pancreas. However, the liver sustains damage when it's forced to store excess iron for a prolonged period of time. The longer the excess iron sits in the liver, the more free radicals are produced, causing liver dysfunction and injury, and over time, leading to diseases, including fatty liver disease, cirrhosis, fibrosis, and even liver cancer.

Fatty Liver Disease

Fatty liver disease (FLD) is reaching epidemic proportions in the United States, affecting as much as 20 percent of the adult population, most of whom are over age forty. Your liver stores excess fat much as it stores excesses of other toxic substances in your body. When the total weight of your liver is more than 5 percent fat, you have fatty liver disease. Causes of this disease include

- Heavy alcohol intake: 100 percent of heavy drinkers have FLD and up to 80 percent of moderate drinkers are affected. The US Department of Agriculture defines heavy drinking for adults over age sixty-five as four or more drinks daily, or eight or more drinks over a period of one week.
- Excess refined sugar and high-fructose corn syrup in the diet
- Obesity
- Diabetes: The risk of nonalcoholic fatty liver disease in patients with type 1 diabetes is almost 50 to 70 percent. For those with type 2 diabetes, the risk is about 50 percent. These patients are at high risk of developing advanced stages of nonalcoholic FLD and progressing to end-stage liver disease.
- Hyperlipidemia: High levels of circulating fats (lipids) in your blood contribute to FLD.
- Genetics
- Some medications that harm the liver, including acetaminophen (an OTC pain reliever), tetracycline (a common antibiotic), and tamoxifen (for breast cancer)
- Toxin exposure
- Iron overload

FLD is a silent disease; you may notice fatigue, right upper quadrant abdominal fullness, bloating after meals, and trouble digesting fats as bile production decreases in the liver.

How can you tell your liver is accumulating iron? Believe it or not, your liver is so desperate to rid itself of toxic accumulations that it's attempting to rid itself through your skin. The skin is the second liver of the body. Liver spots, commonly known as age spots, are those brown blotches (that are too big to be freckles) that appear on your skin as you age. The brown pigment in those spots, called lipofuscin (commonly known as the aging pigment), is a mixture of fats, proteins, and—you guessed it—iron. These liver spots are a sign that toxic cellular waste products (including iron) are building up faster than your liver can eliminate them.

HOW TO DUMP THE IRON

It's a complete paradigm shift to think of off-loading excess iron when you've been told your whole life that anemia is the enemy. But the truth is, excess iron is the silent killer running rampant among our unknowing seniors.

TARGETED IRON-BINDING SOLUTIONS

Once your balanced diet keeps iron from accumulating, and you have received your results from a ferritin blood test, the next step is to pull the excess iron from your tissues. The process of removing heavy metals from the tissues in your body is known as chelation. We look to concentrated nutrients and oxygen therapies for this important task.

- **Vitamin C optimizes iron levels.** Famous for increasing the absorption of iron, there is no research to show that in the case of iron overload vitamin C continues to increase iron absorption. In fact, the contrary is true, making vitamin C the only known vitamin to optimize iron levels, whether high or low. The suggested dosage is 3,000 to 5,000 mg daily of a time-released or buffered C.
- **Supplement with IP6.** Inositol hexaphosphate (IP6), also known as phytic acid, is a fabulous yet often overlooked natural chelator and my supplement of choice for gentle iron reduction. It not only binds excess free iron but also blocks iron from making free radicals. I recommend taking 3 g twice daily for six months, while supplementing with an iron-free multivitamin.
- **Quercetin is effective.** Quercetin, a bioflavonoid, is a powerful iron chelator. For those with elevated ferritin levels, the suggested dosage is 500 mg two or three times per day.
- **Curcumin is a potent iron chelator.** Curcumin, the major chemical component of turmeric, reduces iron stores throughout the body, including the liver. Do know that when taken in excess, it can cause anemia. For those with elevated ferritin levels, the suggested dosage is 500 mg three times daily with meals. Consult your health-care practitioner for your particular needs.
- **Oxygen therapies decrease iron stores.** A veteran functional medicine practitioner will tell you that IV administration of hydrogen peroxide with

DMSO (dimethyl sulfoxide, a sulfur-based compound) and manganese given twice weekly can decrease iron stores and optimize iron levels.

Sweating is a great iron detoxifier. Small amounts of iron are excreted through the skin while sweating. I personally use the Influence FAR Infrared Sauna (see Resources) on a regular basis, for detoxing. Far infrared increases your core temperature, mobilizing toxins from the cellular level.

NUTRITION AND SUPPLEMENT SOLUTIONS: COPPER AND IRON

NAC. Taking 600 mg of amino acid N-acetylcysteine (NAC) one or two times daily and 500 mg of methionine two times daily has been shown to have broad-based chelating effects for just about every metal.

Antioxidants. In addition to NAC, vitamin E (400 IU) taken one to three times per day; beta-carotene (25,000 to 50,000 IU per day); and liposomal glutathione (100 mg, or 1 teaspoon taken twice a day on an empty stomach) are extremely beneficial.

Healing agents. CoQ10, iodine, Modifilan Brown Seaweed Extract, PQQ, taurine, colloidal silver, and zeolite can protect mitochondria from oxidative damage and bind to metals.

Carbonized bamboo. Takesumi Supreme is a relatively new kid on the block, made from carbonized bamboo. It is highly effective for detoxing heavy metals, chemicals, and mold. It grabs onto toxins so they can be transported out of the body through the bowel. The suggested dosage is 600 mg one to three times a day, two hours away from food.

Redox signaling molecules. By naturally generating glutathione and reestablishing cellular communication, these substances clear out heavy metals, chemicals, and wastes. The only verified source for them is ASEA, whose flagship product is composed of trillions of stable, perfectly balanced redox signaling molecules suspended in a saline solution. (For information on purchasing ASEA products, please see the Resources section at the back of this book.)

Minerals can certainly be a double-edged sword, and too much of a good thing definitely applies when it comes to copper and iron. Switching out your cast-iron pots and pans, installing a copper blocking water filtration system, cleaning up your supplements, and donating blood periodically are simple tweaks that should be on your longevity checklist.

CHAPTER 7

NEW RULE #7: OPTIMIZE THE GUT-BRAIN CONNECTION

In this chapter, you'll learn . . .

- How your microbiome influences optimal healthy aging
- About far-reaching cellular effects of probiotics on your body, mind, and spirit
- How your body keeps score by storing emotions in organs, negatively impacting longevity
- Why community is so critical for life extension

FROM MOODS TO METABOLISM, THE HUNDRED TRILLION OR SO INTESTINAL BACTERIA you have are behind the scenes orchestrating a wide variety of your body's crucial functions. Over time, you've collected an assortment of microorganisms from your environment that live primarily in your gut. These "gut bugs" have created their own ecosystem inside you, called your microbiome, and the balance among the over ten thousand different beneficial and disease-causing bacteria is so sensitive that if it changes by even one strain, it can, for example, change your brain chemistry and lead to anxiety.

Probiotics (friendly bacteria) inhabit the walls of the small intestine and the colon, fortifying them, forming a protective barrier that makes it harder for pathogenic bugs to take root and multiply. Ideally, beneficial probiotic bacteria make up about 85 percent of bacteria living in our gut and keep the other 15 percent of harmful bacteria in check. However, when this balance starts to shift, "bad" bacteria overgrow and can cause serious health risks, including changing our gene expression.

We can't look at the health of our cells and our DNA without looking at our mitochondria, the energy-producing "power plants" of each of our cells—their importance can't be overemphasized. These cellular powerhouses produce the energy our body needs and are vital for health and longevity. Mitochondrial dysfunction, caused primarily by free radicals, has been implicated in aging and nearly all diseases.

Common medications, such as pain relievers, antidepressants, benzodiazepine anti-anxiety medications, diabetes medications, Parkinson's medications, and dementia medications, as well as stress, a sedentary lifestyle, and poor diet, can also damage the health of our mitochondria.

WHAT YOUR GUT BACTERIA CAN DO FOR YOU

Your microbiome is a key player in your immune response, digestion and absorption of nutrients, blood sugar regulation, hormone balance, ability to get a good night's sleep, stress-handling capacity, moods, how quickly you lose weight, when you're hungry, and the production of enzymes, vitamins, hormones, and neurotransmitters.

Your microbiome has a symbiotic relationship with your mitochondria and feeds them the fuel they need to give you—and every single one of your cells—the energy needed to stay alive. This partnership is so powerful that your microbiome communicates with the mitochondria of *each* cell in your body, which tell the microbiome what they need for fuel. The microbiome responds with how much energy it needs for your body to function optimally.

This relationship is key to your metabolism. Such probiotics as *Lactobacilli* and *Bifidobacteria* produce the exact fuel (butyrate) your mitochondria need to make ATP, the energy molecule. This means when you eat something, the probiotics go to work helping your digestive system break the food down to extract the nutrients; then, through their own digestive processes, they make additional nutrients for your body to use.

BUILD UP YOUR MICROBIOME'S PROBIOTIC POPULATION

Whether you are looking to beat belly bloat, fight fatigue, lose weight, boost your immune system, lift your moods, or simply stay healthy, minding your microbiome and building up your population of "good guys" is an essential first step. Overuse of antibiotics, sugar, stress, medications, and "bad bugs" can all kill off the healthy bacteria and upset the delicate balance of your microbiome.

Although fermented foods are gaining popularity as a good source of probiotics, it's easy to overeat or undereat them. A good probiotic supplement, either on its own or in addition to eating fermented foods, is really the best option when you are looking to increase your numbers.

The three probiotics that have been in use the longest and have the most research behind them are *Lactobacillus acidophilus*, *Bifidobacterium bifidum*, and

Bifidobacterium longum. These are beneficial bacteria that should colonize us from birth and are the go-to strains to repopulate after antibiotic use. *Lactobacillus plantarum* has impressive research behind it, increasing oxygenation of muscles and stimulating the growth of new mitochondria to fight fatigue, while at the same time fighting fungi, such as *Candida.* And *Lactobacillus reuteri* shows promise with intestinal discomforts and diseases, from infant colic to irritable bowel syndrome (IBS) and inflammatory bowel disease (IBD).

THE POWER OF THE GUT-BRAIN CONNECTION

If you've ever felt butterflies in your stomach just thinking of a new love, then you understand the power of the gut-brain connection. Your intestinal flora produce and respond to the hundreds of neurochemicals that your brain uses to regulate your moods, mental processes, and physiology. Such brain chemicals as GABA, serotonin, norepinephrine, and dopamine are neurotransmitters familiar to those who struggle with depression and anxiety, and all are made by your intestinal flora. Over 90 percent of your neurotransmitters are created and used by your gut.

These probiotics carry on a constant two-way communication with your brain and nervous system, directly affecting your moods, emotions, how you respond to stress, and more. Changes to even one strain of bacteria in your microbiome can directly lead to anxiety. This communication goes both ways. Even mild stress can change your brain chemistry, and subsequently, the balance of the microbiome, affecting the immune system and leading to infectious disease. Roughly 80 percent of your immune system tissue is located in your digestive tract, and for good reason. The air you breathe and what you put in your mouth are the main routes for foreign hitchhikers to try to get inside your body and wreak havoc.

Your intestines are the barrier between your bloodstream and the outside world. The probiotics that populate them not only come to your defense by attacking pathogens directly, but also make antibiotic-like compounds that guard against dangerous microbes while building and maintaining the integrity of the intestinal walls and their mucosal lining. (This ecological balance is also essential for protecting the colon from cancer and inflammatory bowel conditions.)

YOUR MENTAL HEALTH ISN'T ALL IN YOUR HEAD

The environment outside our body has a direct impact on what's going on inside it, including our mental health. Invisible threats to our health wear us down over time. In our twenty-first-century lives, these include radiation and EMFs, lack of exposure to sunlight, not enough time in nature and the outdoors, artificial light at night disrupting our sleep, over eighty thousand untested chemicals in our homes and environment, digestive issues that impair our immunity and block our ability to absorb nutrients, and so much more. All of these environmental factors work their way into our DNA, and in my experience, mental health issues can be red flags for DNA damage.

Fatigue not relieved by rest, low moods, and a low tolerance for stress are all signs your body has become toxic. Your liver is your biggest ally when it comes to detoxification, and once your colon has been cleansed and your microbiome balanced, it's smooth sailing for your liver to eliminate these toxins from your body. Bile—liquid gold made by the liver and stored by the gallbladder—binds fat-soluble toxins and escorts them out from your body through your colon. If your gallbladder has been removed, this function may be impaired, and you may need help to build better bile.

YOUR BODY FEELS EMOTIONS

It is all too true that your body keeps a score, remembering every trauma it has experienced, and it will not forget any suppressed emotion. Every culture has common phrases that show us emotions have a profound effect on our physical health. In the United States, we say we have "butterflies in my stomach" or "my heart was pounding out of my chest." We're familiar with tension causing headaches, and on the positive side, we've experienced how passionate emotions and visual stimuli lead to sexual arousal.

Physiologically, emotional suffering and physical pain share similarities in their neural pathways. They are both perceived as threats and activate the sympathetic nervous system, known as the "fight or flight" response.

When emotions stay suppressed and tensions run high, we shift into sympathetic dominance, where cortisol levels run high and our normal hormone balance is disrupted. For instance, this means you can develop belly fat from having chronic pain. One study showed that, over time, chronic physiological stress not only changes our hormone balance but also suppresses the immune system and contributes to the development and progression of heart disease and even cancer.

Suppressed emotions affect the health of every cell in your body. More than twenty years ago, Candace Pert, PhD, discovered that every cell in your body is capable of experiencing pleasure, pain, emotions, and memory. For more than three hundred years, the scientific community has considered the brain to be the seat of all our emotions and intelligence, and the nerves from the brain have been pictured as controlling all conscious action. In fact, the scientists who study the brain are often not even located in the same building as scientists who study emotions, so the idea of them sharing their findings is not only a mental leap but a physical one as well. It's rare to find a scientist like Dr. Pert who integrates the findings of her research into every part of a person. So, imagine the shock the scientific community experienced when her research showed that even moving a muscle produces emotion!

When you suppress an emotion, such as grief, it is effectively stored in your cells and changes everything from the mitochondrial energy production to the cell's ability to receive nutrients. You experience fatigue and pain, both physical and emotional, because each cell has the capability to experience all levels of emotion, including pleasure and pain. You open your cells up to free radicals and disease by holding in distressing emotions and not expressing them. This stress, in turn, leads to shortened telomeres and DNA damage. Reprogramming our DNA includes learning how to express all our emotions.

THE MANY WAYS GRIEF MANIFESTS IN YOUR BODY

Even with the best support system, an emotional stress like grief can take its toll on us physically, especially when we are already dealing with health issues. Grief is a risk factor for high blood pressure, heart attack, heart illnesses, cancer, and depression. There is a heart condition known as Takotsubo cardiomyopathy, also known as broken heart syndrome, whereby a chamber in the heart temporarily dilates like a balloon and mimics the symptoms of a heart attack. Any chest pain during mourning needs to be taken seriously because there is a twenty-one-fold increase in the risk of heart attack in the twenty-four hours following the loss of a loved one.

Grief also affects your immune system. Your primary stress hormone, cortisol, rises, which suppresses your immune system by reducing neutrophil immune cell function. Normally, the hormone DHEA balances out this effect, but if you are over thirty years old or have been under prolonged stress, your levels have decreased, making your immune system more vulnerable. The longer you grieve, the more your immune system is suppressed, which can lead to chronic diseases and even cancer. This is compounded by the loss of appetite that comes with bereavement and depression, which leads to nutrient deficiencies.

Because the stress of mourning increases your cortisol levels, it also decreases your pH, and a more acidic body is more prone to disease. This increase in stress hormone production can be a drain on your adrenals, and the first signs of adrenal fatigue include exhaustion, insomnia, and low moods. Combined with nutrient deficiencies from changing eating habits, anxiety, depression, and loneliness are often not far behind.

DETOXING YOUR EMOTIONS

Regardless of what the experts say, it's important to know how your own body reacts to your emotions. Start noticing how your body feels when unpleasant emotions arise. Whether you choose to talk about them with a trusted friend or therapist, journal them, meditate on them, or work them out through yoga or other practices, it's vital to your success to release the backlog of stored emotions and avoid toxic buildup in the future.

The solution is simple: the Radical Longevity 5-Day Detox every spring and autumn—a nutrient-rich diet that is high in fermented foods and low-glycemic without all the processed foods and sugars, proactively managing stress, and supplementing with probiotics to keep healthy populations at optimal levels.

Throughout the year, my go-to solution is Bach Flower Remedies. For me, they're like psychotherapy in a bottle. I personally have found centaury (for boundary issues and overgiving), walnut (for cutting ties to the past), impatiens (for lack of patience and irritability), and rock rose (for being hard on yourself) to be the most helpful remedies for my clients and me.

Keep in mind that as you start eliminating toxins from your food, water, and air and begin detoxing your body, all those emotions stuffed in your cells, tissues, and organs may begin to surface for release and transformation.

THE STRESS OF LONELINESS

Even with social media, video calls, texting, and other means of keeping in touch with family and friends, research indicates that we are lonelier than ever. As we get older, we face isolation. Social circles shrink when friends and family members move or pass away. Retirement, though often eagerly anticipated, can prove to be difficult as the day-to-day comradeship of work companions and reliability of a daily schedule becomes a thing of the past.

Beyond the research of how our mental health affects the health of every cell in our body, studies from the University of California at San Francisco concluded that mental health is directly connected to physical health. Participants aged sixty and older who reported feeling lonely had a 45 percent increase in their risk of death. Those reporting feeling isolated had a nearly 60 percent greater risk of both mental and physical decline than others their age. The opposite is also true. According to the National Institute on Aging, older men and women who had positive indicators of social well-being had lower levels of inflammatory chemicals responsible for the onset of such chronic diseases as Alzheimer's and rheumatoid arthritis.

SHOULD YOU LIVE ALONE OR IN COMMUNITY?

Today, 90 percent of people aged sixty-five and older say they want to spend their senior years in their home, continuing to make independent choices and maintain control of their lives. Aging in place has psychological benefits in that it allows you to remain involved in activities of daily living in a familiar environment.

It also has financial benefits, as assisted living facilities cost an average of $50,000 annually. You can do a lot of natural and nutritional therapies for the "wellderly" for that amount of money. Integrative care and a healing diet are also very good options if you no longer want to take so many meds, are finding side effects unbearable, and are seeking more natural alternatives. Preserving independence at home is essential to maintaining access to these complementary therapies.

No one expects to get sick until they get sick, or to become injured until they fall. Practical considerations of living in a communal setting primarily include health and safety, but the savings on living expenses are often an additional plus, especially for those who are single or widowed. If you feel unsteady when you go outside to check the mail, or you find your long-lost car keys in the refrigerator, it may be time for you to consider living with a companion in a cohousing situation.

SAGE-ING, NOT AGING: THE VALUE OF MENTORING

We are the wisdom keepers. As we think back on our life experiences, the wealth of information we've collected in our lifetime, as well as what we might do differently in hindsight, there is much to be contemplated . . . and much that might be shared. We also stand on the shoulders of those who mentored us. Most of us can point to someone influential who helped shape who we are today. I know I certainly can. These mentors, working behind the scenes with us, generously share their time, expertise, and insights to help us grow. Much as you may have wished for someone to counsel and advise you in your formative years, I invite you to consider that it may be the very best thing you could do to help someone in need of the precious insights you have gleaned through your personal life experience.

TARGETED EMOTIONAL SOLUTIONS

Understand the connection between emotions and your body. I highly recommend the work of Gabor Maté, MD, presented in his book *When the Body Says No.*

Revive your adrenals. A good adrenal support is needed to replenish the nutrients you use most during stress while providing glandular support to your hardworking adrenals. I recommend the Adrenal Formula from UNI KEY Health, which is formulated with B vitamins and such immunity-boosting nutrients as vitamins A and C, and zinc. Take as directed.

Nourish your brain and your heart with omega-3 essential fats. UNI KEY Health's Super-EPA is the cleanest omega-3 fish oil I've found, with the right blend of fish oils and balance of essential fats. Combine

Super-EPA with 100 to 200 mg daily of a good-quality CoQ10 supplement, which has been shown to be heart protective in clinical studies. If you take a statin cholesterol medicine, increase your CoQ10 to 300 mg daily and supplement with red yeast rice as well. CAUTION: Because both red yeast rice and statins have similar ingredients, they also may have similar side effects. Red yeast rice contains monacolin K, the same active ingredient that lovastatin has. So, if you don't take CoQ10 with it, you can have the same side effects as you get with a statin, depending on the dose you're taking. Be sure to source red yeast rice from a trusted manufacturer. Consult your health-care practitioner for dosage recommendations.

Enhance your mood with 5-HTP. If your moods are low and you are having trouble coping with grief, then, in addition to counseling, consider taking 50 to 200 mg of 5-HTP daily. This natural amino acid supplement is a precursor to such neurotransmitters as serotonin that boost your mood and increase your sense of well-being.

Rely on flower power. Flower remedies are a kind of vibrational or energy medicine, similar to homeopathics, that offset the emotional turbulence often at the root of physical disorders. Rescue Remedy is a five-flower combo that is used to help alleviate trauma, whether physical, psychological, or emotional. I have also found these other remedies to be of help:

Water Violet helps when you desire a warmer relationship with other people.

Heather helps when you are unhappy being alone for any length of time.

Star of Bethlehem helps with grief, trauma, the after-effect of shock, post-traumatic stress, sadness, sorrow, grief, and loss.

Wild Oat helps with purpose and direction in life.

The homeopathic Ignatia Amara is especially powerful for fresh grief. Ignatia 30c seems to be the most appropriate homeopathic for recent or fresh grief. It is also good for uncontrollable crying and deep sadness.

Natrum Muriaticum 30c, a homeopathic, can be helpful in overcoming unusually sustained, chronic grief.

To relieve depression, try lavender essential oil. Apply a few drops of pure lavender oil to your temples to relieve depression, nervous tension, and emotional stress. Add a few drops to your bath to relieve restlessness and nervous exhaustion.

Orange blossom essential oil can calm you down. This essential oil has proven helpful when treating hysteria. When you are dealing with insomnia, it can be helpful in promoting deep, calm sleep.

Patchouli essential oil helps elevate your mood. You may find patchouli essential oil to be helpful if you are experiencing depression. Just a drop of this essential oil placed on the bottom of each foot or on the inside wrists can help soothe emotions.

COMMUNITY SOLUTIONS

Consider communal living opportunities. If you don't have family nearby, communal living can be a good option. Women in particular often benefit from the support of others in being able to handle all aspects of life—approximately 75 percent of communal living is currently among women. The movement for cohousing—where occupants have private living spaces while sharing common areas, such as dining rooms, and tasks, such as cooking—started in Denmark and is catching on in the United States.

Join an online community. A forum community can be one of the most nurturing, supportive, and encouraging places to call home. If you don't have an online community, consider joining one of my private Facebook groups: Radical Longevity, Inner Circle, Fat Flush, or Radical Metabolism (see Resources).

Participate in faith-based services. When it comes to matters of faith, research shows that attending faith-based services regularly (four times a month) can add an extra four to fourteen years to your life. Denomination doesn't seem to matter.

Volunteer in your community. Find and develop your purpose by volunteering in your community. People who volunteer regularly tend to not only be happier but also have lower rates of heart disease.

Mentor someone. Use the wisdom you have gained throughout your lifetime and pass it along to someone else. They will benefit, and so will you!

Now that you know the 7 New Rules of Radical Longevity, let's put them together in a powerful plan of the core longevity strategies that you can begin to implement today.

PART TWO

THE RADICAL LONGEVITY POWER PLAN

PUTTING RADICAL LONGEVITY TO WORK IN YOUR LIFE

Turn your wishbone into a tailbone and get to work.

—Dr. Hazel Parcells

THIS POWER-PACKED PROGRAM COMBINES TESTING, LIFESTYLE, NUTRIENT, AND PERsonal environment strategies with important food preparation techniques. It's an easy yet innovative eating plan to fortify your body and melt the years away, and serves as a base as you add targeted strategies to address your specific health goals.

CHAPTER 8

ENVIRONMENT, TESTING, NUTRIENT, AND LIFESTYLE STRATEGIES

In this chapter, you'll learn . . .

- How to put together all the recommendations in the 7 New Rules
- About the core of the Radical Longevity Plan that lies in these actions
- An exciting and more youthful way to live
- How to protect your indoor environment

YOU JUST LEARNED A LOT OF INFORMATION ABOUT HOW OUR ENVIRONMENT, FROM what we eat to how we cook it, to the water we drink and the air we breathe, as well as our own individual past, can accelerate aging. I've given you a lot of concrete suggestions in the 7 New Rules. Now that you know the 7 New Rules, here is a way to put all of my recommendations together. While I suggest you follow as many of the targeted solutions as you can (paying special attention to the Rules that are most relevant to your life, as you've gauged from the assessment on page 8, or just from recognizing yourself in these pages), the following solutions really compose the essential core of the Radical Longevity Plan. You will truly find a more youthful way to live by implementing these, as well as the eating plan that follows.

HOME ENVIRONMENT

In Rule #2, Take On Toxic Overload, detoxing your external environment is as essential as detoxing your body. The 7 New Rules are designed to provide a balanced approach, ridding your body of things that accelerate aging and can thwart your efforts while bolstering it to begin reversing damage already done. Your environment is key since it can either enhance or detract from healing and thriving.

Invest in a good air purifier. Here are some tips to help you get the most effective one:

→ Do make sure it captures toxins less than 0.1 microns in size. Toxic mold spores can be as small as 0.9 microns; mycotoxins are even smaller at 0.1 microns.

→ Don't choose one that emits or uses hydroxyls. These are free radicals and can be harmful when released into the air.

→ Don't choose one that emits ozone. I'm a big fan of ozone therapies, but breathing ozone can bring on asthma attacks and cause breathing issues.

→ Don't choose one with photocatalytic oxidation, which generates highly reactive free radicals.

→ Avoid such terms as "oxidizes pollutants." This means it produces ozone.

Consider such trusted brands as AirDoctor, Austin Air, and Blueair.

Improve your lung health with a humidifier. Adding a humidifier to your home environment, especially in the room where you sleep, can help decrease the risk for respiratory infection. The optimal range for humidity in your room/home is 40 to 60 percent. Look for a model with a humidistat that will automatically measure the moisture in the air and can be set to a desired humidity level. You might also consider adding personal humidifiers to your office, kitchen, and other areas where you spend significant amounts of time.

Filter your water. Consider installing a whole-house water filter. I recommend the CWR Ultra-Ceramic Water Filter, the most effective water filtration system available on the market today. The filter is made of ultrafine ceramic with pores so small that they trap bacteria, parasites, and particles down to 0.8 microns in size (see Resources).

If whole-house filtration is a big step for you, I highly recommend filtration systems that can be installed under-counter or countertop water filters with Metal Gon that remove chlorine, parasites, and lead for safe drinking water straight out of the tap (see Resources). And, as a first step, add a filter to your showerhead, which is essential to avoid chlorine and fluoridated water (see Resources).

ESSENTIAL TESTING

Ask for a ferritin blood test. This test can reveal an iron overload and is one case where a simple blood test can save your life. The blood test for ferritin isn't typically part of your standard annual blood work, but it should be. You can request this test from your health-care provider as part of your annual physical or at any time, or you can order it for yourself (for more information, please see Resources). Ferritin, in both men and postmenopausal women, is optimally between 50 and 70 ng/ml. Ferritin levels below this warrant further blood testing to rule out iron-deficiency anemia, whereas levels above the threshold are a sign you are accumulating excess iron. A ferritin test should be repeated at least every two years, and more often if your ferritin levels are above the optimal range.

Check your vitamin D level. Ideally, you want to strive for levels of 50 to 80 ng/ml. Vitamin D levels should be checked at least twice a year and more often if results are abnormal. Ask your health practitioner to test your vitamin D level with a blood test.

Know your zinc status. It is important to test your zinc levels with the most accurate testing, which is an RBC (red blood cell) zinc rather than plasma or serum blood test. Ideally, your zinc level should be in the upper half of normal. Work with a qualified health-care professional to order this test and monitor your zinc levels on an ongoing basis.

Take a hair tissue mineral analysis. This test is one of the most available, sensitive, and inexpensive indicators of exposure to heavy metals. Hair analysis is a reliable heavy-metal screening tool when you consider that hair follicles are washed by blood, lymph, and extracellular fluids that deposit tiny fragments of any metal contaminants they contain. As the hair emerges from its follicle, it hardens and fossilizes the metabolic products within it. Tissue mineral analysis uses this record to show what toxic metals you have been exposed to, as well as the current levels and ratios of nutrient minerals.

Most hair analysis reports contain a two- to three-month nutrition supplement program specifically designed to balance biochemistry, after which a retest is recommended to monitor progress (see Resources).

NUTRIENT STRATEGIES

All the Rules are bolstered by nutritional strategies. These are essential to vibrant health and a strong immune system. Here are the Radical Longevity superstars:

Vitamin D. I recommend a daily intake of 2,000 to 5,000 IU of the D_3 version. Ideally, vitamin D should be taken along with vitamin K_2 to be sure that the increased level of calcium that is being absorbed is directed to your bones and not your arteries.

Vitamin C. This needs to be taken daily as our body does not store vitamin C. I recommend a time-release vitamin C, with a recommended daily dosage of 2 to 5 g of time-released or buffered form daily.

Zinc. Although I typically recommend anywhere from 15 to 45 mg of zinc daily, many people over the age of fifty are highly deficient and need to take more. Once your zinc levels have been drawn (see testing, page 103), you can work with a qualified health-care professional to adjust your zinc intake. Zinc needs to be balanced with copper in an 8:1 ratio of zinc to copper.

Melatonin. Melatonin bolsters your immune system in an amazing way. It increases the antioxidant activity of two powerful chemicals: superoxide dismutase (SOD) and glutathione perioxidase. SOD, which is an anti-inflammatory, helps repair cells, specifically the damage they incur from the most common free radical in the body—superoxide. Much like SOD, glutathione is a powerful antioxidant and detoxifier. Like a resident handyman, it can repair free radical damage on the spot as well as clean up any toxins and the injury they cause. Melatonin keeps both of these in the fight. Recommended dosage is 1 to 3 mg daily, preferably in a time-release form.

Take a daily multivitamin/multimineral formula. Be sure to choose one that is both iron- and copper-free, such as the ones available through UNI KEY Health (see Resources), for which I am a nutritional consultant and brand ambassador. You can check the label of any multi to see whether it includes the individual nutrients listed in this section at the recommended levels.

Vitamin E. It has been shown to scavenge free radicals, increase internal antioxidation, and inhibit blood platelets from becoming sticky. Vitamin E is also protective of two other antioxidant vitamins, A and C. It is important to note that recent studies indicate that although natural vitamin E supplements are good for you, the synthetic form of vitamin E may actually *increase* your heart disease risk. Always source a natural, nonsynthetic vitamin E, such as Jarrow. Aim for 400 mg daily.

Quercetin. This powerful bioflavonoid binds to iron in the digestive tract. It also acts as an antioxidant inflammatory that inhibits histamine release and is valued for its antiviral effect. Quercetin supplementation is recommended at 500 mg, two or three times a day.

Hydrochloric acid (HCl). This is our body's front line of defense against hostile gas-producing bacteria and parasites, so when it is low, we are more susceptible to infections, malabsorption, poor assimilation, and ineffective distribution of essential nutrients. Increase the level of HCl with UNI KEY's HCL+2. Take one to two HCL+2 (hydrochloric acid with pepsin and bile salts for added fat digestion) with each meal.

Magnesium. Recognized as the most important mineral for heart health and protection against EMFs. Aim for 5 mg of magnesium per pound of body weight (500 to 1,000 mg) daily. If you are also supplementing with calcium, your magnesium to calcium ratio should be 2:1 and take your magnesium at a different time of day from when you take a calcium supplement. Avoid taking magnesium with meals because it neutralizes stomach acids that you need for digestion and calcium absorption. If you experience diarrhea, reduce your magnesium intake. If you have kidney disease, you are advised not to take magnesium supplements.

Hemp seed oil. The omega-6 fats found in hemp seed oil make this a superstar for cellular strength as well as skin and joint health. The omega fats fuel the mitochondria, form the structure of the cellular membrane, and reduce the amount total inflammation present in the body. Take at least 1 tablespoon daily or eat 3 tablespoons of hemp seeds daily.

In the next two chapters, we will translate all that you've learned into a rejuvenating five-day reset and delicious diet program that will empower you to look and feel younger, healthier, and more vibrant now and for the rest of your life.

CHAPTER 9

STOCK YOUR KITCHEN

> **In this chapter, you'll learn . . .**
>
> - Why your kitchen should be the laboratory of long life
> - 11 awesome transition tips for living longer in good health
> - The best foods and beverages to enhance healthy aging
> - About the all-star Radical Longevity protectors

HERE IS WHERE YOU WILL LEARN HOW TO IMPLEMENT THE PRACTICAL DAY-TO-DAY secrets of Radical Longevity. My mission in this section is to connect all the dots and put into play a whole new and fresh lifestyle approach for vitality and overall health well into your golden years. I have shared with you the very best tried-and-true ways to put the brakes on the aging process based upon my decades of personal experience and leading-edge, science-based research so that now you can emerge into a new phase of life with vitality, dignity, style, and grace.

RADICAL LONGEVITY FULL SPEED AHEAD!

Reclaiming your youthfulness starts with reducing the toxins you are exposed to while supporting your detoxification systems. The Radical Longevity Program is specifically designed to gently start a cleansing process in the colon and lymphatics and to support liver and gallbladder function at the same time. In addition, the diet provides an eating plan that eliminates all foods that contribute to symptoms of aging.

After you embark on this aspect of longevity, you will have more energy, more clarity, better elimination, and glowing skin. You will look and feel much younger than your biological age. The detox program I am going to share with you has been part and parcel of my own life for the past thirty years; it is the reason I can keep up with the pace of writing blog posts, books, and articles as well as traveling, lecturing, counseling, and doing podcasts, radio, and television—a schedule that would surely exhaust anyone half my age.

The benefits of this plan go far beyond just detoxification. First of all, you will be delighted to find that the Radical Longevity Program is an effective stand-alone program for effortless weight loss. If you need to lose a good 10 to 20 pounds, you can stay on the basic principles of the program as long as necessary to achieve your desired results. We all know that excess weight puts additional stress on weight-bearing joints—the knees and ankles are prime examples. Losing a few pounds can go a long way toward protecting your joints as you age.

The Radical Longevity Program can also serve as a food sensitivity identification program. The most prominent foods that cause sensitivity—wheat, corn, yeast, sugar, and peanuts—are purposefully omitted from this program. You will also find that nightshades—tomatoes, potatoes (except sweet potatoes and yams, which are not nightshades), bell and hot peppers (though black pepper, not a nightshade, is fine), paprika, eggplant, goji berries, and ashwagandha—are purposely excluded. Many people who suffer from any form of arthritis or a rheumatic disorder, such as lupus, find that consuming nightshades exacerbates their symptoms. This program will make you feel more energetic, both physically and mentally, allow you to lose water weight quickly, and reduce the appearance of aging.

11 Essentials to Radical Health

Adopt these 11 Essentials to get on the path to Radical Longevity and long-term health and well-being.

1. Use slow cookers, clay bakeware, and all-natural, nontoxic ceramic nonstick pans (e.g., Xtrema), so you only need a tablespoon or two of oil.
2. Trade in your charcoal or gas grill for a nontoxic, nonstick surface tabletop grill, such as the new generation of George Foreman grills.
3. Marinate your meat, fish, chicken, and even veggies before grilling.
4. Embrace parchment baking paper and get rid of aluminum-leaching foil.

(continues)

(continued)

5. Stew, poach, braise, simmer, and slow-cook instead of grilling, broiling, browning, or roasting.

6. Ditch or decrease most dairy with the exception of Greek-style or full-fat yogurt. Substitute coconut cream for dairy cream, and avocado for cream cheese. For the limited cheese you do use, select lower-fat varieties. If you choose to consume dairy, select dairy products that come from Jersey cows, as they produce the highly sought-after A2 beta-casein (milk protein). Milk from Holstein cows contains the A1 type beta-casein, which is especially inflammatory and most connected to many autoimmune disorders, including rheumatoid arthritis, MS, and even type 2 diabetes. Even better, if you have the option, choose sheep's milk, which seems to be better digested.

7. Only use cold-pressed oils and avoid heating them as much as possible, even higher-smoke-point oils, such as macadamia nut and avocado oils.

8. With iron-rich meals, such as meat and poultry, enjoy a cup of iron-blocking tea or coffee or an occasional glass of red wine. Tea polyphenols bind iron. EGCG from green tea and theaflavin from black tea both bind iron molecules in the blood and scavenge harmful free radicals. EGCG is unique in its ability to cross the blood-brain barrier; its iron chelating effects on the brain may reduce the rate and severity of such neurodegenerative diseases as Alzheimer's and Parkinson's, though further research is needed.

9. Try to give up crispy, crunchy processed snack foods, such as chips, crackers, and pretzels. The high/dry cooking process greatly increases AGEs. Avoid any and all fried foods.

10. Eat your nuts and seeds raw or sprouted, soaked or lightly toasted.

11. Don't bring home the bacon. This Paleo and keto favorite is one of the highest on the AGE chart. Save it for special occasions.

STOCKING YOUR LONGEVITY KITCHEN

As I learned from Dr. Parcells many years ago, we must "span the distance between the test tube and the laboratory and pots and pans in the kitchen." As the biochemist works in his laboratory, so must the cook assume the role of chemist in their laboratory: the kitchen. Properly stocking your kitchen is an absolute priority before you even start to think about foods.

LONGEVITY COOKWARE ESSENTIALS

Although you can find replacements for iron, aluminum, stainless steel, and copper-clad cookware, the best way to combat AGEs in your diet is to go "slow and low" rather than "high and dry." This means bringing back your slow cooker and clay pots for everyday use. My favorite slow cooker is the VitaClay. It's made from zisha clay, an all-natural material and is one of the healthiest, tastiest ways to cook.

Choose glass or glazed ceramic earthenware for baking. The German-made Römer-topf is my favorite. It is a covered, glazed clay cooking pot that increases the infrared heat to the food and helps it retain its own juices, making food more flavorful. Make sure clay bakeware is glazed with a nontoxic glaze to keep any impurities in the clay from leaching into your food. Use a George Foreman grill, which can cut AGEs by 50 percent over standard charcoal and gas grills.

When selecting skillets and saucepans, I am most impressed with such ceramic non-stick brands as Xtrema, This company produces a line of pure ceramic cooking utensils that are free of all toxic metals (including lead and cadmium), and have no PFOA or PTFE with Sol-Gel Ceramic coatings sprayed onto the surface, making them an ideal choice for your kitchen laboratory. Stainless-steel or bamboo steamers are also great additions to your kitchen when steaming foods to preserve nutrients and flavor. Choose stainless-steel, wooden, or ceramic cooking utensils over aluminum.

CHANGE YOUR COOKWARE AND CONTAINERS

Aluminum. Replace all aluminum steamers, measuring cups, spoons, bread pans, and cookie sheets with stainless steel, glass, or Pyrex, and avoid aluminum foil, opting for parchment paper. Use a magnet to test for aluminum content; a magnet will not stick if cookware contains aluminum.

Copper. Replace all copper-lined cookware, as this metal has an affinity for vitamin C and can upset the sensitive zinc–copper balance in your system.

Iron. Cast-iron cookware can leach iron into foods. Contrary to common belief, you cannot get the body's requirement of "good" iron from cooking your foods in cast-iron cookware. Enamel-coated cast iron is a good alternative. The enamel forms a barrier to keep iron from leaching into foods, while providing the same wonderful heat induction that made cast iron such a popular choice to begin with.

Plastics. Plastics are endocrine-disrupting substances and have the potential to leach estrogen-like chemicals into your foods. Instead of plastic containers and bags, store food in lidded glass jars, such as mason jars.

CLEAN YOUR VEGGIES WITH THE LONGEVITY FORMULA FRUIT & VEGGIE WASH

In Rule #2, you learned about parasites and the havoc they can wreak; cleaning your produce is one way to avoid them. This is my tried-and-true wash. The recipe makes 1 quart and should be prepared fresh daily.

INGREDIENTS:

18 drops grapefruit seed extract
4 ounces 3% food-grade hydrogen peroxide
1 teaspoon baking soda
1 quart filtered water

DIRECTIONS:

Blend together ingredients and soak produce for a minimum of 15 minutes; then rinse well in fresh water, at least three times. Dry produce thoroughly on paper towels before storing in refrigerator.

TABLE 14.1 STRATEGIES FOR LOWERING AGES IN DIFFERENT FOODS

TYPE OF RECIPE	TO LOWER AGES . . .
Burgers	• Use lean ground meat (at least 93% lean). • Add finely chopped mushrooms, onions, or other vegetables to the burger mixture, to increase moisture and boost nutritional value. • Shape the center of burgers slightly thinner than the edges, to promote faster, more even cooking. • Avoid pressing down on the burgers during cooking.
Casseroles	• If the recipe includes browned ground beef or turkey, use a nonstick skillet and cook the meat just until done. Minimize browning. • If the recipe calls for cooked chicken, use poached chicken instead of grilled or roasted. • Use unprocessed, reduced-fat cheese, and add any cheese toppings during the last minute of cooking. Do not brown.

TYPE OF RECIPE	TO LOWER AGES ...
Grilled Meats and Poultry	· Marinate your food in an acidic marinade before grilling. · Wrap meats or poultry in a parchment paper pouch for the first part of cooking, or precook by poaching or steaming. Then, finish cooking on a grill surface. · Cook steaks medium rare.
Meatballs	· Use lean ground meat (at least 93% lean). · Omit the browning step and simply simmer the meatballs in the sauce until cooked through.
Meat Loaf	· Use lean ground meat (at least 93% lean). · Use fresh untoasted bread crumbs or rolled oats instead of dried, toasted crumbs. · Add lots of finely chopped vegetables such as mushrooms, peppers, spinach, carrots, and onion to boost nutritional value, add moisture and flavor, and make meat portions go further.
Omelets and Frittatas	· Cook omelets and frittatas in a nonstick skillet, using a small amount of avocado oil or macadamia nut oil instead of butter. · Use unprocessed reduced-fat cheese. · When making cheese-topped frittatas, sprinkle the cheese on last and cook just long enough to melt. Do not brown.
Pizza	· Feature vegetable toppings instead of high-fat meats, such as sausage and ground beef. · Use lower-fat mozzarella cheese and add it only during the last minute or two of baking—just long enough to melt it.
Salads	· Add poached chicken, steamed seafood, or legumes instead of grilled or roasted chicken and meat. · Use unprocessed reduced-fat cheeses. · Use olive oil for dressings. · Substitute canned chickpeas or kidney beans for croutons.
Sandwiches, Spreads, and Dressings	· Use lettuce wraps for sandwiches. · Use lower-AGE fillings, such as poached chicken, canned tuna or salmon, grilled or fresh vegetables, or eggs, instead of roasted or grilled meats. · Add bulk with lots of lettuce, onion, and other vegetables. · Use spreads and dressings made with hummus, mashed avocado, or safflower mayonnaise. · Use lower-fat, unprocessed cheeses.
Soups and Stews	· Include acidic ingredients, such as tomatoes or wine, in the cooking liquid. · Minimize or omit the browning step.

COMPONENTS OF THE RADICAL LONGEVITY PROGRAM

Basically, you will be eating whole, unprocessed organic foods: fresh fruits, vegetables, pasture-raised protein, properly prepared legumes, and essential fats, especially from the omega-6-rich family. Choose foods high in bitters (coffee, cacao, arugula, watercress, ginger, apple cider vinegar, and more), colorful, polyphenol-rich fruits and vegetables, seeds, raw nuts, and avocados to dial back those cravings, keep your metabolism in check, and assist digestion. Select fresh herbs to enhance flavor, primarily dill, rosemary, fennel, sage, thyme, oregano, and cumin, which have digestive, antibacterial, anticancer, and fat-burning properties.

The program is simple to follow. It consists of these six basic elements:

1. Wholesome, non-GMO, AGE-less, and mold-free organic unprocessed foods
2. All-Star Radical Longevity protectors
3. Balancing beverages
4. Live Longer Cocktail
5. Cranberry Elixir
6. Healing oils, especially omega-6s

Here are the detailed guidelines for each of these elements.

1. WHOLESOME UNPROCESSED FOODS

The foods that you eat should be organic and non-GMO. It is essential to give the liver a rest from toxic pesticides, weed killers, and sprays found, unfortunately, in our modern food supply.

> **Protein.** In our older years, we are often increasingly at risk of sarcopenia (loss of muscle mass and strength) as we can lose 1 percent of our muscle mass per year starting at age forty. Men and women aged sixty-five years and older are recommended to eat up to 100 g of protein daily, which is about *double* the RDA for adults *under* sixty-five years of age. To get to 100 g of protein daily, build meals around easily digestible protein powders (A2 milk–derived whey protein drinks or vegan blends of rice, pea, hemp, or pumpkin seeds), as protein digestion can become impaired with the lack of hydrochloric acid as we age. Grass-fed whey protein powder is a sulfur-rich antiaging protein

that is one of nature's most effective foods for boosting collagen production. Non-GMO, New Zealand–sourced A2 Whey Protein doesn't contain the chemicals, antibiotics, pesticides, or heavy metals found in conventional bone broth supplements (see Resources). Eggs are high in avidin, a protein that tightly binds iron, which can reduce iron absorption by almost 30 percent when eaten with iron-containing foods. Always select farm-fresh, pastured, free-range eggs.

Lean beef, veal, or lamb; skinless chicken or turkey; all kinds of fish; non-GMO tempeh and tofu, as well as legumes are all highly recommended, provided they are all prepared by the AGE-less cooking methods. Choose wild-caught fish, organic meat, and free-range chicken.

If you are a vegetarian, try to aim for at least one to two servings of vegan protein powder each day, tempeh, or ½ cup of cooked legumes that are relatively low in carbohydrates (e.g., lentils, chickpeas, or adzuki beans). Find protein powders that contain at least 20 g of protein per serving with negligible carbohydrate grams (fewer than 5 g). My personal favorites are Fat Flush Whey Protein and Fat Flush Body Protein (vegan pea and rice protein powder) from UNI KEY (see Resources).

> **Phytonutrient-rich vegetables.** As they are naturally low in AGEs unless you grill, broil, or roast them, you can eat unlimited amounts of raw or steamed vegetables. The only exceptions are the starchier squash (e.g., acorn, butternut, or kabocha), peas, and sweet potato, which should be portion-controlled to ½ cup per meal.

Choose vegetables for their high fiber and bitter content. Use starchy veggies as your grain substitute: ½ cup peas, winter squash, or sweet potato once or twice a day, weight permitting. Three cups of organic popcorn are allowed as the only grain-based snack that is low in AGEs.

Your body needs antioxidants to remove excess AGEs and to balance your oxidation process so they stop accumulating in the first place. Pack your diet with these all-star Radical Longevity vegetables that are rich in vitamins A, C, D, and E and brimming with two core longevity-supporting minerals—zinc and selenium.

Vitamins A, C, and E, along with such minerals as selenium and zinc, should be plentiful in the diet.

Reminder: Don't forget to include those liver-lovin' bitters (marked with an asterisk [*])!

*Alfalfa sprouts

*Artichokes

*Arugula (rocket)

*Asparagus

Bamboo shoots

*Beet greens

*Beets

*Broccoli and broccoli
  sprouts

*Brussels sprouts

*Burdock

*Cabbage

Carrots (raw)

*Cauliflower

Celery

Chives

*Collards

*Cucumber

*Daikon radish

*Dandelion greens

*Endive

*Escarole

*Frisée

Green beans

Hearts of palm

*Jerusalem artichoke

*Jicama

*Kale

Leafy greens

Leeks

Lemon grass

Mushrooms

*Mustard greens

*Nettles

Peas

*Pumpkin

*Radicchio

*Radish

*Rapini

*Red leaf lettuce

*Rhubarb

*Romaine lettuce

Scallions

Shallots

*Spinach

Squash (acorn,
  butternut, kabocha,
  spaghetti, summer,
  zucchini)

Sweet potatoes

*Swiss chard

*Thistle

*Turnip greens

Water chestnuts

*Watercress

*Wild lettuce

Fruit. Fruits high in vitamin C help stimulate glutathione, our body's most prevalent antioxidant. Do pay special attention to the powerful prune. Thanks to its high source of bone-building boron, essential in staving off age-related bone-thinning, it's an unsung hero.

The following examples will give you an idea of the kinds and amounts of fruits recommended for your daily longevity diet. Each of these equals a single serving.

Recommended servings: 1 to 2 servings per day

Apple (1 small)

Apricots (2 medium)

Avocado (½ small)

Banana (½ small)

Berries (seasonal) (½ cup)

*Bitter melon

Cherries (10)

*Grapefruit (½)

Grapes (12)

Kiwi (1 medium)

*Lemon (including peel/
  rind)

*Lime (including peel/
  rind)

Mango (½ cup)

Melon (1 cup watermelon,
  or ⅛ honeydew,
  cantaloupe, others)

Nectarine (1 small)   Pear (1 small)   Strawberry (2)
Orange (1 small)   Pineapple (½ cup)   Tangerine (1 large)
*Orange peel/rind   Plum (2 medium)   *Tangerine peel/rind
Papaya (½)   Pomegranate (1)
Peach (1 medium)   Prunes (2)

Sweets and sweeteners. Mounting research has shown that sugar is a major culprit in diseases such as obesity, diabetes, and dementia. It also plays a role in triggering inflammation. When looking for a sweetener, choose from one of the following low-glycemic and healthy options.

Lakanto Monk Fruit   Monk fruit   Stevia (from Sweet Leaf
  Maple Flavored   Pure maple syrup   or NutraMedix)
  Syrup   Raw honey   Yacón syrup

Herbs, spices, and condiments. Carefully chosen herbs, spices, and condiments are definite flavor enhancers. Fragrant rosemary, for example, is widely used throughout the Blue Zones where people frequently live to over a hundred. Miso's probiotic, gut-healing properties add rich flavor to soups and even salad dressings. And to create that delicious smoky flavor we all love without the harmful effects of AGEs from grilling, try adding a little liquid smoke to your recipes. Choose from the following list.

Cumin   Rosemary   Gluten-free tamari
Dill   Sage   sauce
Fennel   Thyme   Miso
Oregano   Coconut aminos   Wright's Liquid Smoke

2. ALL-STAR RADICAL LONGEVITY PROTECTORS

Incorporate at least one of these longevity foods from each group (which target the liver) into your daily diet. This amazing organ has more than earned its name, which is derived from an old English word for *life*. The liver is truly key to your body's ability to renew itself. These foods all support the liver's two detox pathways. Remember that the liver clears your system of toxins, which enables all other body systems and organs to operate more efficiently. These foods also have restorative benefits for the heart, fortify your immune system, and support your lymph integrity.

LIVER HEALERS

Artichokes. Do not be intimidated by these prickly vegetables and member of the thistle family. The artichoke is a close relative of milk thistle, queen of the liver protectors, which offers major defense against free radicals and is especially good for people with compromised immunity or alcohol-related liver problems. Artichokes, especially the hearts, contain powerful antioxidants known as flavonoids that protect the liver's cells and tissues. Even more, artichokes are good for the secretion of bile, which aids the body in digesting and assimilating fats. Just 1 cup of cooked artichoke hearts has an antioxidant capacity that earns it the number one spot on the USDA's vegetable list. And you'll find them quite tasty! Toss artichoke hearts in salads or add them to soups (I love chicken soup with artichokes). Recommended serving size is one medium-size whole artichoke or ½ cup of artichoke hearts.

Asparagus. Asparagus, that harbinger of spring, contains more glutathione (quite probably the most important antioxidant in the body) than does any other food. Avocado comes in second, and watermelon third, but you'd have to eat at least 2 pounds of them to get the same amount of glutathione in only five (count them) delicate and delicious asparagus spears! Increasing glutathione in your diet can help you detox from a multitude of sins, including heavy metals, pesticides, and other chemicals in the environment. In addition, asparagus contains high amounts of vitamin A and potassium, another mineral on which the liver depends. Steam, roast, or sauté these delicacies with olive oil and fresh lemon. A standard serving size is ½ cup of pieces, or six medium-size spears.

Whey. Little Miss Muffet may not have known how important whey is to keep her glutathione supplies high—but now *you* do! Don't say I didn't tell you! Whey is a rich source of the amino acid L-cysteine, which, like vitamin C, is a precursor to glutathione, the master antioxidant that every cell in your body is crying out for. The liver's two-phase detox process uses up huge amounts of glutathione, so it's up to us to replenish it daily. Whey also contains methionine, glycine, glutamine, and taurine—amino acids crucial to the liver's detox process. My choice? UNI KEY Health's 100 percent natural hormone-, pesticide-, and chemical-free, nondenatured type A2 milk–derived whey concentrate sourced from New Zealand (see Resources). One scoop is the recommended serving size.

SULFUR-RICH GEMS

Sulfur, the third most abundant mineral in the body, and arguably one of the most overlooked, is vital in the day-to-day function of blood vessels and—*hello*—your hard-working heart. Learn to love these tasty sulfur-rich foods and enjoy their hard-to-match health promoting benefits. Where to start? Incorporate at least one of these longevity protectors into your diet daily.

> **Garlic.** The potent compound contained in garlic is allicin, and its powerful antibacterial and antifungal properties may even ward off our number one and number two killers here in the United States: heart disease and cancer. In addition, some say that a clove a day keeps wrinkles at bay. There may be something to that theory, as the three active compounds in the pungent herb (CA, SAC, and uracil) are known to inhibit wrinkle formation. The daily recommended serving for raw garlic is one clove.

> **Onions.** Rich in antioxidants and flavonoids, it's the quercetin in onions that protects against atherosclerosis and high blood pressure. Their other sulfur compounds, such as allicin and allyl disulfide, are also beneficial in decreasing the risk of vascular diseases. The nucleotides they contain, crucial for detox, help our body repair itself, creating new tissue and maintaining a strong immune system. One serving is equal to approximately three-quarters of a large onion.

> **Daikon radish.** Radishes are another great sulfur-rich food and source of age-reversing nucleotides. This long white radish, with its crisp texture and pungent taste, also acts as a diuretic and decongestant. Recommended serving size is 1 cup.

YOUTH-BOOSTING CITRUS

Fresh vitamin-packed citrus with its longevity protecting antioxidants is a perfect addition to your daily diet.

> **Lemons.** Lemons provide more than four times the vitamin C of oranges, and they're antimicrobial too. Limonene, a substance contained in lemons, can detoxify carcinogens in the body, shrink cancerous tumors, and stimulate the healthy flow of lymph fluids. Citrus pith and peels are equally as

beneficial as the main fruit. Roughly half their vitamin C hides in the peel along with fiber and calcium. I recommend consuming some of the pith (the white stringy tissue under the skin), since this is packed with bioflavonoids. Just ¼ cup of lemon juice contains almost one-third the recommended daily intake of vitamin C.

GLORIOUS GREENS

Vital for providing purifying chlorophyll, these healthy greens can be added to your favorite recipes daily.

Broccoli sprouts. If you add anything new to your daily salad, make it broccoli sprouts! The highest known source of vital phytonutrients, indole-3-carbinol and sulforaphane, aids the liver in its ability to process and neutralize the toxins your body desperately wants to rid itself of. Sulforaphane acts like a "signaling molecule" to communicate with other cells. With the ability to affect over two thousand genes, activating numerous defense mechanisms and neutralizing free radicals, sulforaphane is one potent toxicity zapper. The recommended serving size is 1 cup.

Cilantro. This tasty herb packed with vitamins A, C, and K is a simple and delicious way to tame the toxins and mobilize heavy metals in preparation to be carried out of the body, primarily from adipose (fat) tissue. Make yours organic and add a handful in salads, soups, or your favorite guacamole or pesto recipe. Enjoy daily and reap the benefits! The recommended serving size is ¼ cup of the fresh herb.

3. BALANCING BEVERAGES

The beverages in this section are especially beneficial when enjoyed with meat dishes or other high iron-containing foods.

Coffee. America's favorite beverage is a true champion. Coffee beans carry the highest level of antioxidants of any other staple in the American diet, making a cup of coffee a delicious way to get your daily dose of bitters. Chlorogenic acid, a powerful polyphenol antioxidant found in coffee, revs up your metabolism to burn more fat while still retaining your muscle mass. The latest scientific research also shows that coffee drinkers have lower rates of type 2 diabetes, Parkinson's, MS, and liver cancer. Coffee consumed with your meal or shortly after will lower iron absorption by as much as 80 percent. Be sure to source a high-quality, mold-free, nontoxic coffee, I recommend the cleanest, most antioxidant-rich coffee I've found: Purity Coffee. It is organic, mold-free, and lab-tested for purity (see Resources).

Teas. Be sure your teas are organic and come from the highest-quality tea farms, to prevent contamination. Enjoy one to two cups daily. Here are the healthiest longevity teas in my book:

Hibiscus. Of all the beverages you could be drinking, I'd have to count this one as among the best antiaging and liver-loving beverages known to humanity. With its unprecedented ability to rid your body of toxins (a main factor in aging as you now know) and its ability to both help lower cholesterol levels and prevent clogged arteries, this delicious tea makes a great alternative to potentially harmful pharmaceutical alternatives. The biologically active compounds in hibiscus include tannins, anthraquinones, quinines, phenols, flavonoides, alkaloids, terpenoids, saponins, cardiac glycosides, protein, and free amino acids, making it an ideal source of anti-inflammatory, antimicrobial, and neuroprotective benefits.

While hibiscus comes in many varieties, it is the roselle flowers that are harvested as a natural herbal remedy. Prepare a decoction of red hibiscus with the dried flower calyces with 30 g (about an ounce) of cut and sifted flowers in a liter of water. Drink one cup once or twice daily and refrigerate the remainder (see Resources).

Earl Grey. Earl Grey tea combines the benefits of bergamot (a citrus fruit native to the Calabria region of Italy, which has superior antibacterial and antifungal properties) and black tea. It is great for the immune system and is an excellent natural aid for anyone suffering from anxiety, stress, or depression.

Oolong. Oolong, which refers to tea partially fermented prior to firing, is richer in polyphenols and easier on the stomach than green tea while still containing many of the health-enhancing catechins and their derivatives: ECG, EGCG, and the like.

Herbal teas. Herbal teas also inhibit iron, although to perhaps two-thirds of the degree that coffee and black or green tea do. Their antioxidants help rid the body of free radicals.

Red wine. Madiran wine is made from Tannat grapes grown in southwest France. It has the highest levels in any wine of a plant chemical, procyanadin, which has a beneficial effect on the blood vessels. I recommend drinking one glass (3 to 4 ounces) only on special occasions.

NOTE: As Madiran wine can be difficult to find in some places of the United States, I recommend Dry Farms wine as an alternative. Its wines are all natural, additive-free, lab tested for purity, sugar-free, low in sulfites, and have low alcohol content (12.5 percent or less).

4. LIVE LONGER COCKTAIL

Twice a day, when you rise and when you go to bed, be sure to enjoy this liver-cleansing drink, made up of cranberries, chia seeds, and greens. Unsweetened pure cranberry juice, a known cleanser of the urinary tract and lymphatic system, is the main component. High antioxidant rich cranberries contain several digestive enzymes not found in other foods that are therefore helpful for cleaning out the lymphatic system—the waste transport system of all the toxins you will be loosening from the liver.

The chia seeds form a gel that will help prevent dehydration and act as a time-released and sustained source of water for the entire system. They will also soften and lift waste buildup from the intestinal walls to be carried out of the body. The scoop of daily greens provides purifying chlorophyll, vitamins, minerals, and plenty of phytonutrients in a concentrated form. You'll find the recipe on page 132.

5. CRANBERRY ELIXIR

Apart from the two Live Longer Cocktails a day, my Cranberry Elixir between meals is a real home run. This phenomenal blend of cranberry juice spiked with key antiaging ingredients will help flush the intestines, liver, and kidneys—the organs that are involved most in the detox process—while staving off hunger, balancing blood sugar, and revving up metabolism.

So, how does it work? Orange and lemon juice are key liver-loving foods and are rich in vitamin C, or ascorbic acid. Among its many benefits, ascorbic acid thins and decongests the bile, making it easier for the liver to emulsify (break down) fat at peak efficiency. This combination is also very refreshing and "cleansing" to the palate, offering a satisfying experience that helps mitigate hunger pangs.

Their vitamin C also stimulates the production of glutathione, the major antioxidant on which the liver relies to progress through the two-phase detox process. Vitamin C also helps bind heavy metals and eliminate potentially toxic sulfa drugs.

Cranberries are rich in vitamins A, B_1, B_2, B_3, B_5, B_6, B_9 (folic acid), C, and E, as well as boron, calcium, chromium, copper, iron, magnesium, manganese, molybdenum, phosphorus, potassium, selenium, sodium, and sulfur, all crucial vitamins and minerals for liver activity, as well as for many other bodily functions. These potent red berries are also vital aids to liver detox because they contain exceedingly high levels of lifesaving antioxidants that provide crucial support for both Phase 1 and Phase 2 detox pathways.

Furthermore, their high content of organic acids—such as benzoic, malic, quinic, citric, and ellagic acids—have outstanding therapeutic qualities for many bodily functions. Malic acid, for example, is a potent digestion regulator and helps protect against diarrhea, whereas ellagic acid has been proven to inhibit the initiation of cancer.

Among the most potent elements in cranberries are polyphenols, a kind of plant-based antioxidant that has powerful health-inducing effects. Laboratory studies have shown that 8 ounces of cranberry juice contain 567 mg of polyphenols—even more than the 400 mg of polyphenols from the same amount of red wine. Just 2 ounces of fresh cranberries contain 373 mg of polyphenols—more than much larger servings of oranges, broccoli, blueberries, strawberries, bananas, apples, or white grapes.

The aromatic spices all help us in our quest for long life. Ginger is an especially friendly longevity herb due to its ability to cleanse the body by stimulating digestion, circulation, and sweating. Its digestive actions may serve to cleanse the buildup of waste and toxins in the colon, liver, and other organs. Likewise, cinnamon's natural insulin-like properties will help maintain your blood sugar level, which, in turn, will work to reduce your hunger and cravings. Some researchers even believe that cinnamon is promising as a means of preventing type 2 diabetes.

The warming effects of nutmeg make this spice an aid to digestion, fighting off free radicals and helping to fight hunger and combat cravings. You may also be interested to know that nutmeg is a powerful aphrodisiac.

Ginger is a peppery and pungent natural vasodilator—a substance that causes the blood vessels to expand. As blood flows more freely through the expanded vessels, your body heat rises, and your metabolism revs up along with it. According to an Australian study published in the *Journal of Obesity*, ginger can cause a metabolic boost of as much as 20 percent.

You'll find the recipe on page 132.

6. HEALING OILS

Healing oils include the highly advantageous omega-6s from unrefined and unheated hemp, safflower, sunflower, sesame, and walnuts. Cold-pressed healing oils are beneficial to alleviate arthritis, inflammatory bowel disease, kidney disease, infections, allergies, fatigue, and depression. Besides the benefits, these oils can increase metabolism, as well as attract oil-soluble poisons that have been lodged in fatty tissues of the body and carry them out of the system for elimination. For these reasons, my Radical Longevity Program includes at least 1 to 2 tablespoons of hemp seed oil or hemp seeds a day for omega-6, a couple of tablespoons of omega-3-rich chia seeds, flaxseeds, fish oil, or krill oil dietary supplements, and at least 1 tablespoon of extra-virgin olive oil for omega-9. I have also added coconut oil for its brain boosting ability and to help rev up an aging metabolism while also enhancing immunity. Animal fats, such as butter and cream, are severely limited due to their AGE content. You will note that I have not emphasized nuts and seeds here because their fat and protein content makes them difficult for some "seasoned" systems to digest.

Keep in mind that if you have light-colored stools, are constipated, or have had your gallbladder removed, any of these may be a strong indication that you need bile support. Bile is essential to metabolize fat and eliminate toxic waste. A bile-supporting product that contains choline, lipase, taurine, beet root, and ox bile would be helpful in assisting fat metabolism and helping to carry and store fat-soluble vitamins for optimal immunity (see Resources).

CHAPTER 10

FUEL YOUR SYSTEM

> **In this chapter, you'll learn . . .**
>
> - How to incorporate the 5-Day Radical Longevity Reset into your new Radical Longevity Program
> - What makes up the 7-Day Radical Longevity Menu Plan that will guide you to a new way of eating
> - Delicious new AGE-less recipes for living the radiant life

5-DAY RADICAL LONGEVITY RESET

This easy gut-healing reset not only works rapidly, but it also acts as a transition to soothe the system as you detox and give your liver and gallbladder a well-deserved rest. Fast and simple, this is a great beginning for those who want to wipe the slate clean and feel immediate results. It can also be used at any time to refocus or get back on track on your Radical Longevity journey.

This gently cleansing reset contains all the right ingredients to keep you well hydrated, full, and satisfied. It contains the richest sources of healthy fats, such as coconut oil and omega-6s, that act as membrane medicine to strengthen cell walls, fuel the mitochondria, and kick-start weight loss.

HOW IT WORKS

Factor #1: Fabulous fluids. You will be consuming a Longevity Blaster and two servings of delicious Radical Longevity Soup per day. Between meals, you should drink an additional 64 ounces of water, plus up to two cups of liver-cleansing dandelion root tea and yerba maté. Keeping properly hydrated will accelerate the cleansing process.

Factor #2: Herbs and spices. The Radical Longevity Soup contains just the right amounts of sulfur-based compounds, including garlic, to help with the cleansing process. Cumin, with its ability to scavenge for free radicals, enhances the detoxification process in the liver. Cilantro has a unique ability to serve as an eliminator of heavy metals. Cardamom in the Longevity Blaster is rich in antioxidants and promotes the removal of waste products, such as uric acid and urea, from the body. Ginger supports liver function and contains powerful gingerol antioxidants.

Factor #3: No grain for no pain. For an increasing number of individuals, grains can trigger inflammation as well as hunger-producing insulin and immunity-impacting mycotoxins. Instead of grains, you will be starting your day with the protein-rich Longevity Blaster and filling up on satisfying, protein-rich Radical Longevity Soup. Protein encourages the release of glucagon, which accesses stored body fat for energy. It will also stimulate metabolism by nearly 25 percent.

Factor #4: Detox daily. Ingesting Mother Nature's most purifying cleansing elements—especially chlorophyll-rich green leafy veggies and sunflower lecithin—can help your body eliminate toxins. Since many of the toxins from pollution and pesticides in food are ultimately stored in the liver, the more we can cleanse, the more effectively the liver can detox. Lecithin is an underappreciated fat-melting food that fuels the brain and the myelin sheaths.

You can also snack on raw celery and jicama sticks for even more veggie and fiber power, as well as black olives for satiety and antioxidants. Jicama is a prebiotic that will feed your microbiome, ensuring plenty of friendly bacteria, which reduce pathogens that can negatively impact your health.

To better assist the detoxification organs in the cleansing process, between meals and snacks, drink pure water, hibiscus tea, or dandelion root tea. You can also drink one or two cups of mugwort tea every day. It's been used for generations to kill intestinal parasites.

I also suggest eliminating cold drinks. These act as a shock to the body and cause the intestinal tract to contract and hold on to waste materials.

Factor #5: Skinny fats. The Longevity Blaster and Radical Longevity Soup include two of the most powerful smart fats—coconut oil and hemp seed oil—that you need to satisfy hunger, increase metabolism, and nourish the skin.

What follows is your daily Radical Longevity Menu Plan. These fast, liquid-based meals will help rest your digestive tract since your body doesn't have to digest lots of solid food. This will allow your body to have more available energy for cleansing and detox, especially of the liver and gallbladder.

NOTE: All recipes noted with an asterisk (*) appear in the Recipe section.

The 5-Day Reset Protocol

Daily Menu

Upon Arising: Longevity Blaster*

Midmorning Snack: 2 raw jicama or celery sticks (your choice) or 4 black olives

Lunch: Radical Longevity Soup*

Midafternoon Snack: 2 raw jicama or celery sticks (your choice) or 4 black olives

Dinner: Radical Longevity Soup*

Between all meals and snacks, drink pure water, or dandelion root or yerba maté tea.

RADICAL LONGEVITY LIFELONG PLAN FEATURING A 7-DAY MENU SAMPLER

Congrats to you. You have successfully completed the 5-Day Reset protocol, and you have rested your digestive tract, stabilized your cell membranes, and amped up your metabolic engines. Now that your system is primed, pumped, and purified, it's time to rebuild every cell, tissue, and organ for the Radical Longevity Lifelong Plan ahead.

The following 7-Day Menu Sampler will show you how easy it is to whip up nourishing, tasty, and age-defying meals. Creativity is encouraged! For example, the salads mentioned are up to you to mix and match with the age-defying ingredients you prefer. If you are a vegetarian, feel free to make the recommended substitutions, such as vegetable broth for bone broth. You'll see that sweet treats are not off-limits and can be enjoyed one to three times a week.

And now that you have rested your digestive tract, it is important to note that ongoing liver and gallbladder-bile support is crucial to breaking down toxins and fats and lessening the toxic load, which is a major and ongoing factor in the aging process. Depending upon your personal needs, the recommended supplements in previous and subsequent chapters (and in the handy reference chart on pages 254–260) will be paramount for your own personal strategy as you manage, control, enhance, and overcome many of your more targeted and personalized health concerns in the later chapters in this book.

7-Day Menu Sampler

You'll find the recipes for items followed by an asterisk (*) in the Recipe section later in this chapter, organized by category and providing bonus recipes that give you a great start to following this plan for life.

DAY 1

On arising	Live Longer Cocktail*
Breakfast	Longevity Blaster*
Midmorning	16 ounces Cranberry Elixir*
Lunch	Mediterranean Lentil Soup*
	Large leafy green salad with 2 hard-boiled eggs, green onions, broccoli sprouts, shredded cabbage, ¼ cup grated goat cheese, ¼ cup pomegranate seeds (arils), and water chestnuts
	1 tablespoon Cilantro Lime Dressing*
Midafternoon	16 ounces Cranberry Elixir*
4:00 p.m.	2–4 organic prunes
20 minutes before dinner	8 ounces filtered water
Dinner	Tempting Tempeh*
	4 ounces steamed broccoli and cauliflower topped with 1 tablespoon hemp seeds
	Arugula, endive, radicchio, and hearts of palm salad
	1 tablespoon Tangy Tahini and Herb Vinaigrette*
Before bed	Live Longer Cocktail*

DAY 2

On arising	Live Longer Cocktail*
Breakfast	Longevity Blaster*
Midmorning	16 ounces Cranberry Elixir*

Lunch	Greek salad with 3 ounces feta cheese, 2 chopped hard-boiled eggs, chopped romaine lettuce, black olives, chopped scallions, parsley, radishes, and cucumber
	1 tablespoon hemp seed oil dressing
Midafternoon	16 ounces Cranberry Elixir*
4:00 p.m.	½ cup blueberries
20 minutes before dinner	8 ounces filtered water
Dinner	White Bean and Spinach Soup* (Slow Cooker)
	Mixed green salad with Bibb lettuce, watercress, and sliced daikon radish
	1 tablespoon Hemp Hemp Hooray Dressing*
	1 cup coffee or tea
Before bed	Live Longer Cocktail*

DAY 3

On arising	Live Longer Cocktail*
Breakfast	Longevity Blaster*
Midmorning	16 ounces Cranberry Elixir*
Lunch	Tofu Egg Drop Soup*
	Bok choy simmered in bone broth and drizzled with 1 tablespoon hemp seed oil, fresh squeezed lemon juice, and a sprinkle of garlic powder or 1 chopped garlic clove
Midafternoon	16 ounces Cranberry Elixir*
4:00 p.m.	1 small green apple
20 minutes before dinner	8 ounces filtered water
Dinner	Braised Coconut Milk Chicken*
	½ cup steamed green peas or 6 steamed or lightly sautéed asparagus spears
	Collard greens sautéed in 2 tablespoons of bone broth
	1 slice Mocha Chocolate Surprise Cake*
	1 cup coffee or tea
Before bed	Live Longer Cocktail*

DAY 4

On arising	Live Longer Cocktail*
Breakfast	Longevity Blaster*
Midmorning	16 ounces Cranberry Elixir*

Lunch	Chicken salad with 3–4 ounces shredded chicken with 1 tablespoon safflower mayo, 1 chopped garlic clove, celery, scallions, and water chestnuts. Served on bed of lettuce.
	Drizzle with 1 tablespoon French Riviera Dressing*
	Sprinkle with sesame seeds
Midafternoon	16 ounces Cranberry Elixir*
4:00 p.m.	1 cup full-fat plain yogurt with ½ cup mixed berries
20 minutes before dinner	8 ounces filtered water
Dinner	Salmon en Papillote*
	Riced cauliflower with carrots and snow peas and chopped garlic sautéed in bone broth
	1 cup coffee or tea
Before bed	Live Longer Cocktail*

DAY 5

On arising	Live Longer Cocktail*
Breakfast	Longevity Blaster*
Midmorning	16 ounces Cranberry Elixir*
Lunch	Wild Mushroom Turkey Miso Soup*
	Mixed greens medley made with shaved fennel, grated carrot, and artichoke hearts
	Drizzle with 1 tablespoon olive oil
	Sprinkle with 1 or 2 tablespoons flaxseeds
Midafternoon	16 ounces Cranberry Elixir*
4:00 p.m.	½ cup blackberries
20 minutes before dinner	8 ounces filtered water
Dinner	Red Wine and Rosemary Marinated Lamb Chops*
	Creamy Coconut Collard Greens*
	½ steamed sweet potato sprinkled with hemp seeds
	1 cup coffee or tea
Before bed	Live Longer Cocktail*

DAY 6

On arising	Live Longer Cocktail*
Breakfast	Longevity Blaster*
Midmorning	16 ounces Cranberry Elixir*

Lunch	Radical niçoise salad: cored and sliced fennel bulb, cucumber, chopped scallions, artichoke hearts, ½ cup beans (pinto, fava, or lima), minced garlic, fresh basil leaves, and 2 sliced hard-boiled eggs
	Drizzle with 1 tablespoon olive oil and a splash of red wine vinegar
	Top with 1 tablespoon hemp seeds
Midafternoon	16 ounces Cranberry Elixir*
4:00 p.m.	2 tablespoons Macadamia Nut Crème* with 4 walnuts
20 minutes before dinner	8 ounces filtered water
Dinner	Smoky Black Bean Burger*
	Mixed greens salad with grated carrot, jicama matchsticks, mushrooms, and chopped olives topped with 1 tablespoon Cilantro Lime Dressing*
	Sprinkle with 1 tablespoon sesame seeds
Before bed	Live Longer Cocktail*

DAY 7

On arising	Live Longer Cocktail*
Breakfast	Longevity Blaster*
Midmorning	16 ounces Cranberry Elixir*
Lunch	Edamame spinach salad with ½ cup steamed and cooled frozen organic shelled edamame and 1 cup drained, cubed, firm tofu. Served over a bed of fresh spinach, grated carrot, and sliced scallions with 1 tablespoon French Riviera Dressing.*
	Sprinkle with 1 tablespoon hemp seeds
Midafternoon	16 ounces Cranberry Elixir*
4:00 p.m.	Pomegranate Gelatin*
20 minutes before dinner	8 ounces filtered water
Dinner	Meatball Soup*
	Leafy green salad with grated beet, carrot, and sliced hearts of palm
	1 tablespoon Hemp Hemp Hooray Dressing*
	Sprinkle with 1–2 tablespoons flax- or sesame seeds
	1 cup coffee or tea
Before bed	Live Longer Cocktail*

WHAT'S NEXT?

As your food list can expand to include more friendly starches, such as sweet potatoes, yams, and squash, you can also double up on nuts and seeds as well as introduce more nut butters. Just be sure to keep your daily detox going with the Longevity Blaster, Live Longer Cocktail, and Cranberry Elixir as part of your daily routine. Keep high-AGE butter, cream, cheese, and bacon to a bare minimum or eliminate altogether. Modify all your favorite recipes to include high-moisture, low-heat cooking techniques and avoid high, dry heat, such as baking, grilling, and frying, unless you marinate, marinate, marinate!

RADICAL LONGEVITY RECIPES

BEVERAGES

LONGEVITY BLASTER

If coffee isn't your thing, use dandelion root or oolong tea.

Makes 1 serving

- 8 ounces coffee (regular or decaf) from Purity Coffee (see Resources)
- 1 scoop whey protein, such as Fat Flush A2-derived whey (see Resources)
- Up to 1 tablespoon cacao powder, to taste
- 1 tablespoon coconut oil
- 1 scoop Vitality C (supplying up to 4 grams of the best absorbed powdered vitamin C)
- 1 scoop sunflower lecithin
- ¼ teaspoon ground Ceylon cinnamon, cardamom, and/or ginger
- Touch of stevia or monk fruit, to taste

Whisk all ingredients in a small bowl or shake in a lidded jar. Pour into your favorite glass and enjoy!

LIVE LONGER COCKTAIL

Start and end your day in cleansing mode. Especially good for the liver and lymph, this cocktail will keep your system well hydrated all day long in one age-defying, lean, green drink!

Makes 1 serving

   2 ounces 100% pure unsweetened cranberry juice
   14 ounces plain filtered water
   1 scoop greens powder (I like UNI KEY Daily Greens)
   1 tablespoon ground chia seeds
   Pinch of Ceylon cinnamon

Stir all ingredients together (or shake in a lidded jar)—drink up!

CRANBERRY ELIXIR

Cleansing, comforting refreshment in every cup!

Makes 4 cups (1 cup per serving)

   1 quart Cranberry Water (recipe follows)
   ¼ teaspoon ground Ceylon cinnamon
   ⅛ teaspoon ground ginger
   ⅛ teaspoon ground nutmeg
   ½ cup freshly squeezed orange juice
   2 tablespoons freshly squeezed lemon juice

Bring Cranberry Water to a light boil; lower heat to low. Place cinnamon, ginger, and nutmeg in a tea ball; add to Cranberry Water. (For a tangier juice, add spices directly to Cranberry Water.) Simmer for 15 to 20 minutes; remove from heat and let cool to room temperature. Stir in orange and lemon juices.

CRANBERRY WATER

The quintessential gentle detox drink to keep you happily flushing.

To make 1 quart (32 ounces), add 4 ounces of unsweetened cranberry juice to 28 ounces purified water *or* 1½ tablespoons of unsweetened cranberry juice concentrate to 30 ounces of purified water.

Recommended brands of unsweetened cranberry juice are Lakewood 100% Organic, Mountain Sun, Trader Joe's, and Knudsen. Recommended brands of unsweetened cranberry juice concentrate are Knudsen and Tree of Life. Be sure to look for juice that has no sugar, corn syrup, or other juices added, including apple or grape.

SOUPS, SIDES, AND SNACKS

RADICAL LONGEVITY SOUP

This savory soup is a satisfying meal for the 5-Day Reset and beyond.

Makes 10 to 12 cups (2 to 3 cups per serving)

46 ounces (5¾ cups) plus 2 tablespoons organic bone broth (Kettle & Fire brand is my favorite) or vegetable broth

1¼ pounds ground or chopped organic, grass-fed beef, turkey, or chicken (can omit, or use 30 ounces of beans if vegetarian or vegan)

1 large onion, peeled and chopped, or 2 large leeks, white and light green parts, chopped (about 2 cups)

1 large zucchini or yellow squash, chopped (about 2 cups)

½ cup grated daikon radish

2 garlic cloves, peeled and minced

1 (12-ounce) package mushrooms, chopped

1¾ cups chopped cabbage

1 tablespoon freshly squeezed lime juice

1 tablespoon ground cumin

½ teaspoon Real Salt, sea salt, or pink Himalayan salt

¼ cup fresh cilantro leaves, chopped

¼ cup fresh parsley leaves, chopped

1 tablespoon hemp seed oil per serving

1 teaspoon South River miso paste (immunity-boosting flavor enhancer) per serving (optional)

In a saucepot over medium heat, cook 2 tablespoons of broth for 30 seconds, or until heated. Add beef. Cook, stirring occasionally, for 5 minutes, or until cooked through. Remove from pot; drain, if desired, and set aside. In same saucepot, cook onion, zucchini, daikon radish, and garlic, stirring occasionally, for 5 minutes, or until vegetables are crisp-tender. Stir in remaining 46 ounces of broth plus mushrooms, cabbage, lime juice, cumin, salt, and cooked meat. Add up to 1 cup water or more broth to thin soup, if desired. Cover; bring soup to a simmer (do not let boil), and lower heat to medium low. Let simmer, stirring occasionally, for 20 minutes. Stir in cilantro and parsley. Cover; let simmer for 5 minutes more. Drizzle in hemp seed oil. Add miso paste to individual bowls when serving, if desired. Soup can be stored up to 3 days in refrigerator.

MEDITERRANEAN LENTIL SOUP

This sunny soup from Greece is high on flavor and loaded with healthy high-fiber benefits.

Makes 4 servings (about 2 cups per serving)

1 cup dried lentils, washed and soaked in 4 cups water overnight

3 cups filtered water

1 tablespoon olive oil

1 tablespoon freshly squeezed lemon juice

1 onion, chopped (about 1 cup)

1 carrot, chopped (about ¾ cup)

½ cup chopped escarole, collards, or arugula

1 celery stalk with leaves, chopped

1 garlic clove, minced

2 tablespoons chopped fresh parsley

½ bay leaf

½ teaspoon mustard seeds

½ teaspoon ground cumin

¾ teaspoon salt (optional)

2 tablespoons finely chopped green onion, for garnish

Place drained lentils in 3 cups of fresh water in a covered pot. Bring to a boil and lower heat to a simmer. Add olive oil and lemon juice. Cook for 30 minutes, or until lentils are tender. Add rest of ingredients, except green onion. Cover and simmer for an additional 20 to 30 minutes, or until vegetables are tender. Serve garnished with green onion.

WHITE BEAN AND SPINACH SOUP (SLOW COOKER)

This satisfying nutrient-rich soup is easy to throw in the slow cooker in the morning before you go about your busy day.

Makes 6 to 8 servings (about 2 cups per serving)

1 pound dried great northern or navy beans

3 carrots, diced (1½ to 2 cups)

2 celery stalks, diced (1½ to 2 cups)

1½ cups diced leek

3 garlic cloves, minced

1 tablespoon diced fresh sage leaves, or 1 teaspoon dried

4 cups vegetable broth

2 cups purified water

3 cups fresh spinach, chopped

½ cup fresh parsley, chopped
Sea salt
2 cups shredded low-fat Cheddar cheese

Sort and rinse beans in a colander. Place in a bowl, cover with water, and soak for at least 4 to 12 hours or overnight. (Soaked is best! See note for alternative directions, in case you're in more of a hurry or forgot.) Combine soaked beans, carrots, celery, leek, garlic, and sage in your slow cooker. Cover with veggie broth and water. Cover and cook on HIGH for 6 to 8 hours. If you've soaked your beans ahead of time, they'll be tender in 3 to 4 hours, but the longer they cook, the creamier your soup will be. Fifteen to 30 minutes before you're ready to serve, stir in spinach and parsley; adding them at the end preserves fresh enzymes and nutrients. Taste and add sea salt to taste. Top each serving with ⅓ cup of cheese.

Note: Soaking beans for a few hours or overnight makes them easier to digest and shortens the cooking time. But if you must skip this step, you can rinse them, add them directly to your slow cooker, and let them cook for at least eight hours. Or you can use the Quick Soak Method: Place beans in a large pot and cover with water to about 2 inches above the beans. Bring to a boil and boil for 20 to 30 minutes. Turn off the heat, cover the pot, and let the beans soak for about an hour. Drain and rinse in a colander, then add them to the slow cooker and follow the rest of the recipe.

MEATBALL SOUP

This hearty soup can be made with ground beef, turkey, or chicken.

Makes 4 to 6 servings (about 2 cups per serving)

MEATBALLS:
1 pound ground beef, turkey, or chicken
1 cup mushrooms, minced
1 carrot, shredded (about ¾ cup)

¼ cup fresh parsley

1 tablespoon prepared horseradish (I like Bubbie's brand)

1 teaspoon Dijon mustard

1 egg, or 1 tablespoon ground flaxseeds soaked in
   3 tablespoons water

1 teaspoon dried Italian seasoning

1 teaspoon garlic powder

1 teaspoon sea salt

SOUP:

32 ounces (4 cups) mushroom, vegetable, beef, or chicken broth

2 carrots, sliced (1½ to 2 cups)

2 celery stalks, sliced (1½ to 2 cups)

½ cup sliced leek

4 garlic cloves, diced

2 teaspoons dried Italian seasoning

1 cup mushrooms, sliced

3 cups chopped fresh greens, such as kale, spinach, arugula,
   or Swiss chard

4 cups water

½ cup fresh parsley, chopped, for garnish

Prepare meatballs: Combine all meatball ingredients in a large bowl and let rest in refrigerator while preparing soup. (Veggies take the place of bread crumbs or cracker crumbs in this healthy version of meatballs, so mixture may seem loose but will work just fine when cooked in soup.)

Prepare soup: Heat a large pot over medium-low heat. Pour about ¼ cup of broth into pot and bring to a simmer. Add carrots, celery, leek, garlic, and Italian seasoning. Sauté for 3 to 5 minutes, or until fragrant and beginning to soften. Stir in mushrooms and greens. Add remaining 3¾ cups broth and the water. Increase heat and bring to a low boil. Take meatball mixture from refrigerator. Using your hands, form into meatballs—about 1 tablespoon each—and drop each meatball into boiling soup as you go along. Meatballs may feel loose, but they don't have to be perfectly round and they'll firm up while cooking. Stir gently, then let meatballs cook in soup on a low boil for at least 20 minutes. Lower heat to low and let simmer for another 30 minutes.

Serve topped with fresh parsley.

TOFU EGG DROP SOUP

So soothing for body and soul!

Makes 2 servings (about 2 cups each)

- 4 cups organic chicken bone broth
- 3 scallions, sliced
- 1½ tablespoons gluten-free tamari sauce
- ½ teaspoon sesame oil
- 8 ounces extra-firm organic tofu, diced into ½-inch cubes
- 1 handful organic baby spinach
- 3 large organic eggs

In a medium-size stockpot, heat broth over medium heat until simmering. Lower heat to medium low to maintain simmering, but not boiling. Set aside some sliced scallions for garnish, then add remaining scallions to broth. Add tamari sauce, sesame oil, tofu, and spinach and let simmer for another minute or so. Crack eggs into a small bowl and whisk together. Turn off heat and then, slowly stirring in one direction, drizzle whisked eggs into soup. Eggs will cook quickly, forming light strands. Garnish with reserved scallions and serve immediately.

CREAMY COCONUT COLLARD GREENS

A new take on creamed greens, this healthy version will have you begging for more! For a twist, try it with spinach or escarole.

Makes 2 servings (about 1 cup each)

2 bunches (about 1 pound total) fresh, organic collard greens
1 tablespoon bone broth
½ cup sliced scallions
1 cup organic coconut milk
½ teaspoon organic ground nutmeg
Sea salt
1 tablespoon freshly squeezed lemon juice

Wash collard greens and remove stems. Slice evenly into 1-inch pieces. Bring a large pot of water to a boil. Add greens and blanch for about 2 minutes. Remove from heat, drain, and set greens aside. Heat bone broth in a large skillet over medium heat. Add scallions and cook for about 2 minutes. Add greens, coconut milk, nutmeg, and sea salt. Simmer for another 3 to 4 minutes. Transfer greens to a serving dish. Drizzle with lemon juice before serving.

BONUS RECIPES: SOUPS, SIDES, AND SNACKS

WILD MUSHROOM TURKEY MISO SOUP

Take a walk on the wild side and indulge your senses in this rich, aromatic soup for lunch or dinner.

Makes 4 servings (about 1½ cups each)

1 (½-ounce) package dried mushrooms, such as shiitake, porcini, or a combination
2 tablespoons bone broth

1 pound ground turkey

1 (8-ounce) package fresh, organic cremini mushrooms, sliced

1 (4-ounce) package fresh, organic shiitake mushrooms, sliced

1 (4-ounce) package fresh, organic oyster mushrooms, sliced

1 (2-ounce) package fresh, organic enoki or beech mushrooms

1 leek, finely sliced (about 1½ cups)

1½ teaspoons minced fresh ginger

1 garlic clove, minced

3 cups organic chicken or mushroom broth

1 tablespoon gluten-free tamari sauce

1 tablespoon organic apple cider vinegar

3 tablespoons organic white miso (see Note)

1 head baby bok choy, sliced

1 scallion, sliced, for garnish

In a small pot, bring a cup of filtered water to a boil, remove from heat, and add dried mushrooms. Let soak for 30 minutes.

Meanwhile, in a 4- to 6-quart Dutch oven or stockpot (with a lid), heat 1 tablespoon of bone broth over medium-low heat. Add ground turkey, breaking up with spoon and stirring occasionally until cooked through. Stir in fresh mushrooms and leek, then cover and cook over medium-low heat, until mushrooms have softened, about 10 minutes. Push turkey and mushroom mixture to one side of the pot and add second tablespoon of bone broth to the cleared space. Add ginger and garlic and stir until fragrant, about 30 seconds. Add chicken broth, tamari sauce, and vinegar. Increase heat and bring soup to a gentle boil, then lower heat to medium low and simmer for 10 minutes.

Drain reconstituted dried mushrooms, adding their liquid to pot. Chop and add mushrooms to pot. Spoon miso into a small bowl and add about one 1 tablespoon of the soup broth. Whisk until smooth, then mix into pot of soup. Add baby bok choy. Serve garnished with scallions.

Note: Be sure not to bring the soup to a boil once the miso has been added so as to retain its health benefits.

SPAGHETTI SQUASH TOSS

Can something this fun be this easy and nutritious? You bet! And it's a great stand-in for grain-based pasta.

Makes 4 large servings (or save half and store in refrigerator for leftovers)

1 medium-size spaghetti squash (about 3 pounds)
Sea salt
2 large garlic cloves, pressed
½ teaspoon ground Ceylon cinnamon
1 to 2 tablespoons extra-virgin olive oil

Place whole squash in a steamer basket in a large pot. Fill pot with water to about 1 inch below steamer basket. Bring to a boil over high heat, then lower heat to medium low, maintaining a simmer. Cover with lid and cook for 25 to 30 minutes, or until a knife easily pierces the squash. Run under cold water until cool enough to handle.

Cut squash in half. Remove seeds with a spoon. With a fork, separate (unthread) spaghetti pulp from skin and place in serving dish. Sprinkle on seasonings and oil, tossing lightly.

SAUTÉED ESCAROLE WITH CHICKPEAS

Escarole is a delicious and versatile bitter green. It's great in soups, stews, and salads. Add protein with chickpeas and voilà—you have a balanced meal. If you can't find escarole, substitute arugula, spinach, or a combination.

Makes 4 servings

2 heads escarole, washed and coarsely chopped
1 tablespoon olive oil
3 garlic cloves, crushed and chopped
2 cups fresh parsley, chopped

1 (14-ounce) can organic chickpeas, drained and rinsed
2 tablespoons vegetable broth
2 tablespoons freshly squeezed lemon juice
Pinch of sea salt (optional)

In a steamer basket over boiling water, lightly steam escarole until just tender, about 6 minutes, then drain. Heat a large skillet over medium heat, then put in olive oil and coat skillet.

Sauté garlic for about 1 minute, or until softened—be careful not to let it burn. Add steamed escarole, parsley, and chickpeas and sauté for 2 minutes. Stir in vegetable broth, lemon juice, and salt (if using). Continue to sauté for about 5 minutes, or until escarole is tender and almost all broth has evaporated.

FLAX OR CHIA "EGGS"

Ground flaxseeds and chia seeds make great egg substitutes and can be used in many recipes to act as binders. The added nutrients and fiber are bonuses!

Makes equivalent of 1 large egg (see Notes)

1 tablespoon ground flaxseeds or chia seeds
3 tablespoons water

Mix seeds and water together in a small bowl or cup and let sit for 5 to 10 minutes, or until thickened, before adding to recipes.

Notes
This recipe can easily be doubled or tripled to substitute for two or three large eggs, respectively.

Flax or chia "eggs" can cause some baked goods to have a heavier and denser texture, but they also add a nutty flavor that works great for pancakes, waffles, muffins, breads, and cookies.

MAIN DISHES

TEMPTING TEMPEH

Here's a recipe the whole family will love. Try it rolled in Bibb lettuce!

Makes 4 servings

1 (8-ounce) package tempeh
1 tablespoon coconut aminos or gluten-free tamari sauce
1 tablespoon monk fruit or yacón syrup
1 cup vegetable broth
½ teaspoon Wright's Hickory Liquid Smoke
½ teaspoon smoked paprika
1 teaspoon dry mustard powder
1 teaspoon ground cumin

Slice tempeh crosswise into ½-inch strips and set aside.

Heat a large, deep skillet over medium-high heat.

Meanwhile, place remaining ingredients in a bowl and stir until combined, to create a sauce.

Place tempeh strips in heated skillet and pour sauce over them.

Once sauce begins to simmer, flip tempeh strips over, using a pair of tongs. In about 3 minutes, flip them over again, then repeat about every 3 minutes, coating strips until sauce thickens, tempeh is coated, and most liquid evaporates.

SMOKY BLACK BEAN BURGERS

Black beans are high in protein and fiber, and these hearty burgers taste great alone, on a bed of lettuce, or in a cauliflower bun. Finely diced mushrooms take the place of bread crumbs and add a moist and chewy texture.

Makes 4 servings

½ cup chopped leek
2 garlic cloves, diced
¼ cup fresh cilantro or parsley
1 tablespoon ground cumin
1 tablespoon Wright's Liquid Smoke (see Note)
½ teaspoon dry mustard powder
½ teaspoon sea salt
1 Flax or Chia "Egg" (page 142), or 1 large egg
1 (15-ounce) can organic black beans, drained and rinsed
¾ cup very finely chopped mushrooms

Place leek, garlic, cilantro, cumin, liquid smoke, mustard powder, and sea salt in a food processor and pulse until veggies have been finely chopped. Alternatively, if you don't have a food processor, just make sure all veggies are finely chopped and mix them together in a large bowl.

Add egg replacer, black beans, and mushrooms and mix well.

Chill mixture in fridge for about 1 hour, to help it hold together.

Preheat oven to 375°F. Line a baking sheet with unbleached parchment paper.

Divide mixture into four equal patties (about ½ cup each) and place them on prepared baking sheet.

Bake for 10 minutes, flip, then bake for an additional 10 minutes.

Note: Wright's Liquid Smoke is offered in three flavors: Hickory, Mesquite, and Applewood. Pick your favorite!

BRAISED COCONUT MILK CHICKEN

This fragrant, delicious recipe sounds exotic but is so easy to make! Save a portion to use in a lunch salad for the next day.

Makes 4 servings

- 1 (13.5-ounce) can unsweetened coconut milk
- 2 tablespoons Thai curry paste
- 2 (4- to 6-inch-long) lemongrass stalks, tough outer layer discarded, lightly crushed and chopped
- 1 (2-inch piece) fresh ginger, peeled, smashed, and chopped
- 6 garlic cloves, smashed and chopped
- ½ cup vegetable broth
- 4 boneless, skinless chicken breasts
- ½ cup fresh cilantro, chopped
- 1 lime, cut into 4 wedges

Preheat oven to 400°F. Combine coconut milk, curry paste, lemongrass, ginger, garlic, and vegetable broth in a bowl and stir until well mixed. Pour into a large baking dish. Place chicken breasts in sauce and turn over so they're completely coated. Bake until chicken is tender and thoroughly cooked throughout (internal temperature should be 165°F), about 30 minutes. If you don't have a thermometer, just pierce chicken breasts with the tip of a sharp knife and, if juices run clear with no hint of pink, they should be done. Spoon sauce over chicken and garnish with cilantro. Serve with lime wedges to squeeze over bites.

RED WINE AND ROSEMARY MARINATED LAMB CHOPS

For a special dinner, why not indulge in this easy Mediterranean treat. Marinating reduces the AGEs in the cooking process and infuses the meat with cognitive-enhancing rosemary bathed in the benefits of savory garlic.

Makes 4 servings (2 lamb chops each)

MARINADE:
- 1 cup organic, dry red wine
- ¼ cup olive oil
- 4 fresh rosemary sprigs
- 4 garlic cloves, minced
- 1 tablespoon Dijon mustard
- 1 teaspoon pink Himalayan or sea salt

- 8 grass-fed loin lamb chops, fat trimmed
- Sea salt, for sprinkling
- Garlic powder, for sprinkling

Whisk together all marinade ingredients in a bowl or large measuring cup. Place lamb chops in a single layer in a Pyrex baking dish and pour marinade over them. Let marinate in refrigerator for 1 to 4 hours or overnight, turning occasionally.

Preheat oven to 350°F. Place lamb chops in a single layer on a parchment-lined baking sheet or broiler pan (discard leftover marinade). Bake for 45 minutes, or until desired doneness. Season lamb chops with salt and garlic powder.

SALMON EN PAPILLOTE

Baking fish in a parchment-wrapped packet makes an elegant, moist dish that is sure to impress your guests and delight your taste buds. Once you've tried it, you'll realize it's actually an easy process well worth the effort.

Makes 2 servings

 2 tablespoons gluten-free tamari sauce
 2 tablespoons apple cider vinegar
 1 (½-inch) piece fresh ginger, finely grated
 1 garlic clove, finely grated
 2 skinless wild-caught salmon fillets
 1 organic carrot, peeled and julienned (about 1 cup)
 ⅓ cup julienned fennel bulb (matchstick-size pieces)
 ⅓ cup julienned leek
 2 heads bok choy, leaves separated

Preheat oven to 375°F. Mix together tamari sauce, vinegar, ginger, and garlic in a large bowl. Add salmon fillets, cover, and marinate for 10 minutes at room temperature. Take two large sheets of baking parchment, big enough to encase salmon and vegetables, and place each sheet on a separate baking pan. Divide vegetables between center of each paper and top each with a marinated salmon fillet (reserve marinade). Bring sides of each sheet parchment over salmon and pour half of remaining marinade over each fillet. Fold each sheet tightly together to seal fish in parchment. Bake for 20 to 25 minutes, or until salmon is just cooked through and flakes into large pieces. Serve salmon in their paper.

BONUS RECIPES: MAIN DISHES

TENDER ROAST BEEF

For the most tender roast beef you've ever tasted, use your VitaClay cooker (or any slow cooker you have in the kitchen). Of course, you should select hormone-free, grass-fed beef. Although grass-fed beef tends to be a bit tougher than grain fed, this no-fail method of cooking brings out the flavor while dramatically reducing AGE content. Enjoy with a celebratory glass of organic red wine to cut the iron absorption.

Makes 8 servings

½ cup beef broth
1 (3- to 3½-pound) beef roast, your choice of cut
Splash of red wine (optional)
6 fresh rosemary sprigs, or 1 tablespoon dried
2 teaspoons ground turmeric
1 teaspoon sea salt

Pour beef broth into bottom of clay pot (this is very important: dry cooking will crack a clay pot eventually). Place roast in pot, cutting and removing any twine or packaging. Add red wine (if using), plus rosemary, turmeric, and salt (or your choice of seasonings). Close cooker, set to STEW setting, and cook for 1 to 2 hours, or until meat is tender.

POACHED WHITE FISH WITH MEDITERRANEAN HERBED SAUCE

This recipe works well with any white fish, but it's spectacular with halibut! White wine and fresh Mediterranean herbs complement the delicate flavor and texture of the fish.

Makes 4 servings

SPICE RUB:

1 teaspoon dried oregano

½ teaspoon dried thyme

1 teaspoon ground coriander

½ teaspoon sea salt

2 pounds fish fillets

1 tablespoon extra-virgin olive oil

½ cup sliced leek

8 garlic cloves, minced

2½ cups chicken broth

½ cup dry white wine

Zest and juice of 2 large lemons

½ cup fresh parsley, chopped

10 to 12 large fresh basil leaves, thinly sliced

1 tablespoon capers

4 scallions, chopped, for garnish

Mix together all spice rub ingredients in a small bowl. Rinse fish fillets and pat dry with paper towels. Coat both sides of each fillet with spice mixture and gently rub into their flesh. Set aside and let rest at room temperature.

Heat a large skillet (with a lid) over medium-low heat and put in olive oil. When oil is shimmering but not smoking, lower heat to low. Add leek and toss gently until softened, about 3 minutes. Add garlic and cook for another 30 seconds. Stir in chicken broth, wine, lemon zest and juice, parsley, basil, and capers. Place fish fillets in skillet, cover, and allow to simmer over low heat for 8 to 10 minutes, or until fish is opaque and flaky—firm to the touch but not dry. Remove from heat, spoon pan juices with capers and herbs over each fillet, and top with chopped scallions to serve.

STEAMED GINGER CHICKEN WITH SESAME GARLIC SAUCE

This fragrant dish is wonderfully satisfying served over steamed brown rice with a side of braised broccolini or bok choy.

Makes 4 servings

- 4 large collard greens or Chinese (napa) cabbage leaves
- 4 chicken breast halves, pounded to ½-inch thickness
- 2 tablespoons chopped fresh ginger

SAUCE:

- 2 tablespoons gluten-free tamari sauce
- 2 teaspoons apple cider vinegar
- Dash of sriracha (optional)
- 1 tablespoon sesame oil
- 4 garlic cloves, smashed and minced
- ½ cup fresh cilantro, chopped

Place a steamer basket in a 6-quart pot and fill with water to about ½ inch below bottom of basket. Lay greens in steamer basket and place chicken on top. Scatter ginger over chicken, cover pot, and bring water to a boil. Steam for about 15 minutes, or until chicken is done (at least 165°F internally). Remove ¼ cup of liquid from pot and set aside to use in sauce. Place chicken back in pot and cover to keep warm.

Prepare sauce: In a small bowl, stir together reserved liquid, tamari, vinegar, and sriracha (if using), then set aside. Heat a small skillet over medium-low heat. Add sesame oil and garlic and cook for about 30 seconds, or until garlic is fragrant and softened. Add tamari mixture, stir, and bring to a boil. Lower heat and let simmer until reduced in volume to about ⅓ cup, about 20 minutes. Add cilantro and cook for about 30 more seconds.

To serve, place greens on plate and top with chicken. Drizzle with sauce.

DRESSINGS AND MARINADES

CILANTRO LIME DRESSING

The perfect (and delicious) way to incorporate the power of hemp into your daily diet. Use this on any greens or vegetables (see this recommended list on page 114).

Makes 4 servings

1 cup packed fresh cilantro leaves
1 garlic clove
Juice of 1 lime
1 teaspoon umeboshi (ume plum) vinegar, or ½ teaspoon sea salt
¼ cup hemp oil
Spring or filtered water

Place all ingredients, except water, in a blender and blend until smooth. Add water, 1 tablespoon at a time, if a thinner dressing is desired.

VARIATIONS
Add 2 tablespoons of toasted pepitas.
Use lemon juice in place of lime juice.
Add some lime zest (up to ½ lime) for extra lime flavor.

HEMP HEMP HOORAY DRESSING

Hooray for all the healing benefits of hemp oil in this tasty dressing!

Makes 4 servings

1 teaspoon freshly squeezed lemon juice
1 tablespoon apple cider vinegar
1 teaspoon Dijon mustard
1 garlic clove, minced
Sea salt
¼ cup organic hemp seed oil

Place all ingredients, except hemp seed oil, in a blender or food processor. Drizzle oil into blender as it mixes to emulsify oil into other ingredients. Serve immediately as a dressing for salads.

ZIPPY GINGER MISO DRESSING

Fresh and flavorful!

Makes 4 servings

3 tablespoons extra-virgin olive oil
2 garlic cloves, minced
2 teaspoons grated fresh ginger
¼ cup freshly squeezed lemon juice
¼ cup freshly squeezed clementine or orange juice
1 tablespoon white miso paste
Sea salt (optional)

Whisk together all ingredients, except salt, in a small bowl or cup. Taste and adjust seasonings, adding more miso (or a pinch of sea salt). This dressing packs a bit of a punch, but it mellows once poured over vegetables.

TANGY TAHINI AND HERB VINAIGRETTE

Goes well with almost everything!

Makes 4 servings

- 1 tablespoon tahini
- 3 tablespoons water
- 2 tablespoons freshly squeezed lemon juice
- 1 tablespoon extra-virgin olive oil
- 1 garlic clove, crushed and minced
- ½ teaspoon sea salt, or to taste
- 1 tablespoon finely chopped fresh chives
- 1 tablespoon finely chopped fresh parsley
- 1 tablespoon finely chopped fennel fronds

In a small bowl, beat tahini and water together with a fork. Stir in lemon juice and olive oil and whisk to emulsify. Stir in garlic, salt, and fresh herbs. For a thinner dressing, simply add more water and/or lemon juice, a little at a time, until desired consistency is attained.

FRENCH RIVIERA DRESSING

Great as a dressing or for flavoring a sauté.

Makes ½ cup dressing

- ⅓ cup extra-virgin olive oil
- 3 tablespoons freshly squeezed lemon juice
- 2 garlic cloves, pressed
- 1 teaspoon chopped fresh tarragon
- 1 teaspoon Dijon mustard
- Sea salt

Place all ingredients in a small, covered jar and shake vigorously for 30 seconds.

BONUS RECIPES: MARINADES

Marinating times for beef, poultry, and lamb: 2 to 24 hours; for fish: 30 minutes to 1 hour; for veggies: 30 minutes. Each basic marinade recipe covers four to six servings but easily can be doubled or tripled for more servings. Never marinate fish longer than one hour as the marinade can partially cook the fish. Unless otherwise noted, to use marinades: Mix the ingredients; pour into a resealable plastic bag or glass dish with a lid. Add meat, fish, or vegetables and let the marinade sit in the refrigerator, turning occasionally. Be sure to discard marinade after marinated animal protein is removed for cooking.

TERESA'S LONGEVITY MARINADE

This is the quintessential marinade for infusing antioxidant-rich health benefits and flavor into your main dishes.

Makes ⅔ cup (enough for 1 pound of meat, poultry, fish, or veggies)

½ cup bone broth
¼ cup apple cider vinegar
1 teaspoon ground cumin
1 teaspoon dry mustard powder
1 teaspoon ground turmeric
1 teaspoon ground ginger
1 tablespoon chopped garlic
6 fresh rosemary sprigs, or 1 tablespoon dried leaves
1 teaspoon sea salt

ZESTY LONGEVITY ROSEMARY MARINADE

Step up your game by combining mushroom vegetable broth with fresh rosemary. The taste is out of this world.

Makes ⅔ cup (enough for 1 pound of meat, poultry, or fish)

⅓ cup red wine vinegar (or white wine vinegar if desired)
¼ cup filtered water

1½ tablespoons Dijon mustard

1½ tablespoons chopped fresh rosemary

⅓ cup mushroom broth or vegetable broth

1 tablespoon crushed garlic

¾ teaspoon sea salt

Place all ingredients in a small bowl and stir to blend. Place meat and marinade in a shallow glass, ceramic, or enamel bowl. Turn food to coat with marinade. Remove meat from marinade, discarding marinade or boiling it for reuse as a sauce. TIP: For a sweeter marinade, add a tablespoon of Lakanto Monk Fruit Maple Syrup or plain monk fruit.

ISLAND BREEZES MARINADE

This tasty tropical marinade is especially good with chicken but would also go just as well with shrimp or fish.

Makes about 1 cup (enough for 1 pound of meat, poultry, or fish)

⅓ cup bone broth

1½ tablespoons macadamia nut oil

⅓ cup coconut vinegar

¼ cup crushed pineapple

1 teaspoon onion powder

1 tablespoon chopped garlic

1 teaspoon sea salt

LONG LIFE MEDITERRANEAN MARINADE

The rich broth and herbs in this marinade add an earthy flavor well suited to lamb, beef, or chicken.

Makes about 1 cup (enough for 1 pound of meat, poultry, or fish)

⅓ cup mushroom broth

⅓ cup red wine

1 tablespoon Dijon mustard

6 fresh rosemary sprigs, or 1 tablespoon dried leaves

1 tablespoon chopped fresh parsley

1 tablespoon chopped fresh thyme

1 tablespoon chopped fresh oregano

1 tablespoon smashed and minced garlic

1 teaspoon sea salt

THAI ONE ON MARINADE

This fresh and fragrant marinade with a touch of heat is wonderful with shrimp, fish, and chicken.

Makes about 1 cup (enough for 1 pound of meat, poultry, or fish)

⅓ cup bone broth

⅓ cup freshly squeezed lime juice

1 tablespoon chopped fresh ginger

1 teaspoon chopped scallion

1 teaspoon chopped garlic

1 tablespoon curry powder

1 teaspoon red pepper flakes (optional)

1 teaspoon sea salt

MARVELOUS MARINADE

This delightfully spicy marinade is great with such veggies as zucchini, Brussels sprouts, or even fresh corn on the cob, and it dances beautifully with a nice cut of beef or chicken breasts.

Makes about 1 cup (enough for 1 pound of meat, poultry, or fish)

⅓ cup bone broth
⅓ cup rice vinegar
Zest and juice of 1 orange
1 tablespoon fresh thyme, chopped, or 1 teaspoon dried
1 teaspoon ground cumin
1 teaspoon sea salt

TASTY TREATS

MOCHA CHOCOLATE SURPRISE CAKE

The surprise in this rich, moistly decadent cake is adzuki beans! They add a healthy punch of protein and moist texture—don't tell anyone the secret ingredient until after they've had a bite and are exclaiming about how good it is.

Makes 6 to 8 servings

2 cups almond or tigernut flour or chestnut flour
½ cup unsweetened cocoa powder
2 teaspoons aluminum-free baking powder
¼ teaspoon sea salt
1 tablespoon instant organic coffee powder, or 1 shot organic espresso
⅓ cup macadamia oil
½ cup Lakanto Monk Fruit Maple Syrup

½ cup unsweetened nondairy milk (such as almond, hemp seed,
   macadamia nut, or coconut)
1 teaspoon pure vanilla extract
1 cup cooked adzuki beans, drained

Preheat oven to 300°F. Line a 7- or 8-inch square baking pan with parchment paper. Combine flour, cocoa powder, baking powder, salt, and coffee powder in a large bowl and mix. (If using liquid espresso instead of coffee powder, add it with wet ingredients.) In a separate bowl, combine macadamia oil, maple syrup, milk, and vanilla and whisk together until fully incorporated. Stir in adzuki beans.

Pour wet mixture into dry and stir until thoroughly mixed together. Spread batter into prepared cake pan and bake for 25 to 35 minutes, or until a toothpick inserted into center comes out clean. Serve with a dollop of Cashew Crème (page 161).

MACADAMIA NUT CRÈME

This healthy dessert topping is rich and creamy and makes a great alternative to whipped cream.

Makes 1 cup (8 servings, 2 tablespoons each)

   1½ cups raw macadamia nuts
   ¼ to ½ cup filtered water
   2 tablespoons Lakanto Monk Fruit Maple Syrup
   Pinch of sea salt
   1 teaspoon pure vanilla extract

Soak macadamia nuts overnight in 2 cups of water. Drain macadamia nuts. Place nuts in ¼ cup of fresh water in a food processor or high-speed blender and process until smooth. Add remaining water as needed. Place pureed macadamia nuts, maple syrup, and salt in a medium sized bowl and stir until well blended. Chill in refrigerator.

POMEGRANATE GELATIN

Remember those sugary (or worse!—sugar-free) gelatin desserts? Whether you recall these concoctions favorably or with a shuddering cringe, this upgraded and updated version bursting with flavor and healthy collagen is sure to become a new favorite.

Makes 4 servings (about ½ cup each)

 Avocado oil spray, for dish
 1 cup unsweetened cranberry juice
 1½ tablespoons grass-fed collagen (such as Great Lakes brand)
 2 tablespoons Lakanto Monk Fruit Maple Syrup or honey, or 2
  teaspoons powdered stevia
 Pinch of sea salt
 1 cup pomegranate seeds (arils)

Lightly oil a casserole dish or glass bowl with avocado oil spray. Pour cranberry juice and 1 cup of water into a saucepan. Sprinkle collagen on top, whisk together, and allow to sit for 5 minutes. Place saucepan over medium heat and whisk mixture until collagen is thoroughly dissolved. Remove from heat and stir in your sweetener of choice. Spread ½ cup of pomegranate seeds in bottom of prepared dish and pour collagen mixture on top. Chill in fridge for 2 to 4 hours, or until fully set and firm to the touch. Sprinkle rest of pomegranate seeds on top and serve with a dollop of Macadamia Nut Crème (page 158) or Cashew Crème (page 161).

BONUS RECIPES: TASTY TREATS

RED WINE CRANBERRY POACHED PEARS

This classic, simply elegant dessert is a great finish to any meal. Choose Anjou, Asian, or Bosc pears for this recipe. Bartlett pears are delicious treats on their own but will become too mushy when poached.

Makes 6 servings

- 1 large piece orange peel
- 8 to 10 whole cloves
- 1 cinnamon stick
- 2 cups red wine (cabernet sauvignon or merlot)
- ½ cup unsweetened cranberry juice
- 2 teaspoons pure vanilla extract
- 3 to 6 medium-size pears

Place all ingredients, except pears, in a large saucepan and bring to a simmer.

Peel pears and lower them into poaching liquid. Let them simmer over medium-low heat for 20 minutes, rotating them every 5 minutes to make sure they are poaching evenly.

Serve pears standing upright on a plate drizzled with poaching liquid or chill pears and reheat liquid to pour over them before serving. A dollop of Macadamia Nut Crème (page 158) is nice on the side.

CASHEW CRÈME

This rich tasty crème makes a wonderful topping or spread for desserts and snacks. Make ahead and store in the fridge in a glass jar for two to three days.

Makes 1½ cups (8 servings, 2 tablespoons each)

1 cup raw cashews
⅓ cup unsweetened nondairy milk (such as cashew, hemp seed, almond, coconut, or macadamia)
2 tablespoons freshly squeezed lemon juice
⅓ cup Lakanto Monk Fruit Maple Syrup
¼ teaspoon umeboshi (ume plum) vinegar
1 teaspoon pure vanilla extract

Soak cashews overnight in 1 cup of water. Drain cashews and place in a blender with all remaining ingredients. Blend until smooth and creamy.

BLUEBERRY CRUMBLE

What a satisfying way to have your fruit serving and eat it too! Try substituting other berries or apples in the recipe to change it up.

Makes 6 to 8 servings

CRUMBLE:
½ cup rolled oats
½ cup nut grain-free flour (such as tigernut or chestnut)
½ cup shredded unsweetened coconut
½ cup coarsely chopped walnuts
⅛ teaspoon sea salt
5 tablespoons macadamia nut oil
3 tablespoons Lakanto Monk Fruit Maple Syrup

FILLING:

    1 tablespoon arrowroot powder

    ¾ cup cranberry water (see page 133)

    1 teaspoon ground cinnamon

    Pinch of sea salt

    1 tablespoon fresh lemon zest

    1 teaspoon freshly squeezed lemon juice

    1 teaspoon pure vanilla extract

    4 cups fresh or frozen blueberries

Preheat oven to 350°F.

Prepare crumble: In a large bowl, mix together oats, flour, coconut, walnuts, and salt. Add macadamia nut oil and maple syrup and use your hands to mix thoroughly to form a crumbly texture.

Prepare filling: Place arrowroot powder in a separate medium-size bowl. Slowly pour cranberry water over arrowroot while whisking until thoroughly smooth. Stir in cinnamon, salt, lemon zest and juice, and vanilla. Place blueberries in a casserole dish. Pour cranberry water mixture over berries.

Spread crumble mixture over berries. Cover casserole dish first with a protective layer of parchment paper and then a layer of aluminum foil, crimping edges over dish to seal. Bake for 45 minutes, or until berries are bubbling and topping is lightly browned. Serve while still warm with a dollop of Macadamia Nut Crème (page 158).

CHOCOLATE-DIPPED STRAWBERRIES

Remember to choose dark chocolate with a 60% or higher cacao content and organic berries only. A delicious way to incorporate this bitter in your diet!

Makes 4 to 6 servings (2 or 3 strawberries each)

4 ounces dark chocolate, chopped

12 medium-large fresh organic strawberries, unhulled, rinsed, and patted dry

¼ cup finely chopped walnuts or hazelnuts

Line a large baking sheet with parchment or waxed paper and set aside. Melt chocolate in a double boiler. Insert a toothpick into stem of a strawberry and dip berry into melted chocolate, coating lower three-fourths of berry. Holding fruit by its toothpick over a plate, rotate while sprinkling its chocolate coating with about 1 teaspoon of nuts. Place berry on prepared baking sheet. Repeat with remaining berries. Chill for at least 1 hour before serving.

PART THREE

RENEW YOUR BODY FROM HEAD TO TOE WITH TARGETED STRATEGIES

CHAPTER 11

RECLAIM YOUR BRAIN

In this chapter, you'll learn . . .

- The many reasons for memory loss
- How medication side effects can masquerade as dementia
- How AGEs impact your brain health
- About the undeniable connection between your blood sugar and your brain
- How to turn back the clock on your aging brain
- The most important exercise you can do to restore your memory

As you know by now, I am not a fan of "antiaging." Advancing in years is something you should feel fortunate to achieve, not something to be ashamed of or dreaded. But, at the same time, I don't believe signs of ill health that are written off as "normal" signs of aging should be tolerated in any way. I don't believe that failing memory and cognitive decline are an inevitable part of aging. So-called senior moments are not something you have to get used to. Memory loss at any age should be taken seriously and investigated to find the root cause.

Alzheimer's is the fastest growing disease of our time, and it reflects the age of our brain, not our chronological age. It is also the most feared disease—even more so than cancer. The memory loss we are seeing now goes far beyond hormonal changes. It's a result of unhealthy brain aging. And Alzheimer's isn't the only concern; Parkinson's disease, ALS, Lewy body dementia, and other neurodegenerative diseases, including those that cause chronic pain and mobility issues, are causing even the bravest among us to fear our advancing years.

This rapid brain and nervous system aging reveals itself through many telltale signs. Perhaps you lose your words when trying to communicate to someone—or you can't articulate your thoughts. Maybe you experience new fears and anxiety and have trouble sleeping. Or perhaps even though you try to keep your hand still, you can still see the tremor when you hold your silverware. Maybe you're losing height, and the shape of your spine changes because the disks between your vertebrae shrink.

But if you consider that there are many factors that can impact your brain health and think of it with optimism, you can begin problem solving, providing a much-needed brain boost. First, let's revisit Rule #3, Stop AGEs, and take a closer look at AGEs' impact on the brain and our impressive ability to reverse their deeply damaging effects. AGEs are excess glucose molecules in your bloodstream that attach to proteins, which results in them becoming "sticky," making these proteins more apt to clump together. The proteins then cause major inflammation in organs, causing a breakdown of cell function. Harmful AGEs enter the brain and begin depositing their toxinlike beta-amyloid plaques, which eventually develop into amyloid plaques and neurofibrillary tangles, resulting in cognitive decline, memory loss, and Alzheimer's disease.

Over one hundred years ago, researchers reported that brain cells accumulate a yellow-brown fatty pigment called lipofuscin. Lipofuscin is known as the aging pigment and is described as a composite of oxidized lipids and proteins, formed into a sort of cellular debris. Researchers have discovered that the brain's lipofuscin-like material holds AGE-lipids. As we age, the AGE level in the brain increases.

There are many reasons for memory loss. In fact, Alzheimer's disease is a diagnosis of exclusion. This means that considering all the diagnostic and clinical data that is available, the symptoms aren't consistent with any other known disease. In other words, Alzheimer's is a catchall diagnosis given when nothing else applies. Being diagnosed with Alzheimer's doesn't give you information to go on in terms of the root cause of your memory loss or the key to overcoming it. It can be much more helpful to take a step back and look at the many reasons why you may have memory loss in the first place, such as heavy metal toxicity, DNA damage from cell phone radiation, hormone changes or imbalance, and other factors addressed in the Rules.

MEDICATIONS THAT CAN DRAIN YOUR BRAINPOWER

Although the FDA requires drug fact labels to be included in medication packaging, few of us read them and they often require a medical scholar to understand them. It's quite misleading to call them "side effects" because the truth is that they are unintended effects that are just as important to understand as the issue for which you are taking the medication in the first place. There is one class of medications in particular that you need to look closely at if memory loss or dementia is of concern to you.

The word is *anticholinergic*. Ask your pharmacist if any of your medications—including those that are over the counter (OTC)—fall into this category. This class of medication blocks acetylcholine, an important neurotransmitter your brain needs for proper functioning. As it is, our levels of acetylcholine reduce as we age, so to have its effects blocked on top of the deficiency can cause memory loss, confusion, agitation, and even delirium. All of this together looks a lot like dementia.

Other classes of medications that are known to mimic Alzheimer's dementia include

→ Antianxiety—includes benzodiazepines and other sedatives
→ Insomnia—includes the popular Ambien
→ Antidepressants—especially SSRIs
→ Antihistamines—includes such popular OTC meds as Benadryl
→ Overactive bladder—includes Detrol, among others
→ Seizure—some of these meds are also used for migraines
→ Parkinson's medications
→ Cardiovascular—includes some blood thinners and some blood pressure medications
→ Chemotherapy
→ Steroids—especially prednisone
→ Narcotic pain medications

WHAT'S GOTTEN INTO YOU MAY BE AFFECTING YOUR MEMORY

In your quest to find the cause of your memory loss, if you've ruled out medications, then look to ticks, fleas, and other biting insects as a possible cause. Only 50 percent of people with Lyme disease ever recall being bitten by a tick or exhibit the telltale rash.

In addition to Lyme, there are co-infections, such as *Bartonella, Babesia, Ehrlichia,* and Rocky Mountain spotted fever, among others. And the testing isn't always reliable, especially if it's been a while since you were infected. These stealth infections can lie dormant for years, subdued by your immune system, until a major stressor suppresses your immunity enough for them to become active and cause brain-related symptoms.

Parasitic infections can also mimic Alzheimer's dementia. Because of the gut-brain connection, anything that affects your gut also affects your brain. The gut makes and uses 90 percent of your body's neurotransmitters, giving the brain the first 10 percent. When a parasite invades, whether it travels to the brain or not, it can be a drain on your neurotransmitters, resulting in confusion and memory loss to such an extent that the wrong diagnosis is made.

THE BASICS OF BUILDING A BETTER BRAIN

We all want to stay mentally sharp and it's scary for anyone of any age to notice a mental decline. But the earlier you address your memory issues and begin repair, the better your chances for recovery and long-term brain health. This is one reason why I recommend starting with neuropsychological testing, done by a qualified professional.

This testing is well researched, with up to 95 percent accuracy for pinpointing any areas of concern in your mental health and memory. What's important is that it gives you a benchmark to know whether the steps you begin taking to restore your memory are actually effective. Neuropsychological testing provides an objective point of view of what's really going on and what needs work.

The next step after testing is to take a good look at your diet. Many people with declining memory and Alzheimer's disease are described by their friends and family as "sugar addicts." Sugar is necessary for brain function but is not the preferred fuel for the brain. That preferred fuel is fat. The metabolism of glucose in the brain is essential for memory formation and cognitive function, and when the brain becomes insulin resistant from too much sugar in the diet, it leads to diseases associated with memory loss, including Alzheimer's.

IS ALZHEIMER'S DISEASE TYPE 3 DIABETES?

The typical American eating habits have trained our body to be sugar burners for fuel, needing to eat something every two to four hours, due to changes in our energy level. When you eat a meal or snack high in sugar and refined carbs, your blood sugar spikes quickly. This stimulates the release of insulin, which is good because it escorts that sugar out of the blood and into the cells, where it can be burned for fuel. But high insulin causes the sugar to be taken into the cells more quickly, which causes hypoglycemia, or a sugar low. Low blood sugar causes you to crave sugar; it's a protective mechanism so your sugar doesn't go life-threateningly low.

This is the number one reason you crave sugar. Back in mankind's hunter-gatherer time, this was good because available carbs were healthy. They didn't have the concession stand at the ball game or the racks of candy bars and coolers of soda at the gas station to tempt them into something quick and high in sugar until they could get a real meal.

Just as your body becomes insulin resistant in these conditions, your brain stops responding to insulin as well. It is essential that your brain responds to insulin for such basic tasks as memory and learning. Type 3 diabetes develops when the neurons in your brain become deficient in insulin because they are unable to utilize it in any way. And if you carry the Alzheimer's APOE4 gene, your risk for type 3 diabetes is increased.

According to a study done by Guojun Bu and Mary Lowell Leary at the Mayo Clinic, the APOE4 protein that is produced by the gene can more aggressively bind the insulin receptors on the surfaces of the neurons than does its healthy counterpart, APOE3. Once it outcompetes APOE3, it goes on to do further damage to brain cells by clumping together and becoming toxic. These sticky clumps get inside the neuron and block the insulin receptors from receiving insulin. The end result is starving brain cells, memory loss, and impaired cognition.

The key to getting off this dangerous blood sugar roller-coaster ride and preventing type 3 diabetes is found in protein, healthy fats, and fiber. Each of these slows gastric emptying, which slows the speed of sugar in the diet turning into sugar in the blood.

Start your day by stabilizing your blood sugar with a healthy meal involving protein, healthy fats, and fiber, and you get a slow, steady release of sugar over time instead of a spike, so the highs and lows never come. Protein and fat keep you feeling full and more satisfied for a longer period of time and burning fat for energy retrains your body to have a steadier energy level, allowing you to go up to six hours between meals. This is because 1 g of fat equals 9 calories, and 1 g of carbs or protein equals 4 calories. So, when you burn fat as your primary source of fuel, you can eat less and have a more consistent energy level. Your body stores about 2,000 calories in muscle and the liver, but it can store somewhere between 100,000 and 120,000 calories in your body fat. So, when you burn fat as your primary fuel instead of carbs, you have much more to draw from before you need to refuel.

There are added brain benefits to burning fats as your primary fuel. Ketones are produced when your body breaks down fat for energy. Your brain loves ketones, and increasing their levels can help with brain fog, memory issues, focus, and other cognition, as well as balance and coordination. Because fat burns cleaner than sugar and carbs do for energy, there is also less oxidative stress on the body. This helps decrease cellular inflammation, AGE formation, and other signs of premature aging. Ketosis also helps your cells become more sensitive to hormones, bringing them into balance much more easily and reducing the need for hormone replacement.

THE THIAMINE CONNECTION

Startling new research reports that low blood sugar levels in the brain correspond to low vitamin B_1 (thiamine) tissue levels, and can spark Alzheimer's disease. Your pancreas is a rich storage site for thiamine. Thiamine not only lowers the high blood sugars that lead to insulin resistance in the brain but also raises the low blood sugars inside your brain cells that lead to memory loss. The key to better brain health and balanced blood sugar comes in being proactive and supplementing with benfotiamine, a fat-soluble form of thiamine, before Alzheimer's has time to take hold.

Not only does vitamin B_1 control blood sugar levels, it delivers oxygen to the brain. Although the brain compromises only 2 percent of the body's total weight, it uses 20 percent of the body's oxygen. Proper levels of bioavailable vitamin B_1 that can cross the blood-brain barrier are crucial for vibrant brain health and staving off Alzheimer's disease.

SLEEPLESS NIGHTS DRAIN YOUR BRAIN

Sleep is our primetime for repair and your brain needs sleep more than any other organ in the body. Even the loss of just two hours of sleep per night is enough to dull reflexes, decrease attention, and impair memory. Sleep promotes creativity and out-of-the-box thinking. How many times have you woken up with a great idea or new solution to a problem that's been nagging at you?

While we sleep, our brain is hard at work. Dreaming during REM sleep helps us process emotions and remain more mentally clear during the day. Sleep deprivation makes us more sensitive to anxiety and more prone to depression. Our brain is also consolidating memories into long-term storage and "pruning" the ones it doesn't need. Our lymphatic system is busy detoxing and flushing out beta-amyloid protein, which is the precursor to plaques seen in Alzheimer's disease. Aim to get seven to eight hours of quality sleep each night.

LOVE YOUR LIVER

Traditional Chinese medicine has mapped out a twenty-four-hour clock of when each organ regenerates itself. The liver's "golden hours" are between one a.m. and three a.m., and you must be asleep during that time for optimal restoration. Production of cholesterol by the liver peaks in the evening, then it transitions into detoxifying, breaking down stress hormones, such as adrenaline, and balancing blood sugar levels. Insomnia has been shown in studies to lead to nonalcoholic fatty liver disease (NAFLD), metabolic syndrome, insulin resistance, and type 2 diabetes.

Dance Your Way to Better Brain Health

Whoever likes to cut a rug on the dance floor is doing themselves a world of good. Dancing is more than just a fun time with friends—it actually improves our brain functioning in four important ways:

Dancing enhances neuroplasticity. A study published in the *New England Journal of Medicine* measured mental acuity in aging by monitoring dementia rates. The goal of the study was to discover if physical or cognitive recreational activities had an effect on mental sharpness. The only physical activity that improved mental acuity was frequent dancing, with a 76 percent reduction in dementia. Their conclusion was that dancing helps the brain rewire its neural pathways, thereby increasing neuroplasticity.

Dancing makes you smarter. Dancing is a fast-paced activity that involves quick decision-making, so it is an excellent way to maintain and enhance your intelligence. It increases your muscle memory and integrates your thoughts and responses with your physical movements, a process known as neuromuscular integration, which can align your entire fascia network.

Dancing boosts memory and helps turn back the clock on aging. You can create new neural pathways by learning new things. That way, if one pathway is lost, you have an alternative pathway to access stored information, thus preventing memory loss.

Dancing can improve your balance. If you suffer from dizziness, you'll be glad to know that dancing can be beneficial. That's because the signal going to the part of the brain responsible for the perception of dizziness is reduced.

TARGETED SOLUTIONS
Targeted Diet Solutions

Feed your brain with healthy fats. Essential and healthy fats are the preferred fuel for the brain. These include unheated coconut oil, fatty fish (think: wild-caught salmon and sardines), avocados, nuts (think: walnuts and almonds), seeds (think: hemp, chia, and flax), and their oils. Omega-3, -6, -7, and -9 essential fats boost brainpower; improve energy, memory, and moods; clear clogged arteries; improve cognitive function; aid in cellular repair; and fuel brain cells. Cold-pressed virgin coconut oil improves the body's use of insulin, increases HDL (good cholesterol), helps thyroid function, and acts like an antioxidant and natural antibiotic. Extra-virgin olive oil contains an important substance called oleocanthal that increases the production of key proteins and enzymes that break down the amyloid plaques that can result in the development of Alzheimer's disease.

Enjoy foods high in omega-3 fatty acids. These include salmon, halibut, tuna, mackerel, and sardines. Other foods include beans, nuts, flaxseeds, and perilla oil.

Think of the 3 Bs—blueberries, beets, and broccoli. When it comes to fruits and veggies for brain fuel, these foods are key. Antioxidants in blueberries decrease inflammation, and their flavonoids have been shown to improve memory. Beets are packed with folate, which helps stabilize moods and emotions, while their betaine boosts serotonin production in the brain. Broccoli is packed with antioxidants and vitamin K, which has been shown to improve your ability to comprehend and remember verbal instructions.

Avoid sugar. When the brain becomes insulin resistant from too much sugar in the diet, it leads to diseases associated with memory loss, including Alzheimer's.

Optimize your diet for better brain health. Eat lots of colorful fruits and vegetables, especially leafy greens. Include lean proteins, such as organic poultry, grass-fed beef, and wild-caught seafood. Enjoy berries and dark-colored fruits that are high in antioxidants, especially polyphenols; these include blueberries, blackberries, strawberries, raspberries, plums, oranges, red grapes, and cherries. Follow the food lists on pages 112–115 and incorporate them into your favorite recipes.

Drink your morning coffee and eat dark chocolate for a treat. These both contain important brain-healing antioxidants that may help stave off age-related memory decline. Always be sure to select an organic, nontoxic, mold-free coffee, such as my preferred brand, Purity Coffee (see Resources). Opt for dark chocolate that contains a minimum of 60 percent cacao content and keep servings to one or two squares per day. Avoid milk chocolate.

Change the way you cook, to reduce AGE accumulation in your brain. Choose smart cooking methods, such as stewing, braising, poaching, and steaming, as we learned in Rule #3, Stop AGEs.

TARGETED HERBAL AND NUTRIENT SOLUTIONS

Consider taking lithium orotate. Low-dose lithium has been proven in clinical studies to decrease the onset and progression of dementia and Alzheimer's disease by inhibiting the growth of plaques and amyloid deposits in the brain that can lead to cognitive decline. Because subtle symptoms of Alzheimer's can occur forty years before the actual diagnosis, low-dose lithium started early is a key intervention solution to help prevent cognitive decline. A recommended dose is 20 to 80 mg daily, staggered throughout the day.

Preserve brain health with benfotiamine. Benfotiamine is a fat-soluble form of thiamine. It helps preserve brain and nerve health by protecting the tissues from the effects of oxidative stress. Aim for 300 mg daily.

Slow down brain deterioration with phosphatidylserine. Phosphatidylserine helps keep cell membranes supple. This helps brain cell communication for improved thinking skills and memory. Aim for 300 mg daily.

Turn back time with astragalus. Its neuroprotective properties can significantly improve memory and learning. The recommended dose for enhanced brain function is 2 to 6 g of the powdered root daily.

Green tea extract protects brain cells from oxidative stress. This can help reduce brain damage that could lead to mental decline and such brain diseases as dementia, Parkinson's, and Alzheimer's. Aim for 180 mg daily.

Ginkgo biloba extract helps prevent age-related memory loss. It supports overall mental function by enhancing the delivery of nutrients and oxygen directly to the brain. Aim for 120 mg daily.

Vinpocetine enables the neurotransmitters in your brain to function more efficiently. Vinpocetine helps transport oxygen to the brain by improving blood circulation, helping reduce "brain fatigue." It also enables the neurotransmitters in your brain to function by promoting optimal glucose utilization. Aim for 21 mg daily.

Huperzine A supports memory and concentration. Acetylcholine is one of the most abundant neurotransmitters in the brain. An alkaloid compound that supports an increase in acetylcholine, Huperzine A enhances learning and concentration and protects against age-related memory problems. Aim for 60 mg daily.

Try Ultra H-3 Plus. Ultra H-3 Plus contains all of the top brain-building nutrients, including green tea extract, huperzine A, phosphatidylserine complex with organic soy fiber, Benfotiamine, and ginkgo biloba. Take one capsule three times daily, between meals, or as directed by your health-care professional (see Resources).

OTHER IMPORTANT BRAIN NUTRIENTS

Acetyl-L-carnitine boosts mood, learning, and memory. Some studies show that it slows mental decline in Alzheimer's patients. A recommended dosage is 2,000 mg or less per day.

Resveratrol can slow or even stop the progression of Alzheimer's. A dose of 10 to 100 mg per day is needed to be effective.

EGCG and vitamin C are an unbeatable combination. EGCG, a powerful catechin extracted from green tea, helps protect telomeres while preventing and repairing cell damage throughout your whole body. Vitamin C also slows down the loss of telomere length. I recommend 250 to 500 mg of EGCG daily with vitamin C taken to bowel tolerance (the highest dose that doesn't give digestive discomfort or loose stools). Aim for up to 10 g daily.

MEDICATION SOLUTIONS

Address medication side effects. Check with your health-care practitioner and learn about the meds you are taking—both prescribed and over the counter. In the case of prescription meds, it is important you taper off these medications properly. Quitting them "cold turkey" or tapering too quickly can cause new or worsening of the same symptoms you are trying to improve.

PARASITE SOLUTIONS

Get tested for parasites. Don't assume that because you live in the United States, you are not at risk of contracting parasites. Often, when your symptoms cannot be explained any other way, parasites are eventually discovered to be a root cause (see Resources for recommended parasite testing).

Get tested for Lyme disease. Although it can be difficult to diagnose, you'll want to find a health-care practitioner skilled in dealing with Lyme.

TARGETED LIFESTYLE SOLUTIONS

Get your blood flowing. Just thirty minutes of daily exercise increases your heart rate and gets your blood flowing, which pumps more oxygen and delivers more nutrients to your brain cells. Any activity that increases your heart rate helps your brain, from strength training and weight lifting to swimming and brisk walking or even dancing. Choose the exercise that fits your lifestyle and interests the best. Avoid exercise in the evening hours. Refer to Chapter 13 for simple yet optimum exercise tips.

Make your bedroom a comfortable sleep space. The first key to getting a good night's sleep is setting the stage for slumber in your bedroom: low light, no screens, and no electronics within 3 feet of your comfortable bed. Avoid scrolling through social media or leaving the TV on.

Stay cool. A cooler temperature when you turn out the lights will get you off to a great start. The National Sleep Foundation recommends nighttime bedroom temps between 60° and 67°F.

Avoid stimulants after three p.m. Stimulants, such as caffeine and B vitamins, should be avoided after three p.m., or earlier if you're more sensitive to their effects. Your stress hormones need calming influences in the evening hours to bring them down so you can fall asleep easily.

Mellow out with melatonin. Supplementing with at least 3 mg before bedtime can lead not only to a better night's sleep but also to lower blood pressure, better digestion, and better stress tolerance over time.

ProgestaKey can soothe your hormones and help you sleep. If sleep still eludes you, and you know you're in hormone havoc, then consider applying my specially formulated ProgestaKey at bedtime for natural hormone support. If you're unsure about your existing hormone levels, consider saliva hormone testing to determine them (see Resources).

Rewire your brain with the Dynamic Neural Retraining System. This unique system is a natural, drug-free, neuroplasticity-based healing program. It works by rewiring the limbic system to build more functional neural pathways (see Resources for more information).

Hopefully, you have learned to reawaken your brain and make worrisome memory problems a thing of the past. Now that you're learning how to power through each day with a surge of "young again" energy, let's move on to recharge your heart.

CHAPTER 12

RECHARGE YOUR HEART

> ## In this chapter, you'll learn . . .
>
> - The real truth about cholesterol
> - About overlooked heart markers your doctor may not be assessing
> - How women's heart disease is often misinterpreted
> - How heartbreak is connected to heart disease

FOR OVER FIVE DECADES, WE HAVE BEEN BOMBARDED WITH NUTRITIONAL INFORMAtion and dietary mandates that should have American hearts beating to a healthy rhythm. As a nation, we're eating less trans fat, smoking fewer cigarettes, and trying to exercise more. So it's surprising (or is it?) that heart disease is still the number one cause of death in America. By 2030, it is expected that nearly *25 million* people will die from some type of cardiovascular disease. According to the National Institutes of Health, adults age sixty-five and older account for 80 percent of all deaths attributable to cardiovascular disease.

As I pointed out in Rule #6, Mind Your Minerals, excess stored iron may be one of the most overlooked, common causes of coronary disease that nobody is talking about. Iron is a highly reactive agent, creating big-time oxidative stress that damages the walls of the arteries and causes major inflammation. When excess iron is stored in heart tissue, it contributes to heart muscle damage. Some researchers believe that when the ferritin iron is released from its protein, free radicals are formed that oxidize cholesterol. Oxidized cholesterol clings to artery walls, forming plaques that can block the artery, leading to heart attack and stroke.

People with normal iron metabolism may absorb no more than the amount of iron needed daily, whereas those with hereditary hemochromatosis (HH) absorb it excessively to toxic levels. In the past, HH was thought to be extremely rare, but it is now proving to be quite prevalent, especially among Caucasians. Once HH is diagnosed, it is important that family members be tested, since it can be passed on genetically. Prognosis for HH is good, especially if it is detected early before organ damage results. For this reason, blood profiles are recommended for those men and women showing symptoms that may indicate HH.

Likewise, as you learned in Rule #3 (Stop AGEs), AGEs are a huge cause of heart and blood vessel disease. This is due to an ongoing *inflammatory response* in the vascular system that leads to oxidation, blood clots, calcification, and hypertension—all manageable when you pay attention to what you eat and how you heat your foods (especially protein and fats).

And as we learned in Rule #2 (Take On Toxic Overload), heavy metals and pollutants have a link to an astounding array of aging-related disorders. Lead toxicity is associated with cardiovascular dysfunction, arteriosclerosis, and atherosclerosis; aluminum toxicity can paralyze the heart; mercury can damage the heart as well as other organs; and cadmium toxicity gives rise to hypertension.

This chapter focuses on heart and cardiovascular health, helping you take on the major risk factors for heart disease and fortifying your strong, beating heart for a long lifetime. You'll understand the roles of cholesterol, sugar, insulin, drugs, environmental toxins, homocysteine, and iron overload and the role each play in aging heart health.

UNDERSTANDING YOUR RISK FACTORS

Amazingly, at least 250 factors for heart disease have been identified. Heart health is greatly influenced by epigenetic lifestyle changes and you can begin making changes immediately.

CHOLESTEROL—FACT AND FICTION

Most of us are aware of the connection between cholesterol and heart disease. We know that cholesterol is carried through the bloodstream in two forms: high-density lipoprotein (HDL) and low-density lipoprotein (LDL). The HDL is considered the "good" cholesterol; LDL, the "bad." An excess of "sticky" and oxidized LDL increases our risk of heart attacks and strokes, whereas high levels of HDL protect us. In both men and women, LDL levels should be below 90 mg/dl and optimum HDL levels should be greater than 50 mg/dl. More important than just these single levels, the ratio of total cholesterol to HDL should be below 4:1.

Cholesterol is found naturally in every cell in our body, and each cell also contains enzymes used for cholesterol production. Our brain and spinal cord have about 35 percent of our body's store of cholesterol. It's also found in the skin, bone marrow, and adrenal glands. Cholesterol is essential to good health, and deficiencies have been associated with anemia, acute infection, and excess thyroid function. In our diet, cholesterol is the waxy, fatlike substance found only in products of animal origin, such as beef, poultry, and eggs.

There's no denying that a relationship exists between high dietary cholesterol levels and high levels in the blood, but it's not as straightforward as we were led to believe. How do we explain patients whose blood cholesterol levels are no lower after eating a very low-fat diet? How do we explain a much lower rate of second heart attacks in patients on a typical high-cholesterol diet over patients on a restricted diet?

What the research seems to suggest is the amount of cholesterol in one's blood is related to heart disease, whereas the amount of cholesterol in one's diet is not. What does lead to high blood cholesterol is the lack of other nutrients, such as chromium, magnesium, vitamin B_3, and omega-3 essential fatty acids, which help metabolize cholesterol. Cholesterol also accumulates in arteries only after the arterial wall has been damaged. In fact, approximately 50 percent of Americans who have heart attacks have levels of total cholesterol that are considered normal or only moderately elevated. A US study has shown that nearly 75 percent of patients hospitalized for heart attacks had normal cholesterol levels, which did *not* indicate that they were at high risk for a cardiovascular event.

Almost 75 percent of heart attack patients fell within recommended targets for "bad" LDL cholesterol, according to Dr. Gregg C. Fonarow, professor of cardiovascular medicine and science at UCLA. Researchers also found that more than half of patients hospitalized for heart attacks had *low* levels of "good" HDL cholesterol levels.

Groundbreaking but buried research published over forty years ago in the *American Journal of Nutrition* suggests that pure, fresh cholesterol does not damage arteries, but oxygenated cholesterol does. Cholesterol that has been exposed to oxygen produces toxic substances that decompose into free radicals, a term that has become synonymous with cell and tissue destruction. Free radicals are present in cholesterol that has oxidized as a result of exposure to air, high temperatures, free radical initiators, light, or a combination of these factors. They are unstable and highly reactive oxygen molecules with unpaired electrons, and they search for and steal electrons from other molecules, causing a chemical reaction that creates even more free radicals. It is free radicals that cause damage to our blood vessel walls.

Reexamination of cholesterol studies have found that the cholesterol used was not in the form in which it occurs naturally in food, but as heat-dried egg yolk powder made up in batches to last many days or weeks. This altered cholesterol, because of its exposure to oxygen, formed free radicals.

Oxidized cholesterol can be highly plaque-producing. The processing, packaging, storing, and preparing of foods have a profound effect on oxidation. Animal foods cause problems when they have been exposed to the ravages of oxygen for extended periods of time. For example, improperly stored eggs, milk, or butter that is exposed to room temperature for too long or not kept in tightly sealed containers.

Again, I'm not saying that a diet high in fats and cholesterol is not related to heart disease, but the relationship is different from what we have been led to believe. Fats and cholesterol don't just clog up arteries. They can be a major source of free radicals, which oxidize cells and set off a chain reaction, creating more and more free radicals. To make matters worse, the cholesterol manufactured by our body to fight against the damage done by free radicals is converted into its oxidized form, leading to more free radicals.

So, how do we stop this chain reaction? We need to prevent the oxidation of cholesterol. By avoiding foods that contain oxidized cholesterol and damaged fats and increasing your intake of foods rich in antioxidant vitamins, minerals, and essential fatty acids (EFAs), you can decrease your risk of heart disease. More and more research show that heart disease is related to deficiencies of these nutrients, including vitamins A, C, and E and the minerals selenium, chromium, zinc, and magnesium.

HDL—IS IT REALLY THE "GOOD" CHOLESTEROL?

HDL cholesterol has two important functions that have given it a good reputation. First, it goes through your bloodstream and removes the more dense and "sticky" LDL cholesterol that can clog your arteries. Second, it travels through the blood vessels, constantly repairing the inner lining. This is the cholesterol you want sent to repair injuries to your inflamed arteries.

Normal HDL blood levels are 40 to 90 mg/dl in adults. When this cholesterol is in the normal range, there is plenty available to do these essential jobs. But when your levels are low, which is common with diets that are low in healthy fats and high in sugars, there isn't enough of this cholesterol to go around and LDL cholesterol is sent in its place. Conversely, when HDL cholesterol is too high, it's a sign your liver is congested and having trouble processing cholesterol and may even indicate inflammation.

LDL CHOLESTEROL—THE GOOD,
THE BAD, AND THE UGLY

Many doctors still stand by the myth that all LDL cholesterol is "bad" and should be lowered with dangerous statin drugs. In truth, LDL cholesterol is a transport molecule that's important, not just for your overall health, but especially for the health of your immune system and brain. Current guidelines for "normal" cholesterol levels have dropped so low they are in the range for thalassemia, genetic blood disorders known to enhance consumption of cholesterol and reduce it to dangerous, symptom-producing levels. Normal levels of LDL cholesterol should be <90 mg/dl.

LDL-A is the "good" form of LDL cholesterol. These large, fluffy particles are harmless and contribute the most to overall health. LDL-B is the "bad" form, made up of small, dense particles that contribute to inflammation and plaque formation. The "ugly" form of LDL cholesterol and by far the worst is Lp(a). Most doctors don't test for this fraction—and they should. You can ask your health-care practitioner to include this on your next blood draw. If you are in good overall health, this particle will actually help you repair your damaged cells, but in a body that already has high levels of inflammation, they will build up and accumulate in the injured arteries, causing not only plaque but also blood clots.

TRIGLYCERIDES

Your liver makes triglycerides from refined sugars, and you get additional triglycerides from the fats and oils you eat. In your bloodstream, sticky triglyceride particles act like glue, causing red blood cells to clump and stick together. Your small capillaries become blocked, leading to oxygen starvation of the tissues and organs served by these capillaries. Triglycerides are also the form in which the body stores fat in the connective tissue. The roll above many a middle-aged stomach is actually caused by excess triglycerides.

What we eat and the way we live affect our triglyceride levels. The low-fat, higher-carb diet encouraged by the American Heart Association, the USDA, and others actually raises triglyceride levels and lowers HDL levels in up to one-third of Americans. White sugar, white flour, and such products as white bread, cakes, cookies, candies, soda, and alcohol all increase our triglycerides. Even too much fruit and natural, unsweetened fruit juice can elevate levels.

Not only what we eat, but the way we eat affects our triglyceride levels. If you skip breakfast and/or lunch and make up for it with a heavy evening meal (sound familiar?), you boost your blood triglycerides. Eating a large meal late in the day causes your body to store unused triglycerides in fatty tissue; skipping breakfast the next day results in those triglycerides flooding out of the fatty tissue and sludging up your bloodstream. Our body was designed to be fueled at regular intervals with good, balanced food. If we're not eating regularly, we're damaging our body.

Other behaviors that contribute to high triglyceride levels include lack of physical activity, reaction to emotional stress, and nicotine, certain drugs such as diuretics and birth control pills, and some hormones, including estrogen. Both triglyceride and cholesterol levels increase naturally with age, so have them checked every couple of years as a routine part of your health care. High triglyceride levels are known to increase one's susceptibility to heart disease even when cholesterol levels are normal.

While many experts say that triglyceride levels above 150 mg/dl are cause for concern, I believe you need to monitor levels above 90 closely. More important than your triglyceride level is the ratio between triglycerides and HDL cholesterol. Studies done even in children show when this ratio is elevated, there is a *sixteen times* greater risk of heart disease than those with a lower ratio. Higher ratios are an indicator of stiff, injured arteries. Ideally, you want a <2:1 ratio of triglycerides to HDL.

Women's Heart Attack Symptoms Differ from Men's

A woman's symptoms are much more subtle, often starting weeks or even months before an attack. Women may describe "not feeling quite right," with such symptoms as shortness of breath, unusual weakness or fatigue, sleep disturbances, chest discomfort that may come and go quickly, vision problems, anxiety, and indigestion. The vagueness of these symptoms leads women to ignore them, delaying treatment. When these women do seek treatment, their doctor may misdiagnose their condition.

Heart disease itself develops differently in women. According to researchers at the University of Michigan Cardiovascular Center, significant blockages tend to occur not in major arteries but in smaller, less flexible blood vessels. When diagnostic coronary angiography is performed, the major vessels appear clear. Coronary angioplasty, a procedure to clear blockages, and coronary bypass surgery are both better suited to larger blood vessels.

TRANS FATS

Within the past hundred-plus years, the rate of cardiovascular disease has risen 350 percent, but the cholesterol content of the American diet has remained about the same. During the same hundred-plus years, however, both sugar and processed oil consumption have risen considerably. Hydrogenated polyunsaturated oils, including margarine, have been recommended for years in cholesterol-lowering diets, and while it is true that these oils will reduce cholesterol levels, it is also true that they accelerate arteriosclerosis and other degenerative diseases. Why? Because oils that have been commercially processed to improve shelf life, flavor, smell, and color have been damaged. In the processing, high temperatures convert the polyunsaturated fatty acids from the naturally occurring beneficial "cis" to the unnatural, harmful "trans" form. Cis fats melt at 55°F, well below the normal body temperature of 98.6°F, which makes them fully available to the system. Trans fats melt at up to 111°F, so they remain solid and therefore unmetabolized in the human body.

The process of hydrogenation, which converts liquid oils into such hardened fats as margarine and vegetable shortening, destroys natural fatty acids in even greater numbers, converting them into the biologically impaired trans form. Trans fats cannot be used by the body to produce prostaglandins, hormonelike compounds that regulate every function in the human body at the molecular level. These trans fats interfere with normal cell membrane function and structure and block the good healthy fats, such as raw natural oils that make prostaglandins, from being taken in. In addition to these trans fats, the hydrogenation process also removes the very nutrients that are essential for healthy hearts: vitamins B_6 and E, chromium, and magnesium.

C-REACTIVE PROTEIN LEVELS

C-reactive protein (CRP) may be more important than cholesterol in some individuals when it comes to identifying risk of heart disease. CRP is a natural chemical produced in the liver in response to chronic or acute inflammation. What researchers now know is that atherosclerosis is an inflammatory disease that sets off your body's immune response. Whether plaque builds up on the inside of your arteries, causing blockages, or grows into the vessel walls, causing them to bulge outward, the immune response sends thousands of special cells to attack the plaque. At the same time, your liver produces CRP to help rid your body of the plaque. Unfortunately, this process destabilizes the plaque, which can break apart and cause blood clots that can lead to heart attack or stroke.

How do you know whether the inflammation you have is the type to cause heart disease? The answer lies in a specific measurement of C-reactive protein in your blood, called the cardio CRP or hs-CRP test. This is an early marker of inflammation that is specific to cardiovascular disease. Studies show this test is an accurate predictor of heart disease, whether it runs in your family or you have no history of it at all.

The laboratory normal range for this test is 0 to 3 mg/dl. The optimal range is much narrower and is different for men and women. For women, you want less than 1.5 mg/dl, and for men, it should be less than 0.55 mg/dl. This test won't be accurate if you have high levels of other types of inflammation, such as uncontrolled autoimmune disease or an active acute illness, for instance, influenza.

HOMOCYSTEINE LEVELS

Homocysteine, an amino acid, levels as indicators of heart disease risk are still being studied. Over fifty years ago, Kilmer McCully, MD, proposed homocysteine as a factor in blood vessel damage and heart disease, but it took many years for substantial research to overcome medical skepticism. Researchers are still trying to identify the exact role of homocysteine in not only heart disease but also rheumatoid arthritis, diabetes, and possibly osteoporosis.

Here's what we know: Methionine is an amino acid present in red meat, poultry, legumes, eggs, avocado, and grains, which helps prevent cholesterol from clogging your arteries. During methionine metabolism, homocysteine forms. Under ideal circumstances, the homocysteine is broken down into other chemicals and used or eventually excreted. If conditions are less than ideal, however, blood homocysteine levels rise, damaging cell membranes, destabilizing collagen, and paving the way for cholesterol to form plaques. Among the factors known to increase homocysteine levels are

→ Deficiencies in vitamins B_6, B_9 (folate), and B_{12}
→ Smoking
→ Excessive coffee consumption (8 cups a day or more)
→ Taking anticonvulsant, antibacterial, diuretic, and some chemotherapy medications
→ Having kidney failure or hypothyroidism

MTHFR, a defect present in as high as 30 to 50 percent of the population, leads to high homocysteine levels. If you have high blood pressure and high homocysteine levels, you have twenty-five times the risk of having a heart attack or stroke than those with normal readings of both. Follow the Radical Longevity approach to heart disease to be sure you're getting the nutrients you need. Talk with your doctor about evaluating your homocysteine levels with blood tests currently available.

HIGH BLOOD PRESSURE

The causes of high blood pressure, called hypertension, are now known, including everything from renal disease to electrolyte imbalance to thyroid disease. In cases of hypertension, the repetitive excess force of the blood eventually weakens the artery walls, allowing LDL cholesterol and excess calcium, along with rogue toxins, to form deposits that eventually block the arteries. According to the Centers for Disease Control and Prevention (CDC), one in every three American adults has the condition, though most are unaware of it because it usually produces no physical symptoms. Routine blood pressure checks are helpful in detecting potential hypertension.

Many studies have shown a direct relationship between high salt intake and hypertension, as sodium causes fluid retention, which adds stress to the circulatory system. But salt has only been shown to raise blood pressure in 10 percent of cases, and the all-important trace minerals in such products as Real Salt, sea salt, or pink Himalayan salt can actually *lower* blood pressure in many cases. The natural salts typically consist of trace minerals, such as potassium, magnesium, and calcium.

MAGNESIUM DEFICIENCY

Magnesium is the most important mineral for the heart, and deficiencies can result in irregular and rapid heartbeat, high blood pressure, and sudden death. Magnesium deficiency may also be the cause of idiopathic mitral valve prolapse, a heart valve disorder whose symptoms include palpitations, chest pain, fatigue, panic attacks, and hyperventilation. Low levels of both blood and cellular magnesium have been reported in individuals with high blood pressure and hypertension, and biopsies reveal that individuals who die from a heart attack have lower magnesium levels in their heart muscle than do those who died of other causes. To add to the problem, many people with high blood pressure are prescribed diuretics or fluid pills to treat swelling and fluid retention; these medications actually cause both magnesium and potassium deficiencies, which can exacerbate their heart condition. Many cardiac drugs are known to induce a magnesium deficiency.

Magnesium deficiencies can actually hasten the development of atherosclerosis, also known as hardening of the arteries. If you have a calcium-magnesium imbalance, calcium doesn't become part of the bone. This unused calcium then gets dumped into the arteries and becomes part of the "hardened" artery. With the food industry pumping supplemental calcium into every possible food and beverage, many of us have excess calcium, out of balance with magnesium and other minerals, deposited in our arteries. We must bring magnesium levels back into balance with calcium to keep this excess calcium out of our blood vessels.

Instead of assessing magnesium levels and increasing this important mineral to its proper ratio with calcium, the doctors of many heart patients with potential magnesium deficiencies prescribe calcium channel blockers. A natural calcium channel blocker, magnesium dilates coronary arteries and peripheral arteries when available in sufficient levels.

Magnesium is not just essential for bone health and osteoporosis prevention; it is equally vital to muscle health and in the prevention and treatment of heart disease. Calcium helps make muscles contract, but magnesium helps them relax. In fact, hard water, which is high in magnesium and calcium content, has been linked to low rates of serious heart disease. Intravenous magnesium has been successfully used for over fifty years in the treatment of coronary spasms and heart attacks.

Sufficient magnesium also has been shown to lower total cholesterol, LDL cholesterol, and triglyceride levels while raising HDL cholesterol. Magnesium also reduces platelet aggregation, the stickiness of blood cells, which contributes to their clumping in your arteries.

INSULIN

The insulin response from a diet too high in carbohydrates also produces harmful eicosanoids (tissuelike hormones) that can lead to high blood pressure, heart attack, atherosclerosis, increased fat storage, and unstable sugar levels. Eating foods high in cholesterol does not increase blood cholesterol, but overeating carbohydrates (particularly refined carbs) can. Foods that raise insulin levels are the ones that cause obesity, high blood pressure, high cholesterol, and heart disease.

Research is showing a direct relationship between sugar and heart disease because of insulin. The more sugar you eat, the more insulin your pancreas will produce, and the higher your triglyceride levels are likely to be. Insulin resistance can cause arterial stiffness and deletes nitric oxide, which triggers oxidative stress and inflammation.

HEART MARKERS YOUR DOCTOR
MAY NOT BE ASSESSING

When you go in for your routine physical, make sure you're getting the most up-to-date blood testing done to measure the health of your heart. TIP: For greater accuracy, make sure you are well hydrated for at least a week before having any blood work done. Here are the tests I recommend; optimal ranges are listed, where applicable.

> **Ferritin.** As a measure of your iron stores, this test has a normal range that varies wildly from lab to lab, and from male to female. While the range of 15 to 300 ng/ml can be considered normal, research supports optimal levels in the range of 50 to 70 ng/ml for both men and women.

Complete blood count (CBC). Not only does this test give you an idea of your blood iron levels, it can also show when you're fighting a low-grade infection you may not be aware of.

Comprehensive metabolic panel (CMP). This test is comprehensive, and abnormal results can be used to signal the need for more testing. The optimal range for a fasting glucose level is 82 to 88 mg/dl, as compared to the laboratory normal range of 70 to 100 mg/dl.

Fasting insulin. Insulin resistance causes heart disease by triggering inflammation in your arteries. The laboratory normal range is 2.5 to 25 mg/dl, but the true optimal range is <5 mg/dl.

Cardio-CRP. This is a high-sensitivity measure of C-reactive protein, which is a marker for inflammation. More than thirty studies have shown a direct correlation between high cardio-CRP levels and future heart attacks. The lab's normal range is 0 to 3 mg/dl for both men and women. However, the optimal ranges are <0.8 mg/dl.

Homocysteine. This test is a marker for inflammation and heart disease. The optimal range is 7 to 10 umol/l.

Fibrinogen. This protein regulates clots and gauges viscosity and stickiness of blood. A level over 350 mg/dl is a major risk factor for heart disease.

Lipoprotein (a). Lipoprotein (a), abbreviated as Lp(a), is believed to play a role in the mechanism of plaque rupture, the initiating event of a heart attack. If your other risk factors are normal, but your Lp(a) level is high, your risk for heart disease is greater.

SMOKING

Let's face facts that you already know: If you smoke, your chances of dying from heart disease are almost three times greater than those of dying from lung cancer. The CDC states that the average life expectancy for smokers is at least ten years shorter than for nonsmokers. Nicotine increases plaque formation. Smoking increases LDL cholesterol while decreasing levels of HDL cholesterol. As we learned in Rule #2 (Take On Toxic Overload), cigarettes are high in cadmium, a toxic mineral that damages heart tissue, and e-cigarettes are proving to be equally as harmful.

OBESITY

This may not be news to most of us, but it still bears repeating. As published in the July 23, 2018, cover story of *Cardiology Magazine*, "an increase in body fat can directly contribute to heart disease through atrial enlargement, ventricular enlargement, and atherosclerosis."

Weight appears to be a more significant risk factor for women than it is for men. A study by Harvard researcher JoAnn Manson, MD, found that in obese women, seven in ten cases of heart disease resulted from their excess weight. Even women who are the high end of their "normal" range seem to have an increased risk. To compound the problem, overweight women tend to be sedentary; they are also more likely to develop hypertension, high LDL cholesterol and triglycerides, and type 2 diabetes, all of which increase the likelihood of heart disease.

How the weight is distributed on your body also seems to have an impact. Men or women with an apple body shape, with a proportionally higher amount of fat around their abdomen than elsewhere on their body, have a higher rate of heart disease, hypertension, and diabetes than their pear-shaped peers, who carry their excess fat in their hips and thighs. Scientists believe this association relates to the hormone cortisol, which causes fatty acids to be released into the bloodstream from the central fat cells. These cells are located close to your liver; the released fatty acids stress the liver, causing cholesterol, blood pressure, and insulin levels to rise.

FALSE ALERT: The Great Heart Attack Imitator

As hiatal hernias are most common in overweight men and women, do take note of this heart attack imitator. You may feel you are having a heart attack when, in fact, it is a hiatal hernia with similar symptoms. A hiatal hernia can be asymptomatic for several years or have symptoms so severe you feel you are having a heart attack. It's estimated that up to half the adult population is affected, though it is most common in overweight women over fifty years old.

A hernia happens when an organ pushes through an opening that a muscle is holding in place. In the case of a hiatal hernia, the muscle involved is the diaphragm. Normally, the esophagus and stomach join together right at the hiatus, which is an opening in the diaphragm that allows these digestive organs and the vagus nerve to pass through. When the diaphragm muscle becomes weak, a portion of the stomach protrudes up through the hiatus, resulting in a hiatal hernia.

(continues)

(continued)

Where the stomach and esophagus join together, a sphincter closes so the stomach acid doesn't wash up into the esophagus. When you have a hiatal hernia, that sphincter is mechanically forced open, allowing acid to enter the esophagus, causing acid reflux symptoms. At the same time, this displacement irritates the vagus nerve, which can cause troubling symptoms that imitate other illnesses. Because the vagus nerve travels from the brain to the heart, lungs, esophagus, stomach, small intestine, liver, gallbladder, pancreas, colon, kidneys, bladder, and external genitals, once a hiatal hernia irritates it, the effects can be seen downstream in any of these organs and their functions. Symptoms can include chest pain, heartburn, acid reflux, bloating after meals, nausea or vomiting, excessive belching and gas, frequent hiccups, TMJ disorder, shallow breathing and difficulty taking a deep breath, asthma, and decreased stomach acid.

One way to tell if you might have this condition is to place the fingers of one hand on your solar plexus, located just below your breastbone. Take a deep abdominal breath in. What you should feel is the solar plexus expanding and moving your fingers outward. If you have to lift your chest and shoulders to get a deep breath in, you may have a hiatal hernia. If you see minimal movement of your fingers or no movement at all, then your breathing is shallow and may be a sign of a hiatal hernia.

A SEDENTARY LIFESTYLE

All our muscles, including our heart, need exercise. Exercise helps lower LDL cholesterol and raise HDL. Regular aerobic exercise, such as walking, running, jumping rope, and dancing, reduces the risk of heart disease by about 30 percent in postmenopausal women. It also influences several other risk factors. People who exercise regularly have a 35 percent lower risk of hypertension, as well as a lower risk of diabetes. Exercise stimulates the production of serotonin, endorphins, and other brain chemicals that reduce anxiety and stress and create a balanced sleep-wake cycle, helping to control cortisol levels. When you exercise, you also aid calcium metabolism, triggering the calcification process within your bones so excess calcium does not build up in your blood vessels.

HOW HEARTBREAK IS CONNECTED TO HEART DISEASE

An unexpected emotional hidden risk factor is related to heart disease: heartbreak. The startling truth is that you are at a heightened risk of a heart attack in the twenty-four hours following the death of a loved one.

As mentioned in Chapter 7, Takotsubo cardiomyopathy, "broken heart syndrome," is a condition in which extreme emotional or physical distress temporarily causes the left ventricle in the heart to balloon and mimics the symptoms of a heart attack. It is interesting to note that Takotsubo cardiomyopathy typically affects more women than men: more than 90 percent of reported cases concern women aged fifty-eight to seventy-five.

Grief is highly individualized and healthy grieving takes work. Although the initial stages of grieving can feel overwhelming, just as we must begin to address any needed change in life, we all can learn how to experience grief in a healthy way. This is not a time for retreat. In the initial stages of grief, you need the love, care, and support of others. Long term, you may need to step out of your comfort zone and even find new interests, adventures, and activities. It is important to approach grieving as a process rather than a fixed state. And know that you can deeply miss someone to the point of heartbreak, but that your life must go on.

TARGETED SOLUTIONS
Targeted Dietary Solutions

Enjoy anti-inflammatory heart-healthy fats. As we learned in Rule #5 (Activate Cellular Rejuvenation), oils provide essential fatty acids (EFAs) that support the cell membrane and assist in the transport of calcium into the soft tissues. Enjoy unheated hemp seed oil, safflower oil, sesame oil, and pine nut oil, as well as other oils, such as flaxseed, macadamia nut, coconut, MCT, and olive oil, in no-heat recipes or drizzled onto veggies and starches after cooking, to avoid AGEs. Avoid unnatural fats—such as margarine, vegetable shortening, and processed and hydrogenated vegetable oils—due to their trans fat content.

Adopt an anti-inflammatory AGE-less diet. Foods rich in the antioxidant nutrients—vitamins A, C, and E, beta-carotene, and selenium—are a *must* for healthy hearts. Fresh fruits, leafy green vegetables, freshly squeezed vegetable juices, sea vegetables, garlic, and onions are good sources of these important nutrients.

Make phytonutrient-rich foods a priority. Cranberries are a particularly rich source of phytonutrients that act as antioxidants, blocking the absorption of fat and lowering LDL cholesterol and triglycerides while raising HDL cholesterol. Maintain sufficient levels of vitamin D to lessen your risk of inflammation by including sardines, tuna, sweet potatoes and yams, alfalfa, and egg yolks in your diet; get plenty of sunshine and consider taking 2,000 to 5,000 IU of vitamin D as a supplement daily.

Lower your sodium intake. Avoid foods high in sodium to help prevent high blood pressure and stroke. Start by removing most processed foods from your diet. This means limiting or eliminating most canned, pickled, smoked, instant, and snack foods. Avoid anything that includes the term *sodium* in its ingredients list, such as monosodium glutamate and sodium benzoate.

Mind your Bs. To control your homocysteine levels, be sure to get enough vitamins B_6, B_9 (folate), and B_{12}. Among the best food sources for vitamin B_6 are bananas, carrots, onions, asparagus, peas, sunflower seeds, and walnuts. The best food sources of vitamin B_9 are green leafy vegetables, fortified yeast flakes, blue-green algae, salmon, cheese, brown rice, beef, beans, and barley. Foods high in vitamin B_{12} include liver (beef and chicken), oysters, sardines, cheese, eggs, trout, salmon, and tuna. If you are vegetarian, you will have difficulty getting adequate vitamin B_{12} from your diet and may need to supplement. Because many people over age fifty have inadequate levels of hydrochloric acid—needed to utilize vitamins B_{12}, magnesium, and other nutrients—consider taking a hydrochloric acid supplement, especially if you have symptoms of gastric distress after eating. Look for one that includes pepsin.

Power up with protein. Good sources of protein include poultry, fish, beef, lamb, eggs, and legumes. Avoid most cheeses with the exception of naturally lower-fat, unaged varieties, as the processing and natural aging used in making certain cheeses can contribute heavily to their AGE content. (Please refer to Chapter 3 for proper cooking methods of these proteins.)

Fiber is important too. Fiber—particularly the soluble fiber found in flaxseeds, fruits, and vegetables—helps lower cholesterol levels and assists in eliminating toxins and carcinogens from the digestive tract.

LIFESTYLE SOLUTIONS

Quit smoking. Smoking is one of the most famous risk factors for heart disease, stiffening arterial walls and making them more prone to injury while also decreasing HDL cholesterol levels. Breaking the addiction is challenging, but there are many innovative techniques available to help, from acupuncture to hypnotherapy. Make the commitment and follow up with action.

Drop the weight. If you're overweight, losing weight is a powerful tool in the fight against heart disease. My national best seller *Radical Metabolism* will not only help you lose weight and feel great but also eliminates processed foods, high sugar foods, and trans fats—the "triple threat" of inflammatory foods that lead to unhealthy cholesterol levels.

Exercise daily. The best way to raise a low HDL cholesterol level (and lower triglycerides) is through regular aerobic exercise for at least thirty minutes each day. You'll find great ideas for exercising in Chapter 13.

BLOOD TEST SOLUTIONS

Know which tests to take and what the optimal levels are. Make sure your cholesterol panel includes the Lp(a) test. If the panel doesn't calculate your triglyceride/HDL ratio, it's important you do that yourself (the optimal triglycerides: HDL ratio is lower than 2:1).

Here are the optimally healthy ranges according to functional medicine standards. I strongly encourage you to follow up with your own enlightened cardiologist.

- → Total cholesterol: 180–240 mg/dl
- → Total HDL: 40–90 mg/dl for women; 35–90 mg/dl for men
- → HDL cholesterol subtypes: >25 mg/dl HDL2; >15 mg/dl HDL3
- → Total LDL: 80–130 mg/dl
- → Lp(a): <30 mg/dl
- → Triglycerides: 50–100 mg/dl
- → Triglycerides: HDL ratio: <2:1

Inflammation Markers:
- → Cardio-CRP: <0.8 mg/dl
- → Ferritin: 50 to 70 ng/ml

TARGETED CHOLESTEROL SOLUTIONS

Increase your fiber intake. Fiber (ground flaxseeds, oat bran, and psyllium husks) can help lower LDL levels and increase intake of antioxidants. Flaxseed oil is a buttery, nutty-tasting oil that makes a good butter substitute. It can be drizzled over steamed vegetables, cooked cereals, air-popped popcorn, or as a salad dressing for a rich, satisfying flavor. Flaxseed oil should *not* be used for cooking, as heat destroys its value.

Chromium and vitamin C can help lower cholesterol safely. Both chromium and vitamin C have been shown to lower plasma cholesterol while increasing HDL levels.

TARGETED TRIGLYCERIDE SOLUTIONS

Increase your omega-3s. Make sure that you are taking at least 2 to 4 g of omega-3 essential fatty acids. I handpicked UNI KEY's Super-EPA for the purest daily heart smart protection. Super-EPA contains molecularly distilled fish oil free from PCBs, dioxin, and heavy metals.

Supplement with chromium. This essential trace mineral has been proven to lower triglycerides. Aim for 400 mg daily.

TARGETED HOMOCYSTEINE SOLUTIONS

Boost Bs to lower homocysteine. If levels are elevated (high), you might consider taking 400 to 800 mcg of folate, 100 mg of pyridoxal-5-phosphate vitamin B_6, and 500 to 1,000 mcg of methylated or hydroxylated vitamin B_{12} daily.

TARGETED NUTRIENT SOLUTIONS

Protect your heart with magnesium. I recommend magnesium and taurine as an unbeatable combination for heart health. They team up to create enzymes that contribute to heart muscle contractibility, regulate the amount of calcium moving in and out of the cell to generate nerve impulses, and stabilize the cell membranes by neutralizing free radicals. The most effective way to uncover your unique individual magnesium status is with a simple blood test called RBC magnesium. The most desirable range for magnesium in this test is between 6 and 7 mg/dl, although most reference ranges note 4.0 to 6.8 mg/dl. I typically recommend 5 mg of magnesium per pound of body weight.

I created UNI KEY Health's product Mag-Key (see Resources) as an ideal magnesium supplement designed to deliver all four of the essential magnesium cofactors you are most likely missing. This targeted delivery system focuses broadly on your body and more specifically on your mind and muscles, especially your heart.

Guard your heart with niacin. To lower triglycerides and raise healthy HDL levels, start slowly at 250 mg at bedtime, then increase gradually to 1 to 2 g daily in divided doses. The form best tolerated is inositol hexanicotinate, marketed as Endur-acin.

Increase fatty acids. To lower levels of dangerous Lp(a) cholesterol, take 1 to 2 g of UNI KEY's Super-EPA fish oil daily and get the anti-inflammatory omega-3 essential fatty acids that also help raise healthy HDL levels (see Resources for recommendations).

Make CoQ10 part of your daily routine. Take a 100 to 300 mg softgel of CoQ10 daily—with heart-friendly vitamin E—for preventive maintenance. You may take up to 150 mg of CoQ10 daily if you have insulin resistance or type 2 diabetes; up to 240 mg daily for angina, arrhythmia, high blood pressure, mitral valve prolapse, or periodontal disease; and up to 400 mg of CoQ10 for advanced congestive heart failure. Check with your health-care practitioner to be sure this is right for you.

L-carnitine boosts CoQ10. According to the Mayo Clinic, L-carnitine is effective in reducing the development of angina, as well as reducing the incidence of abnormal heart rate. For best results, take 2 to 3 g per day, spread out through the day.

Alleviate angina with ribose. Ribose is an essential "carbohydrate" or "sugar" that has helped angina more than any other supplement I know. The recommendation is 5 g three times daily.

Consider CoQ10 as a natural alternative to statin drugs. Statin drugs can have devastating side effects. However, some natural alternatives function much like statins. If you do take a statin drug or if you use these natural sources of statins, you must supplement with CoQ10; 100 to 300 mg is recommended daily. As with all products and supplements, please consult your health-care practitioner to see if they are right for you.

Red yeast rice functions similarly to a statin drug by inhibiting cholesterol production. The results of a double-blind, placebo-controlled study of fifty-two physicians and their spouses with a total cholesterol level of greater than 200 mg/dl indicated that by taking red yeast rice, participants lowered their LDL cholesterol levels by 22 percent and total cholesterol by 15 percent. CAUTION: Because both red yeast rice and statins contain similar ingredients, they also may have similar side effects. Take CoQ10 with red yeast to avoid the same side effects that accompany statins. Consult your health-care practitioner for dosage recommendations.

Plant sterols can lower LDL cholesterol. The National Institutes of Health (NIH) Therapeutic Lifestyle Change Guidelines recommend 2,000 mg of plant sterols and stanols per day. Quality supplements, such as Nature Made CholestOff, can help restore proper levels. Check with your health-care provider for recommended dosage.

TARGETED HERBAL SOLUTIONS

Hawthorn is heart healthy. It decreases cholesterol, inhibits atherosclerotic plaque buildup, lowers blood pressure, and dilates coronary vessels, which improve blood flow and increase blood supply to the heart muscle. Although it works well with many heart medications, you should not use hawthorn if you take beta blockers. And do keep in mind that hawthorn contains arginine, which is the antagonist for lysine, so make sure you're taking enough of both. Consult your health-care practitioner to see whether this is right for you.

Garlic can lower cholesterol by 10 percent in less than one month. It also has the ability to prevent blood from clotting. Be aware, however, that raw garlic can lower blood sugar.

Cayenne pepper can play an important role in supporting heart function. It has been used traditionally by herbalists as a crisis herb in coronary and other emergencies. Cayenne is also useful when taken on a regular basis (¼ teaspoon taken three times daily) to stimulate circulation and prevent heart attacks and stroke, but *only if* you are not allergic to nightshades.

Get curious about CBD oil. Cannabidiol (CBD) oil is a natural anti-inflammatory and may prove helpful in relaxing the blood vessels, which allows for more efficient blood flow. The recommended dose is 3 to 30 mg daily. Check with your health-care provider first.

TARGETED BROKEN-HEART SOLUTIONS

Experience your emotions. When you think back on times in your life when you tried to express your sadness and pain, it was often met with

→ Logical reasons you shouldn't feel sad and phrases such as "look on the bright side"

→ Lack of empathy and phrases such as "get over it" and "move on"

→ Shifting the focus off you and onto themselves with "I know just how you feel"

→ Dismissing your feelings with "be strong" and "keep your chin up"

→ One-upping with a story of someone who has it worse than you and "at least it's not as bad as . . . "

Chances are you walked away not feeling any better. When we are grieving, we long for people to listen without analyzing, judging, criticizing, or trying to fix or explain our pain.

We need to allow ourselves to feel our feelings and not let those voices from the past who criticized and judged become our own internal voice. When sadness, anger, fear, and pain rise up, sit with those feelings and avoid judging yourself for having them. It may seem overwhelming, but usually those feelings pass in a matter of minutes.

Have a good cry. Crying is cleansing. My favorite quote from Washington Irving says: "There is a sacredness in tears. They are not the mark of weakness, but of power. They speak more eloquently than ten thousand tongues. They are the messengers of overwhelming grief, of deep contrition, and of unspeakable love."

Simplify your daily routine. When you're in the thick of the pain, confusion, and even chaos of losing a loved one, it's hard to even figure out what's healthy. It's normal to experience a loss of appetite or lack of motivation for your exercise routine, healthy diet, or even going to bed on time. If this is the case, it's fine to simplify your diet and exercise regimens, but don't give them up entirely—this is important self-care. Yoga, meditative walking, dancing, and cooking can all help you work through your grief.

Nurture yourself. In times of grief, you'll want to take extra measures to give yourself some TLC. As published in *Harvard Health*, researchers at the University of North Carolina determined that the hormone oxytocin is released in the experience of a simple hug.

Take all the time you need. Our lives can get so busy and hectic that it seems that there's no time to cope with grief. When you find yourself ignoring or burying your feelings, isolating yourself, pretending your way through the grieving process, setting a time limit for your grief, or trying to numb your pain with alcohol or other destructive habits, these are all warning signs of unhealthy grieving. Grief takes time, and it's different for everyone.

5-HTP can boost your mood. 5-hydroxytryptophan (5-HTP), an amino acid, is often used to treat this condition, as it is known to help raise serotonin levels in the brain. Aim for 100–400 mg daily.

Calm down with CBD oil. CBD oil can help relax, soothe, and reduce anxiety. No wonder it's popular in today's hectic world. Don't worry, this perfectly legal extract does not contain the marijuana component that elicits a "high." Side effects are minimal and may include drowsiness (a plus if you need help sleeping). Discuss with your health-care provider to determine whether CBD oil is right for you.

TARGETED HIATAL HERNIA SOLUTIONS

Increase your stomach acid. Even though you feel the pain of the acid from your stomach washing up into your esophagus, it doesn't mean you have excess acid. In fact, often the opposite problem is to blame. When acid is reduced too low, even though you feel less discomfort in the short term, your food is essentially rotting and fermenting downstream, resulting in gas, bloating, and other digestive issues that back up and put pressure on the diaphragm. When you have optimal stomach acid, you will break down protein more quickly and absorb iron, calcium, vitamin B_{12}, and other nutrients more efficiently, without bloating or fatigue. Taking an HCl supplement (such as UNI KEY's HCL+2) before meals will curb your digestive issues and optimize your liver function. After four weeks, you can experiment with reducing your dosage to once a day. Avoid antacids as they only make the problem worse.

Heal tissue damage with Siberian pine nut oil. Take 1 teaspoon thirty minutes before meals for three weeks. After that, you can reduce the dose to a single teaspoon daily for another three weeks.

Abdominal massage is helpful. A qualified practitioner will target the ileocecal valve and the diaphragm and follow the path of your digestion to relieve physical stress and induce relaxation. This can also help relieve some of the emotional stress associated with hiatal hernia.

Make lifestyle changes. Eat small meals, wear loose clothing, use good posture, practice deep breathing, sit up after eating, avoid alcohol and caffeine, limit fatty foods, and lose excess abdominal weight.

Drink warm water. Warm water relaxes the stomach and weighs it down. After drinking, drop from your tiptoes down to your heels multiple times to bring the stomach down through the hiatus.

Blow up a balloon. Blow up a balloon daily, to both increase lung capacity and to create pressure from the chest cavity that keeps the stomach down and in place. In the beginning, many people can barely blow up one balloon but over time will notice they can blow up several of them per day.

Protecting the heart from the ravages of environmental toxins, persistent oxidative stress, and aging should be a number one priority for all of us. The whole body, mind, and spirit approach presented in this chapter has worked exceedingly well for many of my clients, helping to restore cardiovascular function. In the next chapter, we tackle another prominent aging issue, the care of bones, muscles, and joints.

CHAPTER 13

REPAIR BONES, MUSCLES, AND JOINTS

In this chapter, you'll learn . . .

- The myths about osteoporosis
- Why brittleness, not bone density, is a major sign of osteoporosis
- Bone-building benefits of magnesium and other micronutrients
- About the surprising inhibitors—and enhancers—to bone health
- How to relieve joint pain
- About the regenerative role stem cell therapy plays in joint injury recovery

I WILL ALWAYS REMEMBER THE BONE-CHILLING WORDS OF NUTRITION DETECTIVE Nan Fuchs, PhD:

Magnesium, not calcium, helps prevent osteoporosis. Repeat after me: "High calcium intake causes bones to form that are brittle. Magnesium causes bones to form that are strong and flexible. I need plenty of magnesium and enough, but not too much, calcium."

Here's why. The calcium crystals in bone tissue help determine how brittle or supple your bones will be. Abnormally large, smooth calcium crystals can't grab onto one another and form strong bones. That's why the bone they make is brittle. Magnesium helps form crystals that are smaller and irregular in shape. These crystals bind to one another and create stronger, more flexible bones.

Let's use chalk and ivory to illustrate this bone-building phenomenon. Chalk is pure calcium carbonate, one of the forms of calcium added to many osteoporosis supplements. Ivory, on the other hand, contains calcium with magnesium. If you took a 3-inch-long, thin piece of chalk and dropped it, it would break. The same size piece of ivory would bounce. Do you want your bones to be more like chalk or ivory?

Just like the Nutrition Detective, I want you to have bones more like ivory, not like chalk. Keep in mind that your bones, muscles, and joints, like the rest of your body, are significantly influenced by the Rules. Muscle loss, stiffness, and weakness, for example, are highly subject to AGEs' cross-linking of collagen while osteoporosis (bone thinning) has been connected to the buildup of AGEs in the bone matrix resulting in bone fragility and major oxidative stress in bone cells. Joints are more susceptible to both osteoarthritis (inflammation of the joints and cartilage) as well as rheumatoid arthritis (an autoimmune condition) when you don't consume enough of the lubricating oils from healthy fats, many of which act as nature's most powerful anti-inflammatories.

Platelet-rich plasma (PRP) is very specific in helping to repair many orthopedic conditions ranging from muscle tears, strained tendons, and ligaments to Achilles tendon injuries, chronic tendinitis, fractures, rotator cuff injuries, and even osteoarthritis. As you may recall, platelets are a rich source of hundreds of growth factors so crucial to healing.

The bottom line is that learning how to keep your muscles and bones strong will help you remain independent and active as you age. Strong bones and functioning muscles will keep you mobile, agile, and active. Because we have increased balance issues as we age, remember that our recovery times are longer and less damage is done when our muscles and bones support our framework. Aching joints and muscle atrophy from lack of use become harder to repair and correct over time, so it is important to treat these as we would any other symptoms and put strategies to work when the first discomforts appear. Although your body will experience some wear and tear, remember that osteoporosis is far from inevitable.

ARTHRITIS AND ACHING JOINTS

If you ask any of the fifty million Americans with arthritic joints, conventional therapy, such as nonsteroidal anti-inflammatory drugs (NSAIDs), doesn't work. NSAIDs also inhibit production of regenerative and reparative substances in the joints and further break down cartilage. They also restrict the normal increase in blood flow that bathes damaged tissues in oxygen. Even the smallest dose prevents healing at the cellular level. But that's not all—some NSAIDs may even prevent collagen formation, the "glue" that holds our cells together and is necessary for healing bones, tendons, and joints.

WHAT IS ARTHRITIS, REALLY?

Osteoarthritis is a degenerative disease caused by the breakdown of cartilage, leading to bone rubbing on bone and wearing down. The cushion in your joints between the bones is cartilage, which is made up of a combination of proteins and sugars. When it's healthy, it allows bones to glide over one another and absorbs the shock of any movement. When your joints are inflamed, misaligned, or worn from overuse, this cushion of cartilage thins out, breaks down, and can no longer do its job, causing joint pain and osteoarthritis as the result.

Rheumatoid arthritis is an autoimmune condition that may be related to viruses, parasites, food allergies, or a lack of hydrochloric acid.

Until recently, doctors believed articular cartilage—the cushion in our hip, knee, and ankle joints—could not be repaired once it was injured. Joint replacement surgeries are on the rise, but before you decide on joint replacements of any kind, start by avoiding the medications that inhibit healing while feeding your joints the nutrients they need to heal. All programs dealing with arthritis should address cartilage restoration as well as pain and inflammation.

LOSS OF MUSCLE MASS

After the age of forty, we tend to lose up to 6 pounds of muscle every ten years. Sarcopenia, or age-related muscle loss, is a common, reversible condition. Factors that promote sarcopenia include a sedentary lifestyle, severe stress, a poor diet, and chronic inflammation. A simple handgrip strength test using a grip meter can diagnose sarcopenia. If you notice you're having increased difficulty opening jars or squeezing an orange, it's time to take notice.

Why do we lose muscle mass as we age? There are several causes, including hormone imbalance, AGE induced inflammation, lack of movement (especially excess sitting), and inadequate nutrition from the consumption of poor-quality proteins and impaired protein digestion. Protein digestion requires adequate stomach acid and digestive enzymes, and for most Americans, these are lacking to nonexistent. It's common for people to have a 40 percent decrease in stomach acid production by the time they're in their thirties, and a 50 percent decrease by age seventy. This can lead to such symptoms as gastroesophageal reflux disease (GERD), gas, bloating, nausea, and other symptoms (including crankiness).

THE CALCIUM-MAGNESIUM CONNECTION

The bone benefits of calcium do not come from calcium alone, but from the interaction between calcium and magnesium and a whole host of nutrient helpers. Your bones and teeth, of course, require calcium, but without magnesium and other minerals, your body cannot properly deposit calcium in hard tissue; as a result, the hard tissue will weaken. Excess calcium prevents magnesium from activating thyrocalcitonin, a hormone that directs calcium to the bones, which in turn stops bones from breaking down and aids in bone reformation. Countless studies prove how decisive this magnesium-activated process is. These studies have shown that magnesium, not calcium from the falsely idolized milk, strengthens bones and teeth.

Excess calcium is toxic. It can lead to calcification, the process in which excess calcium is deposited in cells, tissues, and organs. It may sound like a relatively benign mechanism, but imagine the hardening meant for your bones affecting your arterial walls. That's exactly what can and does happen. Instead of strengthening bones, the excess calcium is inappropriately deposited in soft tissue, causing kidney stones, strokes, hardening of the arterial walls (which can raise blood pressure and the risk of heart disease), and stiffening of the lining of the bronchial tubes (which can result in asthma).

Another good reason for avoiding high amounts of dairy products as we age is that the majority of us are lactose intolerant to some extent. Lactose is the sugar in milk, and it is broken down in our intestines by the enzyme lactase. By the age of forty, many of us have stopped producing that enzyme. The undigested lactose moves to the colon, where it ferments and causes bloating, gas, cramps, and sometimes diarrhea. The chances that you are lactose intolerant are particularly high if your ancestry is African, Native American, Greek, Arabian, Ashkenazi or Sephardic Jewish, or Asian.

I'm not saying that calcium is bad for you or that it doesn't help your bones. What I am saying is that to have calcium build your bones, you must have enough magnesium to work with it. Magnesium helps calcium absorption and deposition in the bones, where it belongs.

While we enrich our diet with calcium—we even add the mineral to orange juice and ingest a brand of antacids (Tums) for its calcium content—we eat a magnesium-impoverished diet. We eat less magnesium-rich food—such as leafy green vegetables, nuts, seeds, and sea vegetables—than our Stone Age ancestors did. The magnesium-rich food that we do eat has less magnesium than it did during most of the course of our evolution because it no longer grows in unadulterated nutrient-rich soil. With the best intentions, we have created a magnesium-calcium imbalance.

DIETARY DANGERS: THE INHIBITORS

You can add all the calcium you want, but if you're not aware of the calcium inhibitors, then you'll still be deficient in this important bone builder.

Sugar: the ultimate calcium robber. Sugar is a major cause of calcium imbalance. For calcium to be transported to bone marrow, it needs to be in balance with phosphorus. A healthy calcium-phosphorus level is two parts calcium to one part phosphorus. Without adequate phosphorus for transport, bone marrow doesn't get the calcium it needs, so the body pulls calcium from storage sites in bone. But this acquired calcium cannot be used without adequate phosphorus and results in an excess of calcium that is ultimately just excreted from the body. Eventually, this imbalance of calcium and phosphorus starves the bone marrow of calcium, resulting in osteoporosis.

Because sugar depletes your body of phosphorus, eating sugar can profoundly disturb your calcium-phosphorus ratio, despite your intake of calcium. According to the Department of Agriculture (USDA), Americans eat, on average, between 150 and 170 pounds of sugar in a year. Food labels are the key to controlling our sugar habits. Read those colorful paper labels carefully and search for any of the "-ose" words (glucose, dextrose, sucrose, etc.). Sugar will also be listed as corn syrup, honey, molasses, barley malt, or just sweetener.

Soft drinks. Soft drinks contain phosphoric acid, a phosphorus-containing substance. The soda does not, however, contain an equivalent amount of calcium to maintain the necessary calcium-phosphorus balance. Just how much phosphorus does the average cola contain? A 12-ounce can of cola (with caffeine) comes in first, with 37 mg of phosphorus. In second place is the equivalent 12 ounces of diet cola (with caffeine), with 32 mg of phosphorus. For phosphorus-free drinks, you'd need to consider cream soda, ginger ale, and root beer.

You might be surprised to learn that soft drinks are not the most significant source of phosphorus. Examples are milk and yogurt. An 8-ounce serving of skim milk has 247 mg of phosphorus, and an 8-ounce serving of yogurt has a whopping 385 mg.

Aluminum. Aluminum affects both phosphorus and calcium. According to a seminal article published in *Gastroenterology*, small amounts of aluminum-containing antacids, taken three or four times a day for two to five weeks, caused phosphorus depletion and increased the excretion of calcium in urine and feces, especially in individuals with low calcium intake. This means that when you ingest aluminum, you flush calcium and deplete phosphorus, which leads to bone loss.

Phosphorus. The calcium-phosphorus ratio is a vital factor in the optimal use of calcium. About one-fourth of the mineral content of your body is phosphorus, most of it tied up as calcium phosphate. Excesses in phosphorus build up in a diet high in red meat, poultry, and carbonated soft drinks. Such meats as pork chops and ham contain up to thirty times more phosphorus than calcium.

Oxalates. Some foods contain natural substances that interfere with calcium absorption. For example, spinach may be high in calcium, but it also contains calcium-blocking oxalates. So do cacao, asparagus, sorrel, rhubarb, and dandelion greens. The oxalic acid they contain binds with the calcium to form calcium oxalate, which is indigestible.

Smoking. Smoking more than doubles your risk of developing osteoporosis. Smokers often carry high levels of the toxic mineral cadmium in their blood, and one well-known result of high cadmium levels is a loss of calcium from bone, resulting in osteoporosis. E-cigarettes are proving to be equally as dangerous, as high cadmium levels are associated with e-cigarette vape.

Medications. A number of drugs and medications have been found to interact with calcium or its enhancer, vitamin D; some act to increase excretion; others block absorption. Here are the common ones: Dilantin, phenobarbital, primidone, glutethimide, aluminum hydroxide, Maalox or Mylanta, mineral oil, phenolphthalein, furosemide, ethacrynic acid, triamterene, chlorothiazide, hydrochlorothiazide, thyroid hormone, tetracycline, vitamin A (75,000 IU), cholestyramine, para-aminosalicylic acid, methotrexate, and sulfur-containing amino acids.

Damage from nonsteroidal anti-inflammatory drugs (NSAIDs). Although it can be tempting to reach for medications such as aspirin or ibuprofen to alleviate the pain of arthritis, even the smallest dose of these NSAIDs prevents healing at the cellular level. These medications also interfere with the formation of collagen—the very substance needed for healing our joints, bones, and tendons. A better solution for healing your joints, not simply masking the pain, are supplements and foods.

LIFESTYLE INHIBITORS

Lack of exercise. The familiar adage "use it or lose it" applies to bones. Research has found that when muscles contract, the stress of the contraction is

transmitted to the attached bone. This stress sets off an electrical charge that
stimulates the osteoblasts to build bone.

Staying too thin. Like exercise-induced weight loss, continual, prolonged, or
on-again, off-again dieting habits can severely interfere with hormonal and
calcium function. Obsession with weight and dieting leads too many women
to resort to extremely low-calorie diets that lack sufficient amounts of calcium and other bone-building elements.

Excessive use of alcohol. It appears that alcohol suppresses the growth of
new bone by poisoning bone-forming cells. Nutritional problems resulting
from heavy alcohol use include irritation of the intestinal lining, leading to a
decrease in nutrient absorption and liver damage.

DIETARY DARLINGS: THE ENHANCERS

It isn't enough to just be on the defensive when it comes to bone loss. You definitely want
to fortify your bone strength.

VITAMIN D

Vitamin D is essential to maintain strong bones and reduce the risk of fractures. It
stimulates the absorption of calcium and magnesium and promotes mineralization and
strengthening of the collagen matrix in bone, increasing bone density and overall health
of bone tissue. This process starts in the intestine, then the signal travels to the bones and
the bone marrow, and once the bone marrow is involved, so is the immune system.

The best form of vitamin D is sunshine. Make an effort to get fifteen to twenty minutes at midday with your arms and legs as exposed as possible.

Vitamin D is fat-soluble, so it will typically be found in fatty foods. Sources include
beef liver, egg yolks, fatty fish and fish oil, and even mushrooms, which seem to be the
only nonfat food source rich in vitamin D. Like magnesium, vitamin D supports calcium
absorption, helping to create strong bones.

As it stands, the RDA for vitamin D is 600 IU per day. However, in 2014, research
from the University of Alberta showed that the official RDA of vitamin D from the National Academy of Medicine is significantly lower than needed to maintain a healthy
body. According to the researcher's statistical analysis, the RDA should actually sit at
8,895 IU per day to ensure that the vast majority of the population has adequate vitamin
D in their system. The researchers do note that this dose is higher than any previously
studied dose, and caution should be taken when interpreting this number. I recommend a
daily vitamin D intake of 2,000 to 5,000 IU.

MIGHTY MANGANESE AND SEXY SELENIUM

Selenium deficiency is associated with osteopenia (a preosteoporosis condition of reduced bone mass). This really hits home with me because whenever I review tissue mineral analysis (TMA) reports of those diagnosed with osteopenia, I have consistently found a deficit of selenium. This important trace mineral is deficient in most US soils, with the exception of the Dakotas. Some rich food sources of selenium include Brazil nuts, walnuts, and shiitake mushrooms. I consider the optimum daily dose for adults to be 100 to 200 mcg. (*For information on ordering a tissue mineral analysis, see the Resources section at the back of this book.*)

THE ENHANCING TRACE ELEMENTS

As research into osteoporosis and bone fragility continues, new relationships have emerged, albeit not always clearly defined. For example, researchers at the USDA found that boron plays a key role in maintaining calcium and magnesium levels by helping the body synthesize both estrogen and vitamin D. This is good news for women who want to prevent osteoporosis, arthritis, and other bone-weakening conditions.

Prunes—a High Source of Bone-Building Boron

My friend Dr. Janet Zand shared an extraordinary testimonial from one of her fans about the power of prunes—a high source of bone-building boron: "I am now eighty-two and have had four bone density tests, which have told me I have the bones of a thirty-year-old. I'm told this is very unusual. One clinician told me that at the normal rate of bone loss, I will be a hundred and ten before I have osteopenia. Now I know why. For thirty-five years, I had a house with a plum tree and made prunes. I have continued daily use of four prunes for fifty years, thinking I was doing it for constipation. What a wonderful side effect to get these solid bones!"

Next to oxygen, silicon is the most prevalent element on earth. A UCLA professor, Edith M. Carlisle, PhD, found that silicon in the diet of chicks produced denser bone and faster growth compared to chicks deprived of the mineral. Silicon produced a 100 percent increase in the level of collagen. In rats, those with extra silicon were found to contain 20 percent more calcium and 10 percent more phosphorus than those from control rats fed the same diet without the extra silicon.

PROTEIN POWER

As we age, protein becomes a key nutrient in keeping our bones and muscles strong. Why is that important? It aids in the formation of bone matrix. Strong muscles will help us better maintain our balance and avoid sarcopenia. Don't forget, those with good muscle tone will also have better bone quality.

One study published in 2018 followed 2,900 seniors for over two decades and concluded that those who ate the most protein were 30 percent less likely to suffer from impairment in their routine daily tasks. Another study published in 2017 concluded that seniors who ate the least amount of protein were twice as likely to have mobility problems.

Vegans and vegetarians may not want to hear this, but animal protein contains all nine amino acids, and plant protein does not, so they need to pay extra close attention when planning their meals so as to get the right combination of amino acids for building and maintaining muscle. Vegans and vegetarians can help maintain and can even increase muscle mass through the use of amino acid supplementation that provides the branch-chain amino acids valine, leucine, and isoleucine (see Resources). Others should include proteins from foods high in muscle-building amino acids, such as whey, fish, poultry, and (low AGEs) cheese.

ALL THE RIGHT MOVES

Coupled with the right amino acids and protein, exercise is definitely one of the most important lifestyle habits for those seeking Radical Longevity. Exercise aids mineral metabolism to strengthen existing bone and stimulate the formation of new bone. Activities that are aerobic provide intermittent stress and strain that stretches the bone and helps maintain and build bone mass. The stress causes an electric current to go through the bone, triggering the calcification process known as the piezoelectric effect. This is important to understand because weight-bearing exercise appears to be one vital element of the bone-building formula as bones become stronger with physical stress.

An ideal well-rounded exercise program should include exercises designed to meet the three basic physical fitness components: cardiovascular endurance, muscle strength, and flexibility. The cardiovascular aerobic exercises include swimming, bike riding, rowing, cross-country skiing, brisk walking, jogging, racket sports, jumping rope, aerobic dancing, and high-intensity interval training (HIIT). What all these activities have in common is that they require a sustained supply of oxygen. This conditions the heart and respiratory system pumping oxygen to all parts of the body. For these exercises to be effective, you must sustain them, keeping up your pulse rate for fifteen to thirty minutes. Cardiovascular exercises promote energy and endurance and raise the level of happy hormones in the bloodstream.

For muscle endurance, the best choices include weight training, progressive resistance training on an Inspire or similar brand equipment, push-ups, and sit-ups. These exercises help tighten and tone the muscles, aiding weight loss, because building muscle tissue uses more calories than fat. In addition to building muscles, these exercises build stronger bones, and strong healthy bones are the best prevention for osteoporosis.

Flexibility exercises can be chosen from yoga, dance classes such as Zumba or Nia, special stretch and toning classes, as well as Pilates. Good for developing muscle and joint fitness, these exercises make us bend and stretch. In addition to alleviating physical tightness, flexibility exercises can help relieve stress and tension.

Choosing a variety of exercises that fit into each of these three categories will ensure that the entire body gets a workout. High-caliber routines of all types of exercise are now abundant online, so try a variety and find some you enjoy.

For those who have not been exercising on a regular basis, here is a sample program that you can follow.

→ Cardiovascular exercises three days a week (for at least 20 to 30 minutes each day)
→ Muscle strength exercises: in alternation with cardiovascular exercises three days a week (for at least 30 minutes each day)
→ Flexibility exercises six days per week (for at least 20 minutes)

Since resistance is such a key to building stronger bones, let's delve a little deeper into the nitty gritty of weight-bearing exercise.

KEY EXERCISES TO PREVENT OSTEOPOROSIS

Resistance, or weight-bearing, exercises are especially needed to prevent osteoporosis. When muscles experience resistance, it creates torque—a twisting force—in the muscles equal to the force it is resisting. This torque then sets off a small but critical electrical impulse that triggers calcium deposition, therefore strengthening, in the long run, the exact bones being taxed in the moment.

The Mayo Clinic conducted a study on a type of safe, progressive resistive weight-lifting exercise that produces impressive results in the lower back muscles. In the study, postmenopausal women ranging from fifty-eight to seventy-five years old lie on their stomach wearing weighted backpacks equivalent to 30 percent of the maximum they could lift. They then lifted the backpack by lifting their arms, chest, and chin off the floor a total of ten times. They did this exercise five days a week over the course of two years. The amount of weight they lifted increased as their strength grew, with the total weight of the backpack never exceeding 50 pounds.

The women who completed the exercise regimen not only strengthened their back muscles during the study but also had less muscle loss eight years later compared to the control group. Their ten-year risk of spine fracture was also reduced by 300 percent in comparison to the control group.

To create this necessary resistance for your body, try walking, running, bicycling, aerobics, light weight lifting, or any other form of exercise that makes extensive use of the hips and legs. Twenty minutes to an hour three times a week is adequate. Research has shown that women who did this kind of exercise for an hour three times a week increased their bone density by 2.6 percent in one year.

The Dangers of Overexercising

Overly strenuous exercise (continuous strenuous exercise for two or more hours) can actually damage the body, increasing oxidative stress and throwing estrogen levels out of whack, which leads to bone loss. In contrast, moderate exercise has been shown to encourage bodily processes to stay active and keep toxins moving on out. Exercise gets everything moving—blood, lymph, bile, and bowels.

REBOUNDING FOR BONE HEALTH

A type of exercise called rebounding combines the joys of the trampoline with the joys of good health. This jumping exercise moves and stretches every cell in your body, supporting the influx of nutrients and the elimination of waste as it boosts blood circulation and lymphatic drainage.

It also strengthens bones gently without the jarring impact on the joints that more strenuous exercises, such as jogging, can inflict. In fact, in the early 1980s, NASA conducted research that showed rebounding provides a more even, full-body workout than running, with less impact on the body, while still producing similar cardiovascular results.

You can use rebounding as part of your weekly cardio workouts. Just be sure to warm up first with light, gentle bouncing or marching for at least one minute, and after your workout, cool down gently for another minute.

VIBRATIONAL TRAINING

Supported with research conducted by NASA, whole-body vibrational training uses 3G vibration platforms that vibrate at a specific speed to take advantage of gravity (see Resources). In essence, vibrational training is a one-stop shop in terms of effective exercise. It combines aerobic and resistance training all at once while improving mitochondrial function and body composition like no other forms of exercise.

This vibrational motion triggers muscles to use natural reflexes to respond much as if you were unexpectedly falling and trying to catch yourself. Essentially, this stimulates the strong muscle contraction of bracing against a fall—without actually falling. Simply standing or holding different positions on these platforms sends vibrations throughout the body, which stresses the muscles and generates muscle- and calcium-building torque, but without the risk. One study showed that using vibrational training actually reversed bone loss, increasing hip bone density by 1.5 percent.

SUPER SLOW TRAINING

Super Slow uses a very precise method that delivers noticeable results with short workout times and nominal risk of injury. It uses—as the name implies—extremely slow movement, focusing on proper form. A sample exercise would be a bicep curl, performed by slowly curling up for ten seconds and then slowly curling down for ten seconds. The reduced acceleration and momentum improve muscular loading because they limit the amount of force your body is exposed to during exercise.

BALANCE TRAINING

As we get older, we often get more unsteady on our feet due to injuries, medical conditions, and strokes, as well as the normal aging process. Since falling is the number one cause of death in the elderly, it only makes sense to give attention to better balance. Balance is better addressed before you begin to notice any problems, but balance training can improve balance at any time.

Improve your balance with this simple exercise. The ability to stand on one leg can be a key indicator of your ability to balance. And it's something you can easily improve upon. The single-leg stance is a simple, but very effective exercise to try:

1. Stand upright with your feet together. Position yourself near a stable object such as a chair or kitchen counter so you can grab it if you start to feel unsteady. If you are using an aide such as a cane or walker, do not attempt this without the help of a person as a spotter beside you.
2. Lift one foot off the ground.
3. Time yourself to see how many seconds you are able to stand on one foot.
4. If you are able to stand on one foot for sixty seconds or more, try the single-leg stance test while standing on a soft surface, such as a pillow.
5. If you are unable to stand on one foot for sixty seconds, hold the pose for as long as you can, then repeat using your other leg.
6. Repeat daily and increase the length of time you stand on each foot.

TARGETED SOLUTIONS
Targeted Bones and Muscle Solutions

Eliminate calcium inhibitors. Avoid the calcium robbers, such as sugar, soft drinks, aluminum, certain medications, and avoid being sedentary.

Add calcium enhancers. Adopt a bone-building lifestyle by incorporating regular exercise into your daily routine, getting plenty of sun, and eating adequate amounts of protein—and don't forget the boron-rich, bone-building prunes.

Eat to beat weak bones. Avoid excessive gluten, sugar, processed foods, alcohol, and too much saturated fat. Eat calcium-rich foods from dairy and nondairy sources. Nondairy sources of calcium include collard greens, carob flour, nettles, dandelion greens, watercress, chickweed, and sea vegetables. Two tablespoons of blackstrap molasses daily is a delicious way to incorporate calcium into your diet.

Build your bones with collagen. For the best bone-building, collagen-building bone broth, my favorite brand to buy is Kettle & Fire, which was the only brand I tested that did not have high levels of heavy metals.

If collagen protein powder from gelatin is a better fit for your lifestyle than pure bone broth, then Great Lakes is the only tried-and-true, clean brand I recommend. Great Lakes Gelatin is rich in glycine, the most abundant amino acid present in collagen, and can be used in cooking, baking, and even making healthy gummy snacks, which is a great way to supplement collagen in children and older adults. It is very high in type 1 collagen, which helps build bones, muscles, tendons, and cartilage.

Opt for absorbable forms of calcium. The form of supplemental calcium I recommend is microcrystalline hydroxyapatite (MCHC) because research has shown it to be among the best absorbed of the various calcium compounds. It appears MCHC not only stops bone loss but also regenerates bone. You will want to look for supplements that include these forms of calcium as well as magnesium. The brand Osteo-Key from UNI KEY Health Systems provides calcium and magnesium in a 1:1 ratio, along with other bone-building vitamins and trace minerals. Depending upon how much calcium you are getting in your foods, I recommend anywhere from 500 to 1,000 mg per day of additional calcium from dietary supplements.

If you are experiencing symptoms of magnesium deficiency—such as extreme edginess, muscle cramps or tremors, apathy, sleeping problems, or increased urination—consider adjusting your calcium-magnesium intake so you are taking twice as much magnesium as calcium. Take 500 to 1,000 mg of magnesium (5 mg of magnesium per pound of body weight) at a different time of day from when you take a calcium supplement, and avoid taking magnesium with meals because it neutralizes stomach acids that you need for digestion and calcium absorption. Once you feel a better balance has been achieved, return to the 1:1 ratio of calcium and magnesium. If you experience diarrhea, reduce your magnesium intake. If you have kidney disease, you are advised not to take magnesium supplements.

If you get adequate calcium from your diet and don't need a high-dose calcium supplement, you may want to consider taking a high-quality multiple vitamin supplement that includes all the vitamin and mineral bone nutrients like the Advanced Daily Multivitamin from UNI KEY (see Resources).

Drink your morning joe for strong muscles. It may seem outrageous, but America's favorite beverage, coffee, which is a staple in the Longevity Blaster, can help you maintain your lean muscle mass while revving up your fat-burning metabolism to lose weight. Its secret weapon? *Chlorogenic acid.* This compound signals the cells to burn the fatty acids in your fat cells for fuel. This is especially good news for us as we grow older. And according to Korean researchers, because this powerful polyphenol antioxidant chlorogenic acid (CGA) promotes the regeneration of muscle, adults who drink coffee daily have an almost 60 percent lower risk of muscle loss. Make sure your coffee is rich in chlorogenic acid, high in antioxidants, and free of mold.

Protein plus exercise builds muscle mass. Muscles contain more protein than any other structure of the body. To support your muscles, you must eat adequate amounts of protein daily, or consider amino supplementation, such as PerfectAmino, which contains all the bone-building essential amino acids in a vegan, highly bioavailable form.

Optimize your home to prevent falls. Avoid injury by securing throw rugs or doing away with them altogether. Keep floors clear of electrical wires and all other tripping hazards. Light-colored flooring and walls increase visibility. Install night lights where needed. Sturdy grab bars in the bath or shower are helpful.

TARGETED JOINT SOLUTIONS

Lose weight. The pressure on your knees when you are walking on level ground is 1.5 times your body weight. You can significantly ease the stress on your joints by losing weight and then maintaining a healthy weight.

Avoid NSAIDs. Whenever possible, avoid NSAID medications, such as ibuprofen or aspirin, and turn to supplements and foods to nourish the joint tissues and promote healing.

Avoid nightshades. Nightshades (tomatoes, white potatoes, eggplant, bell and chile peppers, tomatillos, ashwagandha, and goji berries) should be avoided, as they are commonly known to aggravate joint pain and inflammation, possibly due to their alkaloid and lectin content.

Anti-inflammatory fats relieve joint pain. Omega-6 and -3 fats found in hemp seed oil, safflower oil, and black currant seed oil are superstars for joint health. The omega fats reduce the amount of inflammation present in the thick fluid that bathes the joints.

Relieve joint pain and inflammation naturally. The most effective natural choices include turmeric at 200 to 500 mg per day, sea cucumber at 1,000 mg per day, bromelain at 2,000 to 6,000 mg on an empty stomach, and boswellia at 400 to 800 mg daily.

Try supplementation to rebuild cartilage. Consider 1,000 to 1,500 mg per day of glucosamine, and up to 1,200 mg of chondroitin sulfate for healthy cartilage restoration.

Consider hyaluronic acid supplementation. A product called Baxyl, found in most health food stores, contains a patented source of hyaluronic acid that has been shown to be effective in reducing joint pain within a month and increasing hyaluronic acid in the joints.

We all want to maintain an independent and active lifestyle well into our eighties and nineties. We can attain this goal by building up our bones and muscle strength while healing aching joints. A surefire recipe for achieving a more vibrant lifestyle is to follow the recommendations in this chapter. Now, let's talk about how to reveal more radiant skin, a topic of equal importance for those in the age-defying radical mind-set.

CHAPTER 14

REVITALIZE YOUR SKIN

In this chapter, you'll learn . . .

- Why your skin is a visible barometer of the condition of your health
- How *more*, not less, omega-6 results in sexy skin
- Which product you should throw out *today* to practice "safe sun"
- The proper care and feeding of your skin to reduce signs of aging
- Why your skin is critical to detoxing your body

NEVER LET ANYONE TELL YOU THAT WRINKLES, SAGGING SKIN, HYPERPIGMENTATION, or other skin issues are just "normal" signs of aging. They aren't. It's the lack of healthy fats, toxin overload, unrelenting stress, hormone imbalance, sun exposure, and mineral deficiencies that show up as signs of aging.

In the early days of my career, I saw many clients who were following the low-to-no-fat diet model of the 1980s and early '90s, and I began noting how the lack of the right kinds of fats took its toll on the skin first—leaving it more susceptible to redness, extreme dryness, and showing significant moisture loss.

Your skin is a two-way street, not only absorbing chemicals but working to rid the body of toxins too. The skin is a major eliminative organ (considered a "second liver" and "third kidney" by some). When your elimination pathways are clogged elsewhere, your skin helps your body to detoxify through its vast number of sweat glands. When this happens, your skin may also display visible SOS signals in the form of irritation, blemishes, and rashes. This is why you need to look at these as signs of distress and give attention to both what is going on with your skin and deeper within your body.

GET GLOWING WITH GLA

I take pride in my smooth complexion and firmly believe that wrinkles and dry, sagging skin aren't inevitable hallmarks of aging. Beauty is an inside—and outside—job. On the inside, I supplement with lots of omega-6 fats—GLA, CLA, hemp, and pine nut oil are my personal beauty salves.

GLA is a unique healing beautifier that belongs in your skin renewal regimen for soft, glowing skin. It helps trap moisture and prevents water evaporation from the surface of the skin. Without enough GLA, cellular membranes dry out, leaving the skin with a dry, rough appearance. A GLA deficit can cause weakened capillaries and increased moisture loss, resulting in itchy, scaly, and dry, wrinkle-prone skin.

GLA can help both internally and externally:

Internally, I have found that black currant seed oil offers the most balanced form of GLA for long-term use. That's because black currant also contains a hefty dose of omega-3, providing the best of both essential fatty acids. Externally, topical applications help too. Terrific for people of all ages, the topical application of omega-6 essential fatty acids, such as those in GLA, result in a more luminous glow, a smoother texture, and firmer skin. For years, I have applied an opened capsule of GLA to my face and neck both morning and night and let it soak in before adding my moisturizer. It is one of my secrets I am happy to share with you that has given me dewy, glowing skin, and I am in my seventies.

RELIEF FOR ECZEMA OR PSORIASIS

If you are suffering from a more severe condition, such as eczema or psoriasis, research suggests a GLA deficiency may be to blame. Essential fatty acid researcher Artur Klimaszewski, MD, has found that in eczema, the conversion of dietary linoleic acid—found in common vegetable oils—to GLA is impaired. This results in a lower level of healing omega-6 oil to the skin, which causes itching and inflammation.

Twelve-week placebo-controlled human trials at the University of Italy demonstrated a dramatic reduction of eczema symptoms with GLA supplementation. At the end of supplement therapy, itching decreased by 90 percent, and vesicles (watery bubbles) were reduced by 40 percent. In addition, the topical application of GLA results in fast relief for eczema sufferers.

REPLENISH YOUR COLLAGEN

Wrinkles and crepey skin are surefire signs of collagen loss. In fact, we produce about 1 percent less collagen in our skin each year. AGEs further degrade collagen proteins, resulting in skin that becomes thinner and more fragile with age. Although you can't measure your collagen level, you can tell when you're losing fullness and tone. Since collagen makes up 70 percent of the protein in your skin, dietary collagen is a key ingredient in preventing sagging and wrinkles.

NEW KID ON THE BEAUTIFYING BLOCK

One of the hottest new oils for skin health and beauty is broccoli seed oil. Made from cold-pressed broccoli sprout seeds, the oil has a high sulforaphane content. This potent antioxidant helps prevent damage to the skin. Simply apply a light layer of the broccoli seed oil beneath your daily moisturizer. As with all other oils, you'll want to store it in a cool place, out of sunlight. The shelf life is approximately two years.

RESPECT THE SUN

The sun bestows many health benefits, but we must first learn to respect it and develop good sun habits, so that our health isn't negatively impacted. Too much sun and too little sun can both cause problems. Researchers tracked the sun exposure habits of three thousand Swedish women for twenty years. They found that women who strictly avoided the sun during that period had a twofold greater risk of early death than women who received normal amounts of sun exposure.

Not getting enough sun exposure will result in a vitamin D deficiency. Darker-skinned people require more sunlight exposure than those with lighter skin to synthesize the same amount of vitamin D. Optimal sun exposure time varies (depending upon skin type, from about five to thirty minutes) daily. One study in *Health and Nutrition* reported that thirty minutes in the sun provided 300 to 350 IU of vitamin D for the average person. Sun exposure while wearing sunscreen will not prevent vitamin D deficiency. Sunscreen absorbs the ultraviolet rays that are needed for our body to synthesize vitamin D, and continual sunscreen use has been found to *decrease* vitamin D levels in the blood.

All that said, it's critical to learn the right way to avoid sunburn. While we may love our sun-kissed, glowing tan in the summer, we must be careful not to burn. There are numerous studies linking sunburns to melanoma; however, due to a wide range of factors, our skin has become increasingly less resistant to sun exposure. Our body is naturally built to receive sunlight, and the sooner we come into the light, the better. The appropriate amount of regular sun exposure actually protects against skin cancer. Certainly no one questions advice to avoid becoming sunburned, but like everything else involving health, blocking skin exposure to the sun can be carried to extremes.

I want nothing more than to radically change your mind about the toxic biohazardous sunscreen product you may be using. You think you are preventing cancer, without realizing it is actually *increasing* your chances of melanoma. Chemical sunscreens also disrupt both androgens and estrogens, alter male/female sex differentiation, impact brain development, disrupt thyroid function, impact both male and female fertility, *and* lead to a vitamin D deficiency.

Melanoma is up nearly 2,000 percent since the 1930s. At that time, approximately 75 percent of the workforce held jobs that kept them outside during the day, while today that number is only around 10 percent. Sunscreens were introduced in the 1970s, yet the rates of melanoma have been rising for the last forty years. If sunscreens actually worked, the incidences of melanoma should be decreasing.

Many of the chemicals in commonly used sunscreens are known carcinogens and endocrine-disrupting chemicals (EDCs). It's EDCs that disrupt both androgens and estrogens.

To make matters worse, many sunscreen manufacturers use nanoparticles of titanium and zinc oxide in their formulas. Because they are so small, nanoparticles cross the blood-brain barrier and even penetrate cell walls. Unfortunately, this *increases* the possibility of skin cancer as it promotes damage to cells.

Chemical sunscreens absorb UVE radiation, but not all prevent UVA light, which penetrates the farthest into the skin and is involved in the formation of melanoma. UVA light suppresses the immune system, specifically causing a loss of Langerhans cells, which keep the skin healthy and protect it from free radical damage, bacteria, and other pathogens.

It doesn't help that people using sunscreen usually stay in the sun longer than others who don't because they develop a false sense of security when they're not getting sunburned.

YOUR SKIN AND THE ACID MANTLE

While we constantly hear about the protective mantle of the atmosphere known as the ozone mantle, nobody talks about the importance of matching your skin with the proper pH-balanced products consistent with your skin's protective shield, known as the acid mantle. Healthy, glowing skin requires the proper pH balance and it is important to match the acid mantle of your skin. Start testing all your cosmetics and hair and skin care products. It is easy to do. Apply a bit of the product (cream, lotion, serum) to a small strip of nitrazene, or litmus paper, available at drugstores and pharmacies. If the paper turns yellow, the product is on the acidic side, which is what you want. If the paper turns bluish or purple, the product is alkaline, which you don't want.

TARGETED SOLUTIONS
Targeted Diet and Nutrient Solutions

Up your omegas. For a youthful glow, try adding a couple of tablespoons of omega-6 hemp, safflower, sesame, or Siberian pine nut oil to your daily routine.

Keep your skin moist with black currant seed oil. Up to 2 g a day of black currant seed oil will help strengthen your skin and keep it moist by supporting the natural barrier function.

Take vitamin C to repair damaged skin cells. The suggested dosage is up to 7 g per day.

Take proline to promote skin cell regeneration. This amino acid is commonly used in beauty care products due to its ability to pump up skin repair and regeneration. A suggested dosage is 1 to 7 g daily.

Build collagen with lysine. Your body doesn't manufacture lysine, so you need to get it from food sources or from supplements. The recommended dosage is up to 3,000 mg daily.

Glamour up with glycine. Glycine stimulates collagen production and has the ability to reduce the appearance of fine lines and wrinkles, maintain skin firmness, and promote skin repair and regeneration. Glycine is also key in the formation of glutathione, that multitasking antioxidant that prevents all kinds of signs of aging from cellular damage. By adding only 2 tablespoons of collagen to your daily regimen, you will add about 3 g of glycine to your diet.

Stay hydrated. It's a *must* to stay hydrated throughout the day, not only for your skin to look its best, but to help flush out toxins. A little bit of salt in your daily water (a smidge in each 8-ounce glass) will help you retain hydrating fluids. Choose sea salt or pink Himalayan salt instead, rich in minerals, or gray sea salt, such as Celtic.

SKIN DETOX SOLUTIONS

Sweat it out. Sweat not only helps regulate your body temperature, which can fend off a fever, it also helps your body heal faster by getting rid of germs and bacteria that made you sick in the first place. Sweat at least two to four times a week.

Dry brush for invigorated, glowing skin. Dry brushing your skin is a great way to rid your body of dead skin cells, promote lymph flow and blood circulation, stimulate oil-producing glands in your skin, and enhance your immune system. This simple technique also helps lessen the appearance of cellulite, rebuilds new, strong connective tissue, and promotes supple skin. Look for a medium-firm brush with natural bristles. Strive for five minutes, two times a week.

Once a week, soak your brush for thirty minutes in a solution of 1 quart of water and a few drops of chlorine bleach or tea tree oil. Make sure your brush dries before you use it.

Draw out impurities with clay masks. Look for nontoxic, fragrance-free brands, such as Aztec Secret Indian Healing Clay or Dead Sea Mud Mask.

SAFE SUN SOLUTIONS

Don't shun the sun. Get your vitamin D stores to an optimal level and maintain a light, protective skin color by allowing yourself regular, but brief, unprotected sun exposure in the early morning or early evening.

Avoid sunscreen when possible. You don't need to wear sunscreen every minute you are out in the sun, especially if you're only going to be outdoors for no more than twenty minutes.

Read all labels. Always check labels for anything you are considering placing on the skin, especially aluminum and parabens. Then decide whether you really want the chemicals it contains floating around in your bloodstream.

Avoid synthetic body products. You should also be careful to avoid synthetic makeup and conventional deodorants, which contain aluminum and other additives, such as mineral oils, that inhibit your skin's eliminating function.

Be cautious about using mineral-based sunscreens. Keep in mind that many mineral-based sunscreens (zinc oxide and titanium dioxide) are not a safe alternative as they are made from nanoparticles so tiny that they are able to breach cell membranes, nuclear membranes, and the blood-brain barrier. Use nontoxic products instead. Look for products that contain non-nano zinc oxide *only*, such as 3rd Rock Essentials, which has a line of non-toxic products that are completely different than any other sunscreens on the market.

Use Hawaii's best-kept secret. Hawaiian islanders have added microalgae into their diet to protect their eyes and skin from the oxidizing UV rays
that cause sunburn. I take an astaxanthin supplement (12 mg daily) that is
derived from that same microalgae.

The truth is you can read your skin like a book. Outward blemishes, spots, wrinkles,
rashes, and discoloration are all signs of inner imbalance. Once you heal from within,
your skin will reflect your new glow of ageless beauty and radical radiance, but now, what
about your hair?

CHAPTER 15

REVERSE HAIR LOSS

In this chapter, you'll learn . . .

- How specific nutritional deficits and declining hormones impact hair as we age
- The impact that toxins, prescription drugs, and such minerals as copper have on your hair
- About the stomach acid and protein connection
- About the connection between thyroid function and hair loss

OVER THE DECADES OF OUR LIVES, WE SPEND COUNTLESS HOURS PAMPERING, STYLing, and caring for our hair. Why then do we accept hair loss or hair thinning as a classic sign of aging? Our hair, after all, is 99 percent protein, and our body uses protein building blocks of all nine amino acids to rebuild and repair all our bodily hormones, enzymes, and muscle proteins. You can't live without your heart, but you can live without your hair. Our body knows we cannot exist very long without a strong heart muscle, so the hair is the first thing to go when there is not enough protein to maintain our bodily tissues. As we age, thinning hair is so much more than just a cosmetic concern. It puts us on notice that there are far more serious issues going on internally regarding protein utilization.

WHY IS MY HAIR THINNING?

If thinning hair is sending you into panic mode, you are far from alone. Hair loss is a problem shared by men and women alike. Alopecia—abnormal hair loss—is mistakenly believed to be a male disease, but 40 percent of sufferers are actually women.

To properly restore your hair volume requires getting to the root cause of your hair loss. Hormonal fluctuations, medications, toxins, nutritional deficiencies, illness (including diabetes and autoimmune conditions, such as lupus), stress, and other factors may be playing a role. Sometimes hair loss resolves on its own, but many times it will not stop until the underlying cause is identified and corrected.

HAIR TODAY, GONE TOMORROW

Each of your hair follicles grows a strand of hair over the course of four to six years in the anagen phase, then rests for two to four months in the telogen phase. After telogen, a new strand is produced that pushes out the old, causing the hair to be shed. At any one time, about 90 percent of your hair is in the anagen phase and 10 percent is in the telogen. This cycle is what accounts for normal hair loss, but many things can alter the cycle, causing the anagen phase to shorten or sending excess follicles into telogen.

Telogen effluvium (TE) is the term for when as much as 70 percent of your hair follicles "go telogen" at one time. TE can be triggered by such stressors as illness or injury, high fever, surgery, medications, psychological trauma, or the hormonal changes that accompany childbirth and menopause. Hair loss resulting from TE typically occurs two to three months after some major stressor, either mental or physical, produces a "shock" to your system.

Stress is a toxin and both acute and prolonged stress can result in hair loss. Depression and anxiety can affect hormone balance and lower vitamin B_{12} levels. A good deal of research supports the notion that stress and emotional trauma can change hair follicle biochemistry and cause a greater percentage of hair follicles to enter the telogen phase, particularly if you're genetically primed.

Sadly, hair loss generally increases as we age. By age forty, the rate of hair growth slows down in both men and women. But healthy aging can offset the severity of this loss when the body is supported to such a degree that it has the resources to provide for the growth and renewal of your hair.

THE MOST LIKELY NUTRITIONAL CULPRITS

If your hair is visibly thinning or you're noticing more hairs on your hairbrush, the first thing to consider is whether you might have experienced high stress or trauma over the past several months. Have you had a serious illness or surgery? Suffered an injury? Is your stress level over the moon? Are you postmenopausal? If the cause is not obvious, the next thing to consider is a nutritional deficiency. The five most common hair-damaging deficiencies are the following:

→ **Protein:** Protein is critical for strengthening and sustaining hair growth. The body identifies hair growth as nonessential so it can divert protein to other vital body systems when protein levels are inadequate. As constituents of protein all of the amino acids are needed to maintain healthy hair. Hair and nails each consist of 95 to 98 percent protein. The sulfur-containing amino cysteine and methionine are particularly important.

→ **Iron:** Although most women stockpile iron as they grow older, others throughout their lifecycle can actually be deficient. Be careful to supplement with iron only if you are truly deficient as found by a ferritin blood test. If your ferritin is below 30 ng/ml for women, you may in fact need iron supplementation, especially if you are experiencing hair loss (see Resources).

→ **Zinc:** Zinc acts directly on hair follicles, and stress alone can triple zinc loss. Zinc helps metabolize testosterone, which in excess can cause hair loss.

→ **B vitamins, especially biotin:** Biotin (vitamin B_7) promotes growth and helps rebuild damaged hair, which is why it is included in some shampoo formulations.

→ **Essential fatty acids:** Omega-3s promote thicker hair and help reduce body inflammation, which increases hair loss.

THE COPPER CONNECTION

Copper imbalance (a.k.a. copper dysregulation) affects nearly 80 percent of people, and hair loss is but one symptom. *We need copper,* but only in small amounts.

Copper activates more than thirty enzymes and is important for collagen and melanin production, healthy connective tissue, and maintenance of natural hair color. Copper dysregulation causes deterioration of the protein structures in hair by inhibiting lysyl oxidase, a collagen-synthesizing enzyme. Lysyl oxidase is necessary for a healthy scalp, hair follicle function, and hair structure.

The problem is that many diets today, especially those that are plant based, are heavy in copper and low in zinc. Copper is a major component of soybeans, many nuts and seeds, and some of our other favorites, such as coffee, dark tea, and chocolate. If you are zinc deficient, you'll stockpile copper because zinc and copper are antagonistic to each other.

IRON: THE DOUBLE-EDGED SWORD

Low ferritin levels, anything less than 30 ng/ml (the stored form of iron), is a common cause of hair loss. Ferritin is stored throughout your body, including your hair follicles; when you are low in iron, your body "borrows" ferritin hair, which is less vital to your existence. So, while excess iron is a problem, it is really all about balance. And it's another reason to have your ferritin level checked routinely,

THE IMPORTANCE OF BEING ACIDIC

Millions of people are on stomach acid-reducing or -blocking medications that are handed out like candy by many medical professionals and are even available OTC at the pharmacy. And with all the health books out there talking about the importance of our body being alkaline, it would seem that stomach acid is not important. But nothing could be further from the truth!

Your ideal stomach pH is 2, which is very acidic. Hydrochloric acid, which is the acid in your stomach, is the first line of defense against harmful bacteria and parasites that are often ingested with food. It activates pepsin, which is an important enzyme needed for protein digestion, and signals the production and release of pancreatic enzymes for further digestion and absorption of important nutrients. Without this, we can't form collagen, resulting in hair loss, autoimmune diseases, and other serious illnesses.

THE DELICATE DANCE BETWEEN HAIR AND HORMONES

It has long been known that male sex hormones (androgens) contribute to hair loss in both men and women. Male-pattern baldness (MPB) accounts for about 90 percent of hair loss cases. It affects approximately half of all males in Western industrialized countries. MPB is a form of *androgenetic hair loss*, meaning that it is caused by genes and male hormones. Dihydrotestosterone (DHT), a metabolite of testosterone, is also thought to be a primary factor in shrinking hair follicles and subsequent hair loss. So, it is no surprise that DHT levels tend to increase with age.

Women are just as affected; fewer than 45 percent of women go through life with a full head of hair. Before age thirty, 12 percent of women develop hair loss, and by age seventy, 41 percent have detectable thinning. If women with the pattern of a receding hairline all over the crown were to get tested, the results would most likely show a high level of DHT in their blood. One common cause of thinning hair in women is hormone havoc resulting from the environment, stress, and even insufficient dietary fiber. During menopause, testosterone levels can also rise. Low vitamin D levels are also associated with hair loss—particularly alopecia areata, an autoimmune disease in which the body attacks hair follicles.

THE THYROID CONNECTION

Thyroid function is critical—every part of the body requires thyroid hormone for proper functioning, including hair follicles. In fact, human hair follicles are targets of thyroid hormones T3 and T4, regulating everything from cycling to pigmentation. Noticeable hair loss is a red flag of potential problems in regulating your thyroid hormones. Hair loss is one of the first symptoms of low thyroid; one-third of those with hypothyroidism experience hair loss. For your hair's sake, it is vitally important to supply your body with nutrients that will support the thyroid gland. If the thyroid is underactive—and almost 40 percent of Americans are walking around with underactive thyroids—this can lead to hair loss.

Hairs fall out and are replaced by new ones on a regular basis. The loss of fifty to one hundred hairs per day is normal. But problems result when lost hairs aren't replaced right away, aren't replaced at all, or are replaced with inferior-quality hair.

The prothyroid hormone progesterone is another piece of the hair-loss puzzle. If you have hair loss, a low progesterone level may be the culprit. Low progesterone can cause the adrenal cortex to secrete the hormone androstenedione, as an alternative chemical precursor for the manufacture of other hormones, to compensate for the diminished level of progesterone. This steroid hormone is associated with some male characteristics, one of which is male-pattern baldness. When you raise your progesterone level with natural progesterone cream, your androstenedione level will gradually decline, and your hair will grow back normally. Sometimes a blend of natural, compounded progesterone and T3 (a thyroid hormone) prescribed by your health-care practitioner and formulated by a compounding pharmacy can be applied directly to the scalp to stimulate hair follicles. Be patient—hair growth is slow, and it may take several months before you notice a difference.

TARGETED SOLUTIONS
Targeted Diet and Nutrition Solutions

Power up on special amino acids. The amino acid cysteine is involved in maintaining hair strength, supporting liver function, and promoting keratin formation. The preferred form of supplemental cysteine is N-acetylcysteine. Also, 500 mg of methionine taken twice daily keeps hair from falling out. Essential fatty acids from flaxseeds and hemp seeds are essential to healthy hair and a deficiency can cause hair to become extremely dry and thin and can result in hair loss. A 2015 study showed that a supplement of omega-3 fats plus omega-6 and antioxidants decreased hair loss and increased hair thickness in a group of healthy women. Aim for 1 to 2 g of omega-3s daily.

Bone broth is an excellent "hair food." Its abundant minerals, amino acids, proteins, and collagen can help stimulate hair growth.

Bet on the Bs. For lustrous locks, consider 1 to 2 g of pantothenic acid (B_5), 50 to 100 mg of pyridoxine (B_6) or activated pyridoxal-5-phosphate (P5P), and 1,000 to 3,000 mcg of methylated B_{12} daily.

Bolster your biotin. Symptoms of biotin (vitamin B_7) deficiency include thinning hair, weak, brittle nails, and red and scaly skin around the eyes, nose, or mouth. Increase your biotin intake by eating organ meats (such as liver or kidney), egg yolk, nuts, legumes, mushrooms, and cauliflower. Aim for 5 mg of biotin daily.

Restore proper copper-zinc balance. If you are supplementing with zinc, strive for 45 mg of zinc daily. There is no reason to supplement copper, as there is plenty in your diet if you have a well-rounded diet. Make sure your daily multivitamin and mineral supplement is copper free, such as one available through UNI KEY Health, for which I am a nutritional consultant and brand ambassador.

Bump up your vitamin C. Vitamin C helps reduce oxidative stress, which affects hair-damaging AGEs. The recommended amount of vitamin C is 1 to 7 g daily.

Go gluten free. Celiac disease is associated with alopecia areata, which may progress to baldness; gluten intolerance is more typically marked by thinning hair.

Make MSM your friend. MSM (methylsulfonylmethane) is a sulfur-rich compound that aids keratin production. Keratin is one of the primary proteins in hair. Consider at least 1,000 mg daily.

Feed your follicles with silica. As we age, we lose silica, diminishing our once beautiful, silky hair, soft skin, and strong nails. My favorite source of silica is Alta herbal silica, which contains 500 mg of horsetail extract. I recommend one to three tablets per day. Horsetail extract can also rebuild teeth.

Depend on D. Vitamin D stimulates hair follicles to grow! Strive for 2,000 to 5,000 IU daily.

Add aloe vera to your diet regimen. Aloe vera helps reduce sebum. Sebum buildup is a common reason behind slow hair growth. Aim for 1 to 2 ounces in 4 ounces of water.

HORMONE SOLUTIONS

Consider natural DHT blockers. Several natural compounds block the conversion of testosterone into follicle-suppressing DHT. They include saw palmetto, flaxseed, licorice root, stinging nettle, EGCG, pygeum extract, and pumpkin seed oil.

STRESS SOLUTIONS

Root for rhodiola. Just 500 mg daily may help fight stress and reduce hair loss. Best to take it early in the day because it can be too stimulating for some people.

HAIR CARE SOLUTIONS

Avoid chemical-laden hair products. Shampoos, conditioners, dyes, bleaches, and perms are often loaded with harsh chemicals. Eliminate such chemicals as sodium lauryl sulfate, which corrodes hair follicles. Also be on the lookout for diethanolamine DEA and cocamide DEA, which are chemicals that can make your hair dry and unmanageable, and parabens, such as methylparaben and propylparaben, which act as estrogen-like preservatives. Avoid products that contain alcohol as an ingredient, as alcohol is exceedingly drying.

My favorite shampoo brands that are chemical-free include a brand called Seven, available at 7haircare.com. I also like Aveda, Kevin Murphy, Pureology, Chi, and Natulique Organic Hair Care.

Revere rosemary as a topical solution. One way to stimulate follicles is by applying a few drops of rosemary oil to a natural bristle brush, then brushing your hair one hundred strokes just before bed. This is also wonderfully relaxing to the muscles beneath the scalp! Alternately, massage your scalp with your fingertips moistened with a couple of drops of rosemary essential oil in a carrier oil, such as 1 tablespoon of jojoba.

LIFESTYLE SOLUTIONS

Avoid chlorinated and fluoridated water. Chlorinated and fluoridated water can lead to breakage, clogged and irritated follicles, and increased shedding. Consider installing a whole-house water filter or a water filter in your bath or shower (see Resources). Avoid overly hot showers as they can dehydrate hair and strip away oils, leading to brittleness and falling out.

Avoid hair-ravaging drugs. Ask your doctor whether you can take a more gentle alternative that may not have hair-damaging effects. Prescription drugs are notoriously unkind to hair.

Check your ferritin levels. The optimal level for both men and women is 50 to 70 ng/ml. Ask your health-care practitioner to order the test or order it yourself (see Resources).

THYROID SOLUTIONS

Check with your doctor or naturopath about safe alternatives to medications. Thyro-Key, which I helped to develop, contains a number of synergistic glandulars (see Resources). Check with your doctor or naturopath if you suspect a thyroid-related hair loss.

TARGETED STOMACH ACID SOLUTIONS

Increase stomach acid. Take the HCL challenge. Simply take a teaspoon of unpasteurized apple cider vinegar every morning before breakfast. This wakes up your digestion and lowers the pH of your stomach. If you don't have peptic ulcer disease, supplement with UNI KEY Health's HCL+2 or any HCL+2 supplement (hydrochloric acid with bile supplement) with every meal that contains fat and protein. It's best to take it before you eat, but if you forget, take it as soon as you remember.

If you took the acid test and had no burning with one capsule, then increase it to two capsules with each meal. After two days of doing this, if there's no burning, then increase to three capsules per meal. Keep increasing every couple of days until you feel a warmth or burning sensation. Your dose will be one pill *less than* the dose that gave you the burning.

If you are over age sixty-five, have had gastric surgery, or have peptic ulcer disease, then pancreatic enzyme supplementation is a must. I recommend Digesta-Key, taken with meals. If you also have joint inflammation or autoimmune disease, you can take these between meals for their anti-inflammatory properties. Do not take between meals if you have peptic ulcers.

Like glowing skin, lustrous locks are an inside job. The right nutrition, supplements, and even topical agents will go a long way in helping you take charge and bring out your best looks, and that's a good thing because we're on the way to reigniting your sex life.

CHAPTER 16

REIGNITE YOUR SEX LIFE

> **In this chapter, you'll learn . . .**
>
> - Why sex in your seventies and eighties is your natural birthright
> - How environmental chemicals interrupt hormone balance and accelerate aging
> - Why adrenal support is the backup for declining hormone output as we grow older
> - The basics on hormone replacement therapy
> - Radical ways that diet, nutrients, supplements, and lifestyle ramp up hormones

By right, we should all be enjoying sex *far* into our seventies and eighties. In most cases, age is not the real culprit behind dwindling desire; rather, it is the modern-day environment. Hormone-hijacking chemicals and industrial pollutants are flooding the body with endocrine-disrupting chemicals that can inhibit the production of all hormones, including estrogen and testosterone, upsetting our natural balance. To add insult to injury, a high-carb inflammatory diet restricts circulation, which inhibits blood flow to sexual organs. This, in turn, also restricts intimacy.

Rule #2 (Take On Toxic Overload) couldn't be more relevant when it comes to taking on your sex life. A whole new breed of endocrine-disrupting chemicals has come into use; known as *xenoestrogens*, these chemical imposters mimic estrogen in the body. Poisonous infiltrators are spearheading a continual assault on your health in the form of pesticides, plastics, solvents, automobile exhaust, industrial chemicals, food additives, and environmental pollutants. Xenoestrogens are a thousand times more potent than the body's natural estrogen, meaning your liver has to work overtime to eliminate them. Even in the smallest doses, they can wreak havoc with your natural estrogen receptors, and this results in a slew of hormone-driven symptoms, such as diminished sex drive, depression, headaches, brain fog, and accumulation of unwanted body fat that can make us feel less than desirable and that can dampen anyone's sex drive.

But even if your desire is intact, you may find your sexual response and sensitivity are not what they once were. You're less easily aroused and find yourself less sensitive to your partner's touch. Age-related changes in peripheral nerves, blood vessels, and muscle tissue may play a role. Individuals with diabetes or neurological disease may have similar nerve damage affecting their sexual response. Fatigue, from hypothyroidism or insomnia and other sleep problems, or from depression, may be a contributing factor. Taking steps to correct these conditions may be all that is needed to get your juices flowing again.

About 70 percent of healthy seventy-year-olds remain sexually active, and there are a variety of ways you can also. Consider, for example, that a strong pelvic floor improves sexual performance. And the pelvic floor is exactly what it sounds like. It is quite literally a floor of muscle that spreads across the bottom of your pelvic bones, stretching like a trampoline from the pubic bone to the tailbone and from side to side. Strong pelvic floor muscles support the bladder, bowel, and uterus in women and help stabilize the hip joints.

In women, a lack of libido can also be related to vaginal dryness that causes discomfort and lack of response, as well as low testosterone levels. Even the use of sedatives, antihistamines, or other commonly prescribed drugs can dry vaginal tissue. As levels of estrogen decline, the vaginal walls begin to lose their elasticity and become drier and thinner. Mucus secretions from the cervix also decrease, and the vagina itself shrinks, becoming shorter and narrower. The tissues of the bladder and urethra also become more sensitive. These changes may cause pain during intercourse and lead us to wonder whether our days of sexual pleasure are over. Luckily, many things can be done to help you become the radically sexy and sensual goddess you are meant to be throughout life!

For men, *the* leading sexual dysfunction is impotence, which literally means "no strength." Two major factors that contribute to impotence: circulatory insufficiency and hormonal disorders. Circulatory insufficiency is the most common cause of impotence in men. Arteriosclerotic plaque on the walls of penile arteries can result in diminished blood supply to the penis. Clearly, keeping the arteries free of plaque is not only good for the heart, it's also good for sexual performance. For optimal sexual functioning, the adrenal glands in both sexes, as well as testicular function in men, must be supported.

ADRENAL POWER

As we age, nature doesn't simply turn off our hormones and expect us to compensate with synthetic hormone replacement therapy. A natural backup system is in place, consisting of the adrenal glands and our own body fat, both designed to make up for the declining hormone output.

The adrenals also work in tandem with the thyroid to maintain the body's energy levels, and surplus energy is exactly what you are after for peak sexual performance. However, the years of enduring the stress of modern-day living severely compromise the ability of this secondary system to function at optimal levels. When the adrenals burn out, so does your sex drive. If you're tired when you get up and spend the better part of your day spiking your overworked adrenal glands with caffeine, nicotine, and sugar just to get through another day, there's not much energy left to spike you into sexual action in the evening.

Underproduction of thyroid hormones, known as hypothyroidism, can also lead to fatigue and loss of libido. Again, the lack of energy necessary for peak sexual performance and enjoyment is missing in anyone suffering from hypothyroidism.

SEX DE-STRESSES STRESS

A fulfilling sex life enhances physical, as well as emotional, health. Sex is just plain good for us. Plus, as a bonus, sex helps relieve stress. By doing so, it may also enhance the body's immune function. The stress response involves a reduction in T cell count and beta endorphin levels. T cells are immune cells that fight off invading germs or other foreign bodies. Endorphins are brain chemicals that help us tune out pain. They're produced in large numbers during strenuous exercise and during sex. When stress is reduced, endorphin and T cell production increase. Therefore, by alleviating stress, sexual activity can enhance immunity and reduce pain. The increased endorphin production that results from sexual activity may explain why it tends to relieve back pain and arthritis. In addition to blocking pain, endorphins also produce feelings of euphoria and exhilaration.

HORMONE THERAPY PRIMER

Hormones virtually influence everything we think, feel, and do. Despite that, we really don't know much about their intricate workings. The key is to figure out what is "just right" in the most effective forms to defy aging while sustaining energy, maintaining a healthy libido, and feeling an overall sense of well-being. Simply put, we need to restore our hormones to more youthful levels so as to reverse declining hormones as we age, and we need to know how to do it safely.

Regardless of how complicated it may seem; hormone replacement therapy is unquestionably one of the best age-defying strategies. Let's unravel the seemingly mysterious world of hormones because the more you understand, the better you'll be able to utilize them to offset aging.

BIOIDENTICAL HORMONE THERAPY

"Bioidentical" hormones—hormones precisely identical to those found in the human body rather than synthetic hormones extracted from horse urine—include estrogens, progesterone, and testosterone. Bioidentical hormones are becoming increasingly popular because they are considered safer and more effective than the synthetic version. Derived from such plants as wild yams and soybeans, these plant molecules are converted in the lab to testosterone, estrogen, and progesterone. Today, bioidenticals come in many different shapes, sizes, and delivery systems. There are creams, pills, patches, lozenges (sublinguals, such as troches), gels, injections, and pellets. While all these choices are good news for the consumer, they are definitely bad news for Big Pharma. Pharmaceutical companies can't patent bioidentical hormones so there has been a lot of unfounded negative publicity surrounding them.

TESTOSTERONE

Testosterone is the master hormone of desire, or the assertive hormone. It's what gives you your zest and drive. As the principle hormone in the androgen hormone group, it is most often associated with men, though it serves key functions in both sexes. This powerful sex regulator governs sex drive, bone mass, fat distribution, muscle size and strength, and red blood cell production. It also is important for heart health, cognitive function, and overall well-being. And it starts to drop by 1 to 2 percent each year, beginning at age thirty, for both sexes.

In men, "low T" is characterized by erectile dysfunction, libido drop, and weight gain. Without enough testosterone, putting on (and keeping) that lean body mass is much more difficult. In women, flabby muscles, low sex drive, and even osteoporosis can result. Adding insult to injury, low testosterone can also create overall weakness, stiffness, pain, nervous exhaustion, irritability, and profuse sweating, with intolerance to heat. Thankfully, all these conditions and symptoms of low testosterone can easily be resolved.

ESTROGEN

When your estrogen is in balance, it's magic, helping your libido, your complexion, and your brain, and enabling you to feel calm and in focus. We commonly think of estrogen as a single hormone, but it is actually a group of hormones: estrone (E1), estradiol (E2), and estriol (E3). Both sexes produce these various versions of estrogen:

Estrone (E1). The only estrogen the female body makes after menopause; when in excess, estrone has been linked to both endometrial and breast cancer. Low levels of estrone may lead to the development of osteoporosis, and symptoms include fatigue, low libido, and depression.

Estradiol (E2). The most potent of the three estrogens, it's the most common type in women of childbearing age. Although estradiol treatment can be useful as hormone replacement therapy after menopause, the side effects may cause breast tenderness and/or weight gain, and an increased risk of uterine cancers.

Estriol (E3). The weakest form of estrogen in the body, it is known as the anticancer estrogen. Evidence suggests that estriol offers many of the benefits of traditional estrogen-replacement therapies without significantly increasing the risk of breast or ovarian cancer. When taken for more than ten years as a topical treatment, estriol can induce potent antiaging effects. Women using estriol therapy found that it demonstrated remarkable improvement in vaginal dryness as well as improvement in skin quality.

Estrogen deserves credit for serving many functions in maintaining health. It acts as a powerful antioxidant that fends off the growing number of precarious free radicals trying to harm your DNA. Estrogen receptors line the blood vessels, contributing to that rosy, vibrant glow you want by guarding arterial linings, so blood can move along without being impeded. It also helps lower LDL and raise HDL cholesterol levels.

Estrogen also aids in collagen production to keep your skin firm and toned as it supports hyaluronic acid production for moisture-rich skin. Besides giving your bladder tissues elasticity, estrogen has receptors in your bone to enhance your body's use of calcium and to reduce loose teeth, cavities, and soft bones. In salivary hormone testing, estrogen should be in a 30:1 ratio in favor of progesterone. Your estriol levels should be more dominant, typically in an 8:1 ratio over the other two estrogens.

The breaking down process of estradiol into estrone and estrogen metabolites helps the body to maintain estrogen balance. Among the hundreds of jobs of your hardworking liver is to inactivate unneeded estrogen and expel it from the body through the bile, urine, and stool. That's why congested bile and poor digestion can contribute to estrogen dominance.

Adequate estrogen is also a surprising weight-loss catalyst. When your estrogen levels are low, the body cannot synthesize choline, a key slimming nutrient that produces low-density lipoprotein, which escorts fat out of the liver.

PROGESTERONE

Progesterone counters excess estrogen's negative and often irritating side effects. Progesterone is touted as the feel-good hormone because it is up to twenty times more concentrated in the brain than in the bloodstream. Low levels of progesterone are associated with bone thinning, excess facial hair in women, and male-pattern baldness in men. Progesterone is vital for regulating the sleep cycle, as well as boosting immunity and brain function. So, it's no surprise that an imbalance of progesterone can lead to classic symptoms associated with aging, such as "brain fog," mood swings, and a decreased quality (and quantity) of sleep.

As a natural antidepressant and diuretic, progesterone helps stabilize blood sugar levels and for women can prevent those whiskers on your chin. If you've ever wished for a "magic bullet" for your hormone woes, you'll be glad to know that natural progesterone could be your answer. Progesterone is deficient in practically *every* female I test from age eighteen to eighty. Many women simply aren't producing enough in their body because they lack the nutrient precursors zinc and vitamin B_6.

Without sufficient progesterone, the adrenal cortex can secrete the androgen hormone androstenedione as an alternative chemical. This steroid is associated with some male characteristics, one of which is male-pattern baldness. When your progesterone level is raised, your androstenedione level will gradually decline.

Progesterone also contributes to activating osteoblasts, those bone builders critical for a strong stature and graceful appearance. Keeping progesterone in a 300:1 ratio with estrogen is vital. When you have a balance of progesterone in your system, you should have a sense of tranquility and experience less anger and irritability, so common with excess amounts of estrogen.

DEHYDROEPIANDROSTERONE (DHEA)

The adrenal cortex makes small amounts of all the sex hormones but makes large amounts of dehydroepiandrosterone (DHEA) in both men and women. DHEA is intimately tied to the metabolic processes that yield progesterone, estrogen, testosterone, and cortisol. Cholesterol is the originating molecule for all these compounds, including pregnenolone (the grandmother of corticosteroid hormones) and DHEA (the mother of corticosteroid hormones).

Taking nonprescription doses of DHEA or pregnenolone is claimed to confer all kinds of health benefits on users, including protection against aging, burning muscle pain, depression, fatigue, stress, diabetes, lupus, and cancer. The problem with taking *high-dose* DHEA and pregnenolone is that they are hormones involved in little-known biochemical interactions, which means that each has a wealth of potential side effects. The most serious potential side effect is the stimulation of breast cancer because DHEA can raise estrogen levels.

This is why some individuals elect to boost the adrenal glands that secrete these hormones in lieu of taking DHEA.

HUMAN GROWTH HORMONE (HGH)

Human growth hormone (HGH) is secreted by the pituitary gland and plays a crucial role as we age. It is most known for the spurring of growth in both children and adolescents, but there is increasing interest in supplementing with this hormone to decrease the negative effects of aging. HGH strengthens bone density, helps build muscle mass, repair muscle tissue, and is the great white shark of fat burners. HGH also reverses the hormone dihydrotestosterone (DHT), a more potent form of testosterone, often the culprit for thinning gray hair in both sexes, and stimulates the production of growth factors, amino acids, and nutrients—raw materials for the growth of hair from the hair follicles. Symptoms of low HGH include anxiety, depression, low libido, high body fat, muscle loss, and high blood pressure. HGH supplementation is available in sprays, gels, and homeopathic forms.

TARGETED SOLUTIONS
Testing Solutions

When you know what your hormone levels are, you can then seek targeted and appropriate treatment, if you need it, on an individualized basis. The test result also gives you a baseline with which later test results can be compared, so you can monitor your hormone levels over time. Although any individual hormone level can test in the "normal" range, it is your complete hormonal profile that tells the story. You need to work with a knowledgeable health-care practitioner and test your hormones at least every three months. If you can't commit to that, then don't start.

Seek salivary hormone testing. Saliva testing is often considered more convenient than blood testing for establishing accurate hormone level baselines and determining changes in hormone replacement therapy (HRT). When testing for hormones with a salivary hormone test, aim for these optimally healthy ranges:

→ Ratio of progesterone to estradiol. It is most optimal at 30:1 for relief of such symptoms as weight gain, irritability, anxiety, hot flashes, and night sweats.

→ Progesterone levels. Low levels can result in premature aging, bone loss, and weight gain. Ideal level for both men and women is 5 to 95 pg/ml.

→ **Estradiol levels.** High amounts can result in mood swings, memory fog, and anxiety. Ideal range for women is 1 to 4 pg/ml; ideal range for men is 5 to 25 pg/ml.

→ **Testosterone levels.** Important for healthy libido, energy levels, and forming lean muscles. Ideal levels for adults: borderline 6 to 9 pg/ml, normal 10 to 38 pg/ml.

→ **DHEA levels.** Significant in memory function of postmenopausal women. Ideal range for adults: 3 to 10 g/ml.

→ **Morning cortisol levels.** Important as a stress indicator. Ideal range for adults: 13 to 24 nM.

→ **Blood tests can also give a snapshot view of your hormones.** Aim for these optimally healthy ranges:

  → Estradiol 50 to 100 pg/ml
  → Progesterone 1.4 to 2.0 ng/ml
  → Testosterone 270 to 1,070 ng/dl
  → DHEA 160 to 250 ug/dl

DIET AND NUTRIENT SOLUTIONS

Eat to increase sexual satisfaction. The Radical Longevity Program focuses on warming foods rather than cooling foods. Warming foods are believed to nourish sexual energy and support the organs that govern sexual vitality. The plan's ample section of beans, green leafy vegetables, and seeds (such as hemp and flax) also feed sexual energy. These contain the germ of life and are an excellent source of zinc, which is a precursor to progesterone and is found in abundance in seminal fluids. Seafood, especially oysters, are another prime zinc-rich food. Artichokes and mushrooms, which appear in many of the recipes, have been noted to have aphrodisiac properties, most likely due to their high level of phytonutrients. The plan's signature staples (e.g., the Longevity Blaster and the Cranberry Elixir, pages 131 and 132) contain such spices as cinnamon, ginger, and cardamom, which are considered to be aphrodisiacs due to their warming and gentle stimulating nature.

Feast on the right kinds of fats. The omega-6 fats, as detailed in Rule #5: Activate Cellular Rejuvenation, help balance your hormones and keep them in check by producing prostaglandins that regulate sexual response. Insufficient prostaglandins due to lack of the omega-6 essential fatty acid can result in sexual dysfunction. Along with the plan's hemp seed oil, black currant seed oil, evening primrose oil, and borage oil are all excellent sources of gamma linoleic acid (GLA). They provide specific fatty acids that produce heightened sexual response. Spirulina is also rich in GLA and is an excellent source of complete and highly digestible protein. It has been used to treat decreased libido and impotency. Omega-6 is vitally important to both your metabolism and the health of your cell membranes. Our cellular membranes are embedded with thousands of hormone receptors. When these membranes become damaged by processed fats, the hormone receptors also become damaged.

Continue to love your liver. Do keep in mind how important it is to support your liver so that it can produce enough quality bile, which is necessary to transport excess hormones out of the body. Liver-healing foods are found throughout my Radical Longevity Program precisely because of this.

Power up with potent vitamins and minerals. Some of your most powerful allies for sexual vitality are vitamins and minerals, including vitamins A, C, and E and manganese, selenium, and zinc. Many of the proteins, fruits, and vegetables in the plan include excellent sources of all these nutrients, which help in a variety of ways to improve sexual function. Vitamin A is richly found in yellow fruits and vegetables, fish, and dairy products. The best food sources for vitamin B complex are the legumes while foods rich in vitamin C include broccoli, citrus, fruits, and berries. Good food sources of vitamin E are sweet potatoes, organ meats, and cold-pressed oils. Nuts and seeds are rich in manganese; selenium is found in nuts, sesame seeds, and fish. Zinc is an incredibly important mineral for sexual prowess. It is vital to both the production of progesterone and testosterone. The ability to absorb zinc declines with age. Besides being in seafood, it is found in mushrooms, eggs, soybeans, and seeds, especially pumpkin. All these nutrients also support the adrenal and thyroid glands for optimal sexual functioning.

ADRENAL AND THYROID SOLUTIONS

Shake MORE salt. Yes, you read that right. Most of us are sodium deficient and the right type of sodium, such as Celtic and Himalayan salt, can support adrenal function and help your body better cope with stress. It is recommended to take ¼ teaspoon of salt in ½ cup of warm water first thing in the morning.

Sip an adrenal cocktail. I have recommended this for years for my overstressed and overworked clients. Mix together 4 ounces of freshly squeezed orange juice, ¼ teaspoon cream of tartar, and ¼ teaspoon of Celtic sea salt.

Bottoms up! The need for vitamin C skyrockets while under stress. Cream of tartar is rich in potassium and works as a blood cleanser to decrease toxic load and nourish the adrenals. The sea salt is an important electrolyte, which are often depleted in stressed individuals with tired adrenals.

Lights out. Try to be in bed by ten p.m. when your cortisol levels diminish to their lowest levels (three hours after sunset), and to give muscle-building growth hormone a fighting chance to properly release.

Go barefoot. Going barefoot on your lawn or at the beach for at least fifteen minutes a day can help your body get grounded. When you are grounded, you discharge chaotic energies and absorb healing electrons from Mother Nature, soothing adrenal exhaustion and inflammation.

Get the chill pill. Magnesium is your tranquilizer in a bottle. It combats anxiety and stress-related symptoms in both the body and the mind. Notoriously deficient as we grow older, it works in tandem with vitamin B_6.

TESTOSTERONE SOLUTIONS

Who needs Viagra? A variety of herbs have been shown to enhance libido, primarily by stimulating testosterone production. Try to find formulas that include one or more of these ingredients: damiana, horny goat weed, yohimbe, *Mucuna pruriens*, and *Tribulus terrestris*.

Go for ginseng. The testosterone-booster *Panax ginseng* taken over a period of three months can significantly thicken the vaginal mucosal lining. Women have reported no discomfort during sexual intercourse as well as the end of vaginal dryness. The dosage is suggested at 100 mg of a standardized ginseng extract, taken three times daily.

Seek saw palmetto oil. Saw palmetto is a remarkable supplement best known to support prostate health, but it can also even out testosterone. It is filled with beneficial fatty acids and contains chlorophyll, lutein, and lycopene. I recommend a dose of 320 mg per day.

ESTROGEN SOLUTIONS

Eat your estrogen. Flaxseeds help modulate estrogen and can balance either high or low levels. Take 1 to 2 tablespoons of flaxseeds daily.

Vary your veggies. The Radical Longevity Plan's recommended cruciferous vegetables, such as Brussels sprouts, cabbage, cauliflower, broccoli, and kale, contain compounds called indoles that help facilitate estrogen metabolism.

The product dindolylmethane (DIM) can help remove both xenoestrogens and excess estrogens from the system. I suggest 200 to 300 mg daily.

Consider the trifecta of choline, methionine, and inositol. At a dose of 500 mg each per meal, these three lipotropic superstars break down estrogen in the liver to nontoxic estriol. With the proper balance, these powerful B vitamins can accelerate fat burning, as well as decongest a fatty liver.

Fill up on fiber. Aim for at least 35 g a day from your veggies, nuts, seeds, and legumes. Fiber ties up excess estrogens and escorts them out of the system.

Rescue hormones with helpful phytoestrogenetic herbs. Red clover, ginseng, black cohosh, hawthorn berries, wild yam root, chasteberry (*Vitex agnus-castus*), and licorice root all have strong, estrogen-like qualities. Try a blend of Ayurvedic herbs, such as haritaki (a rich source of vitamin C, which also acts as an adaptogen and rejuvenator), licorice, and shatavari (well known as a natural source of estrogen).

Get rid of environmental estrogen mimics. Avoid personal care products that contain endocrine disruptors, such as parabens phthalates. Use glass instead of plastic, waxed paper instead of plastic wrap. Wash your hands after handling gas, cash register, or ATM receipts, which have surprisingly been found to contain high levels of BPA.

PROGESTERONE SOLUTIONS

Balance estrogen with progesterone. This will improve libido, enhance the immune system, increase hair on the scalp, elevate the metabolic rate with resulting weight loss, act as a natural diuretic, boost the thyroid, and stimulate the production of bone, while relaxing smooth muscles and promoting the strength of the myelin sheath. I personally prefer the use of transdermal creams, which can bypass the liver. A bioidentical progesterone cream can help thwart hormonal weight gain, revive vitality, and spark your sex drive by balancing your progesterone/estrogen levels. Look for products that contain the recommended 20 mg of natural USP progesterone from wild yam. Women find it helpful to mimic the natural cycle by taking it from the twelfth to the twenty-fifth day of the calendar month, along with some natural estrogen. Note: As therapeutic as progesterone can be for most women, it may be contraindicated for some. Please check with your healthcare practitioner to be sure it's right for you.

DHEA SOLUTIONS

Get a DHEA boost. Pregnenolone may be helpful as a supplement to your diet because it is a hormonal precursor to DHEA. Once daily with a meal, take 5 mg of pregnenolone along with 5 mg of biotin, which will optimize the conversion of this "mother hormone." You can also try a DHEA supplement. The dosage is anywhere from 5 to 50 mg per day. It is important to go slowly when starting this supplement. Cut back if you experience palpitations or facial hair growth (especially if you are a female).

PRACTICE THESE PLEASURE PRINCIPLES

Use it or lose it. Regular intercourse helps increase blood flow to the vaginal tissues, which improves tone and natural lubrication. Older women who have remained sexually active throughout their lives seem to have fewer problems with vaginal dryness. Loving, relaxed foreplay can increase natural secretions, and the use of unscented lubricants, such as MoisturePom, a natural personal lubricant that contains pomegranate extracts and soothing oils (see Resources), pure aloe gel, vitamin E oil, or even borage oil during foreplay can reduce irritation and pain. Natural progesterone cream applied directly to the vagina can help dryness dramatically. A sensitive, patient lover can be a woman's best friend. Women without sexual partners can use self-stimulation to promote vaginal secretions and reduce dryness.

Take sex to a new level with niacin. Niacin (vitamin B_3) is used to dilate blood vessels, which improves arousal in both women and men. Proper blood flow and circulation in the genitals is necessary for arousal and heightened pleasure. Start slowly at 250 mg at bedtime, then increase gradually to 1 to 2 g daily in divided doses. The form best tolerated is inositol hexanicotinate. Endur-acin, a slow-acting, time-released niacin, is typically available in three strengths—250 mg, 500 mg, and 750 mg—for easy compliance for those that need higher amounts.

Prime your pelvic floor. A massage tool known as the Serenity TMT (see Resources) can help stretch the pelvic floor muscle and release trigger points. This tool can aid in abating bladder, bowel, and sexual dysfunction symptoms while relieving pressure or pain related to the pelvic girdle, tailbone, or genitalia. Kegel exercises can help strengthen the pelvic floor. To identify the right muscles, stop urinating midstream. You just used your pelvic floor muscles! To do Kegels, the Mayo Clinic suggests you contract your pelvic floor, keep it contracted for five seconds, then release and relax the muscles for five seconds. Do this for four or five repetitions. Over time, build up to ten-second periods of pelvic floor contraction, followed by a ten-second period of relaxation.

Enhance the encounter. The sense of smell can be stimulated by the use of essential oils. Aphrodisiac oils include jasmine, ylang-ylang, cinnamon, aniseed, clove buds, ginger, nutmeg, peppermint, pepper, and rose. Drops of these oils can be placed onto the mattress. To further enhance the aromasphere, orange, magenta, and purple decor are said to increase arousal.

The PRP "O-shot" solution for female sexual dysfunction. The PRP Orgasm Shot (O-shot) is a safe, drugless procedure in which one's own platelet-rich plasma is injected in the female genitalia area. Treatments are long lasting, often up to two years. Women who have had the procedure report improved urinary control along with an increase in sexual drive, natural lubrication, and stronger orgasms. Consult your gynecologist or local medi-spa for recommendations.

ThermiVa is a radiofrequency treatment for women. This painless treatment essentially warms the vaginal tissues in a way that induces the tissue to produce and remodel collagen, which firms and strengthens your soft tissues, including those that support the bladder. It remodels the shape and structure of the entire vaginal area and improves blood flow, which in turn improves nerve sensation and perception of both sexual pleasure and the signal for urination. There are typically three treatments that last up to thirty minutes in length, and there's no downtime afterward, so you can resume normal activities immediately following. Once you finish the three initial treatments, a yearly maintenance treatment is often recommended. Consult your gynecologist or health-care practitioner for recommendations.

A satisfying sex life can enhance all aspects of health. When you attain balance in your diet and lifestyle, you restore your body's homeostasis, which ultimately leads to a positive attitude, a fit body, and nurturing intimacy. You've learned how radical longevity can make a dramatic difference in many areas of your life, and believe it or not, there are even more leading-edge enhancements to explore in the next chapter.

CHAPTER 17

TAKING IT TO THE NEXT LEVEL

> **In this chapter, you'll learn . . .**
>
> - Why your biology is not your biography
> - The keys to prolonging the longevity of your cells
> - About safe stem cell therapy you can do in the privacy of your own home
> - Why PRP is an incredible healing elixir for your skin, hair, joints, muscles, and tissues

HERE'S THE THING ABOUT AGING: THE SCARY STATISTICS SHOW THAT AFTER YOU turn sixty, your risk of dying doubles every eight years, so by the time you turn sixty-eight years old, your risk of dying is double what it was when you were sixty, and your risk of dying at seventy-six years old is double what it was at sixty-eight years, and so on. The snowball of changes happening in your life are happening at the cell level as well. Over time, through toxin buildup, glycation, and other factors, your DNA gets damaged, presenting as shortened telomeres, which eventually lead to genetic mutations, malfunctions, diseases, and even death.

But you can stop that snowball before it even starts and get things going in the right direction. In this chapter, we'll go over exactly what your cells need in their environment to thrive and keep your body humming along with drugless solutions, from stimulating your own stem cells to groundbreaking new research on powerful cell level antioxidants.

YOUR GENES ARE NOT YOUR DESTINY

Good or bad, your genes are set in stone. Fortunately, all you've inherited is the *potential* for disease or health. The bottom line is that, despite what you've previously been taught, your genes are not your destiny. Your environment, both inside your cells and outside your body, plays a major role in your gene expression; this is called *epigenetics*. Changing your environment reprograms your DNA for health and radiance, no matter how many years you have under your belt.

GENETIC IMPOSTERS

A young woman who was recently married decided to make a roast to impress her new husband. She carefully cut both ends off the roast before placing it in the roasting pan. Curious, her husband asked her why she did that. She replied that it was the way her mother had always done it. She called her mother and asked her why she cut the ends off her roasts. Her mother explained to her that was the way *her* mother had always done it. When she asked her grandmother why she did it, her grandmother explained that the roasts never fit in the only roasting pan she owned, so she cut the ends off to fit it into the pan.

This example isn't just about the roast. It's about the lifestyle choices and habits that are often handed down for generations without being questioned. When they're unhealthy enough to cause illness and disease, it's assumed the disease was inherited and genetic, which simply isn't the case. For instance, only 5 to 10 percent of all cancers are genetic, which implies that the answers are found in the environment of the cells.

FIND YOUR TRIGGERS

The science of epigenetics says, "If genes load the gun, then environment pulls the trigger." With over eighty-three thousand chemicals in our environment, and only about two hundred of them being studied according to the Environmental Protection Agency's (EPA) standards, it comes as no surprise that there are plenty of triggers for unhealthy aging and disease we unknowingly come in contact with every day.

Stories abound of communities riddled with cancers that have discovered they were built on toxic sites, and the water they drink and bathe in is contaminated with cancer-causing chemicals. The food we rely on to feed our families is being sprayed with chemicals that cause cancer and autoimmune diseases. There are chemicals in every household product, from furniture to toothpaste, that are known to cause cancers, autoimmune diseases, and other "incurables."

The environment your cells are in is affected by your total toxin load, nutrient deficiencies, cellular pH, how much you sleep and exercise, how negative or positive your thoughts are, how much stress you are under (and for how long), and many other factors that can lead to premature aging and chronic diseases that have no known cure. It's up to each of us to find our triggers, disarm them, and reprogram our DNA.

ARE TELOMERES THE KEY TO RADICAL LONGEVITY?

At the heart of every cell in your body is its nucleus, where your genetic code is stored in the form of double-stranded DNA molecules called chromosomes. At the end of each of these chromosomes are your telomeres, which tell us a lot about how well we are aging.

Telomeres are like caps at the end of chromosomes that keep them from fraying or sticking to one another, which would damage or lose valuable genetic information. Each time a cell divides, the telomeres get shorter. Think of a wick on a candle; when it gets too short, it can no longer do its job. When telomeres get too short, the cell can no longer divide, so it becomes inactive or dies. The shorter your telomeres, the higher your risk of unhealthy aging, chronic diseases, such as cancer, and even death. According to research by geneticist Richard Cawthon from the University of Utah, people over age sixty with shortened telomeres are three times more likely to die from heart disease and eight times more likely to die from infectious diseases than are those with longer telomeres.

But how do we preserve our telomeres? One promising option may be with encouraging production of an enzyme called telomerase. This enzyme adds length to the ends of telomeres and protects them from wear.

Telomerase seems to be a double-edged sword, however. After a cell becomes cancerous, it protects itself by making more telomerase enzyme, so it can continue to grow quickly without shortening its telomeres. Scientists are looking at measuring telomerase as a way to detect cancer and are looking at ways to block its activity to encourage cancer cells to die. The unfortunate and dangerous side effects of this type of therapy include premature aging, impaired fertility, slow wound healing, and inhibition of the production of blood cells and immune system cells. Interestingly, when researchers have taken normal cells and caused them to divide beyond their normal limits while giving them ample amounts of telomerase, these cells don't become cancerous.

When chronological age, telomere length, and gender (women statistically live longer than men) are factored in together, it turns out that these combined factors only account for 37 percent of the increased death risk. The other 63 percent is found in the environment.

Scientists believe that chronological age, telomere shortening, gene mutation expression, AGEs, and oxidative stress from free radicals all work together to cause unhealthy aging and premature death. So, it follows that as we change our diet and cooking methods to reduce AGEs and eliminate as many environmental toxins as we can, and supplement with powerful antioxidants, we can naturally increase telomerase and protect our DNA from damage.

STEM CELLS—YOUR BODY'S OWN DNA DAMAGE CONTROL

Your body is constantly renewing and repairing itself, and much of that process is thanks to stem cells. Stem cells have unlimited potential and can be used to build a variety of different tissues, depending on what your body needs at the time. We are focusing only on adult stem cells because they are the focus of the safe, natural therapies available to us for at-home use.

Adult stem cells are made throughout your life, but production slows down as you get older. These cells are undifferentiated and basically lying dormant, waiting until your body calls them into action for a specific purpose.

Once your body calls on the stem cells for a specific purpose, they begin growing and dividing indefinitely, turning into whatever tissue is needed. Scientists have found evidence of stem cells in the brain, liver, skin, muscles, bone marrow, blood, and blood vessels. They heal your skin wounds, and they can even regenerate an entire organ!

WHY I AVOID THE STEM CELL CONTROVERSY

As research into stem cell therapies grows, the controversy around them deepens. The oldest controversy is around embryonic stem cells because harvesting these cells means a fertilized egg cannot continue to develop into a fetus. Once the stem cells are harvested, researchers often put them into animals, which is another ethical issue. These are the reasons why, in many countries, it is illegal to produce embryonic stem cell lines, and why I don't endorse pursuing these avenues.

Some stem cell therapies are expensive, ineffective, illegal, or even dangerous. A variety of antiaging treatments derived from stem cells claim to be the "fountain of youth." I cannot emphasize enough the importance of doing your own research into the safety and effectiveness of those types of therapies, none of which I endorse in this book.

What I see as being most beneficial is to naturally encourage the production of your body's own adult stem cells. Fortunately, this is a process that is safe, effective, and relatively inexpensive. Changing what you eat, how you eat, and taking nutritional supplements nourishes and stimulates your body to heal itself, without risk or harm.

PRP—THE FUTURE OF RESTORATIVE THERAPY

Platelet-rich plasma (PRP) is an exciting new therapy to repair damaged tissues and rejuvenate sagging, wrinkled skin and much more. PRP can repair your joints and relieve back and neck pain—without invasive surgery. Professional athletes are using it to heal from sports injuries at a much faster rate than they would with surgery. Studies show its effectiveness with arthritis, inflamed tendons, torn muscles, injured ligaments, damaged joint cartilage, degenerated disks, and knee osteoarthritis. To me, this isn't even the most exciting part.

There are stem cells circulating in your blood that are captured in PRP that produce high levels of the telomerase enzyme, making it available to the tissues that need them the most.

A small amount of your own blood is drawn, and the tube is placed in a centrifuge to spin it to separate out the red blood cells. What's left is plasma with a high concentration of platelets. As you may be aware, platelets are your blood clotting factors, but they also have another important function. Platelets are rich in about seven different human growth factors, which are critical for repairing wounded tissues. When platelets congregate around an injured area, they attract stem cells, which go to work multiplying at a rapid pace to repair and rejuvenate the damaged tissue.

METHYLATION AND MTHFR MUTATION

Methylation is a big deal; every cell in your body uses it. It's how we repair our damaged cells, process toxins and hormones, keep our DNA healthy, break down and use B vitamins, help the liver to process fats, activate and regulate our immune systems, reduce inflammation, and balance our neurotransmitter levels. Methylene tetrahydrofolate reductase (MTHFR) is an enzyme that is critical for proper methylation.

It is estimated that more than 40 percent of the world's population has at least one MTHFR gene mutation. When the MTHFR gene is mutated and switched on, it affects how well every cell in your body is able to get rid of toxins and repair itself, and whether each cell is able to fight off disease. The more MTHFR mutations you have, the less the MTHFR enzyme is able to do its job, and the more this can negatively impact your health. Depending on how many MTHFR gene mutations you have, your body's ability to detoxify can be impaired by as much as 90 percent.

MTHFR gene defects also have been linked to more than sixty different chronic health conditions, including heart disease, Alzheimer's, depression, blood clotting disorders, birth defects, thyroid diseases, and certain cancers. In the past two decades, the MTHFR gene mutation has been studied for its role in more than six hundred medical disorders. But just because you've been tested and found to have these gene mutations, doesn't mean you'll get these diseases. Changing your cellular environment for the better can change the expression of these gene mutations, effectively muting them or turning them off completely.

THERE'S NO METHYLATION "MAGIC PILL"

Simply having the gene doesn't mean you're in hot water with your health. However, just supplementing with missing vitamins used in methylation doesn't keep you from having the MTHFR gene mutations switched on. There's no magic pill for gene expression.

As MTHFR knowledge has grown, so has misinformation. Countless articles have been published saying it's just folate (vitamin B_9), vitamin B_{12}, vitamin B_6, or riboflavin (vitamin B_2) deficiency, and that getting your levels of these vitamins back to normal will solve the whole problem. While it is true that methylation defects are associated with deficiencies in these vitamins, it doesn't address the underlying reasons for those deficiencies.

If your diet is the reason for the vitamin deficiencies, then you'll also be low in zinc, magnesium, and other minerals essential for proper methylation, not to mention the essential fats needed to rebuild healthy cells. You may also have a high enough toxic load from not being able to detoxify that a cleanse is needed to relieve the toxic burden from your liver and your cells before methylation can take place normally.

TARGETED SOLUTIONS
Diet and Supplement Solutions

Rescue your DNA with resveratrol. We're taking another look here at resveratrol through the lens of DNA. This potent plant antioxidant has been found to slow—or even stop—the progression of Alzheimer's disease in some people. It works by preventing damage to the DNA of brain cells. Resveratrol also reduces the inflammation associated with heart disease and protects the heart and brain during episodes of oxygen deprivation, including heart attack or stroke. Resveratrol works by activating your own antiaging genes, notably the sirtuin 1 DNA repair survival gene.

The big issue is that most resveratrol on the market today has limited (or no) bioavailability in humans. However, according to the results of a twelve-week study published in *Experimental Gerontology*, Longevinex "activates nine-fold more longevity genes than plain resveratrol." When taking Longevinex, a dose of 100 mg per day is recommended (see Resources).

Enjoy the benefits of resveratrol and red wine. Resveratrol is a thousandfold more concentrated in red wine than in grape juice because of fermentation. When selecting red wine, be sure to select only organic, pesticide-free wines.

Give a nod to NAD, the coenzyme you can't live without. Nicotinamide adenine dinucleotide (NAD) delivers the energy released from glucose and fatty acids to your mitochondria. New research shows that NAD fuels the activity of sirtuins and has a unique ability to protect tissues, induce DNA repair, and increase life span. One of the easiest ways to naturally boost NAD levels is exercise, as it induces our muscles to produce more mitochondria. Intermittent fasting as well as eating such foods as fish, cremini mushrooms, and green vegetables are other ways to increase your NAD levels.

Astragalus is awesome for graceful aging. Researchers have discovered that an extract of astragalus, used in Traditional Chinese medicine for centuries, is now used in longevity medicine due to its ability to turn on telomerase activity, thereby effectively lengthening the shorter telomeres. The supplement I like best is Astragaloside IV (AG-IV), with a recommended dose of one capsule once or twice daily.

Protect your telomeres with EGCG. Green tea extract (EGCG) protects telomere length and cell damage by hunting down free radicals. Suggested dosage is 250 to 500 mg daily.

Give yourself a cellular tune-up with antioxidants. As you now know, a major cause of unhealthy aging is still oxidative stress. Look to foods and supplements rich in antioxidants, such as colorful fruits, vegetables, non-irradiated spices, and even mold-free organic coffee. Once again, be sure to avoid processed foods, sugar, flour, trans fats, and grains.

Prevent cell death with NAC. N-acetylcystein (NAC) prevents cell death by activating glutathione and the human telomerase gene. Suggested dosage is 1,800 to 2,400 mg daily.

Guard your telomeres with alpha-tocopherol. Alpha-tocopherol guards against telomere shortening by reducing oxidation from free radicals. Suggested dosage is 400 IU of vitamin E daily.

Lengthen your telomeres with gamma-tocotrienol. One study reported a 16 percent increase in telomere length. The recommended dosage is 20 mg of mixed tocotrienols.

L-carnosine rebuilds tissue and gets rid of toxins. This prolongs the life cycle of your cells. The recommended dosage is 1,000 mg daily.

L-arginine increases oxygen to your cells. This amino acid helps increase nitric-oxide, which relaxes blood vessels, and also increases blood flow and oxygen to your cells. The recommended dosage is 1 to 3 g daily.

Vitamin C is an excellent DNA protector. Vitamin C slows down the shortening of telomeres up to 62 percent. Recommended dosage is up to 10 g daily.

Vitamin D₃ stimulates good immune function. It increases telomerase activity by just over 19 percent. Suggested dosage is 2,000 to 5,000 IU daily.

Milk thistle extract increases telomere activity. Milk thistle (silymarin) is a cell detoxifier, well known for restoring a damaged liver. Suggested dosage is 200 mg twice daily.

Ginkgo biloba stops the loss of telomeres. Ginkgo biloba increases the circulation of oxygen to blood vessels. Suggested dosage is 120 mg once or twice a day, cycling every four to six weeks.

Folate prevents telomere damage. Folate (vitamin B₉) stops the accumulation of homocysteine in your bloodstream, which damages telomere length. Suggested dosage is 2 to 5 mg daily.

Acetyl-L-carnitine turns on telomerase. This amino acid enhances the brain's amount of nerve growth activator, which turns on the human telomerase gene. Suggested dosage is 1,000 mg daily.

LEADING-EDGE SOLUTIONS

Supplement with more targeted stem cell activators that are designed to heal organs, tissues, and bodily systems. In addition to the LifeWave X39 Patches that were introduced in Rule #5 (Activate Cellular Rejuvenation), some of the most promising new products I have found include the line of specific stem cell activators from Medix4Life. Its formulas contain the regulatory proteins that have been extracted at a nano level and used in ultralow doses that activate your body's own stem cells in specialized areas to accelerate the healing response. These nanoceuticals are specific to the tissues and organs they target—heart, lungs, brain, ligaments, joints, tendons, and endocrine system—virtually any part of your body that needs repair and rejuvenation.

Medix4Life offers a variety of stem cell activators to address specific body systems and organs (see Resources for more information on ordering):

ADR Medix supports adrenal insufficiency as well as fatigue, exhaustion, and metabolic imbalance

BLD Medix supports oxygenation, arterial wall damage, and varicose veins

BLDR Medix supports bladder tone, incontinence, urinary urges, and bladder conditions

BRST Medix supports healthy breast tissue

CNSE Medix supports the central nervous system, including depression, anxiety, and cognitive function

CNSN Medix supports tissue and cellular regeneration of the central nervous system as well as neuropathy, nerve damage, and degenerative and pathological conditions

CNT Medix supports scarring, stretch marks, tendons, and ligaments

ENDO Medix supports hormone balance for both men and women

FEM Medix supports the female endocrine system

GB Medix supports all gallbladder conditions, including bile insufficiency, sludge, and gallstones

HRT Medix supports all heart conditions, including a history of myocardial infarctions

HYP Medix supports body temperature, water balance, and sleep and weight issues

IMN Medix supports all autoimmune conditions, including Hashimoto's, lupus, and platelet disorders

KDN Medix supports tissue and cellular regeneration in the kidneys

LGI Medix supports all degenerative digestive tract conditions, including leaky gut, IBS, and constipation

LNG Medix supports all lung and bronchial conditions

LVR Medix supports all conditions of the hepatic system, and the body's detoxification

OST Medix supports all tissue and cellular regeneration of the bones, including osteoporosis, osteopenia, and fractures

PANC Medix supports all blood sugar issues as well as pancreatic insufficiency

PROST Medix supports all prostate issues

SPL Medix supports natural immune response

THYM Medix supports the body's defense against viral and microbial infections

THYR Medix supports tissue and cellular regeneration of all thyroid conditions

METHYLATION SOLUTIONS

Avoid processed foods that contain synthetic folate. When MTHFR is switched on, your body won't process it well and it can build up just like a toxin.

Get your B vitamins from natural sources. Dark, leafy greens are rich in folate; grass-fed dairy products are rich in riboflavin; and grass-fed meats are a good source of vitamins B_6 and B_{12}.

Make sure your multivitamin supports methylation. UNI KEY Health's Advanced Daily Multivitamin contains the methylated forms of the B vitamins your body needs for proper methylation and energy production. Start slowly and work your way up—if methylation has been impaired, too many B vitamins at once may not be tolerated.

Consider a colon cleanse. Cleanse your digestive system of the harmful bugs that release toxins and impair methylation. You also need to repopulate your gut with healthy bacteria that support healthy methylation (see Resources).

Become a toxin detective. Identify and remove as many toxic products as you can from your environment. Gentle daily detox through infrared sauna, deep-breathing exercises, walking, and detox baths will all help lower your toxin load and give your methylation a chance to get back on track.

This final chapter brings us to the end of the book, but hopefully it's just the beginning of your personal quest for Radical Longevity. After reading all the Radical Rules, the Power Plan, and Targeted Strategies, the understanding that we have a choice in how we age should not seem radical at all. The elegant truth is we no longer must accept the debilitating effects of toxic overload, hormonal shifts, and emotional imbalances as inevitable effects of growing older. Instead, we can choose to make positive lifestyle changes and have a miracle mind-set with our diet and supplements. We can clean up our inner ecology as well as our indoor environment. We can choose to replenish our youthful supply of signaling molecules and tap into the peptide power of restorative and regenerative stem cell activators and cutting-edge phototherapy. The choice is ours as we enter this next phase of life with guts, grit, and grace. I hope you'll join me.

MASTER TABLE OF PRESCRIPTIVE ELEMENTS

NOTED BY RULE AND TARGETED STRATEGY

MAKING THE MOST OF THE 7 NEW RULES

RULE	NUTRITION	SUPPLEMENTS	LIFESTYLE	OTHER
Rule #1: Immunity Is Everything	Foods rich in vitamin D; e.g., beef liver, egg yolks, fatty fish and fish oil, mushrooms Zinc-rich foods; e.g., seafood, eggs, pumpkin seeds Foods rich in quercetin; e.g., capers, asparagus, cranberries, apples, kale, okra, spinach, elderberries, red grapes	Vitamin D$_3$ 2,000–5,000 IU daily Vitamin C: 2–5 g daily or Vitality C Zinc: 15–45 mg daily Quercetin: 500 mg, 2x to 3x daily Melatonin: 1–3 mg, time-release form Immune Formula	15–20 minutes sunshine daily Regular quality sleep Therapeutic bath soaks Use real soap, not sanitizers Keep house humidity at 40–60%	Tissue mineral analysis (TMA)

RULE	NUTRITION	SUPPLEMENTS	LIFESTYLE	OTHER
Rule #2: Take On Toxic Overload	Cilantro Fiber-rich diet, including chia, hemp, and flax Fiji brand water	Boron: 3 mg daily Fulvic and humic acid minerals Selenium: 200 mcg daily My Colon Cleanse: Para-Key Verma-Plus Flora-Key Oil of oregano: 1 or 2 gelcaps 2x daily, Y-C Cleanse, and high-dose Vitamin C (to bowel tolerance), along with a binder; e.g., chlorella, charcoal, citrus pectin, zeolite, or bentonite clay Osteo-Key for calcium dysregulation (contains calcium hydroxyapatite)	Avoid aluminum cookware and foil, aluminum in baking powder, deodorants, cosmetics, dental work, antacids Avoid smoking, secondhand smoke, e-cigarettes, vaping Avoid exposure to cadmium found in chocolate, seaweeds, metal containers, cookware, antiseptics Avoid mercury found in dental amalgams, fish and seafood, medications Avoid lead found in pottery, vintage dishware and glassware, and in inferior supplements Remove mold and mycotoxins from home and office Limit use of cell phone, microwave, Wi-Fi	Expanded GI panel Mycotoxin urine test ERMI (Environmental Relative Moldiness Index) Analysis Visual Contrast Sensitivity (VCS) test EMF protectors Smart meter shield EMF-blocking Faraday Bag Shungite Water filters
Rule #3: Stop AGEs (Advanced Glycation End Products)	Emphasize a plant-based diet Reduce consumption of cheese, butter, and bacon Avoid highly processed, dehydrated, and fried foods. Limit AGEs to 8,000 kU daily	Benfotiamine 300 mg Vitamins A, C, and E Selenium and zinc N-acetylcysteine, alpha-lipoic acid, chlorophyll, choline, taurine	Choose low-heat, moist, slow cooking methods: stewing, simmering, braising, or poaching Avoid high, dry cooking methods: grilling, roasting, baking, and air-frying Marinate before grilling	

RULE	NUTRITION	SUPPLEMENTS	LIFESTYLE	OTHER
Rule #4: Free Up Fascia	Bone broth High-quality collagen powders	Rath's Healthy Collagen formula (900 mg vitamin C, 900 mg L-lysine, and 450 mg L-proline) daily L-arginine: 1–3 g daily with equal amounts of lysine Trimethylglycine (TMG): 2,500–6,000 mg taken in 2 divided doses daily Endur-acin: taken as directed by health-care practitioner Gotu kola: taken as herbal tea (2 cups daily); topical paste; tincture (2 teaspoons 2x daily in water); or as a supplement (Gotu Kola Complex by MediHerbs, 1 tablet 3x daily)	Stay hydrated Daily weight-bearing exercise (minimum 30 minutes daily) 5 minutes a day rebounding on mini trampoline Relax daily in a warm Epsom salts bath or detox bath Gentle exercise or Yin Yoga	Cupping therapy Dry brushing Myofascial release massage
Rule #5: Activate Cellular Rejuvenation	Healthy omega-6s: 1 tablespoon hemp seed oil or 3 tablespoons hemp hearts daily Live Longer Cocktail (page 132) Chia seeds, flaxseeds, such herbs as marshmallow root and slippery elm Celtic, Himalayan, or Real Salt Diluted coconut water, cranberry water, citrus, or cucumber added to water Bone broth Organ meats and bone marrow	Resveratrol: Longevinex 100 mg daily ASEA Redox Signaling Molecules: 4 ounces 2x daily Chromium: 200 mg 3x daily, plus core mineral zinc Berberine: 500–1,000 mg 3x daily Vitamin D_3: 2,000–5,000 IU daily	Restorative sleep Intermittent fasting Avoid steroids, if possible Avoid quinolone antibiotics; e.g., Cipro and Levaquin	Stem cell patches

RULE	NUTRITION	SUPPLEMENTS	LIFESTYLE	OTHER
Rule #6: Mind Your Minerals	Balance copper-rich foods (avocado, soy, shellfish, tea, chocolate, nuts, and seeds) with zinc-rich meat, pumpkin, and eggs Drink tea and coffee to block iron absorption	Copper-binding resveratrol: Longevinex 100 mg Vitamin C Iron-chelating inositol hexaphosphate (IP6), 3 g 2x daily for 6 months Copper- and iron-free daily multiple vitamin Quercetin Curcumin: 500 mg 3x daily with meals N-acetylcysteine (NAC): 600 mg 1x or 2x daily	Remove copper products, including copper-lined pots, pans, and other copper kitchen items, and copper dental components Eliminate cast-iron cookware	Oxygen therapies FAR Infrared Sauna
Rule #7: Optimize the Gut-Brain Connection	Fermented foods	Flora-Key Adrenal Formula Combine Super-EPA with 100–200 mg daily of a good quality CoQ10 supplement 5-HTP: 100–200 mg daily	Avoid overuse of antibiotics Bach Flower Remedies Ignatia 30c Natrum Muriaticum 30c Lavender essential oil Orange blossom essential oil Patchouli essential oil	Communal living Online groups and communities Volunteering, attending faith-based services, and mentoring

HOW TO IMPLEMENT THE TARGETED STRATEGIES

TARGETED STRATEGIES	NUTRITION	SUPPLEMENTS	LIFESTYLE	OTHER
Reclaim Your Brain	Omega-3, -6, -7, and -9 essential fats The 3 Bs—blueberries, beets, and broccoli Colorful fruits and vegetables Lean proteins Avoid sugar 1 to 2 cups coffee daily 1 to 2 squares dark chocolate (*minimum* 60% cacao content)	Ultra H-3 Plus (includes benfotiamine, phosphatidylserine, biotin, green tea extract, PABA, ginkgo biloba, vinpocetine, niacin, huperzine A): 1 capsule 3x daily, between meals Lithium orotate: 20–80 mg daily, staggered throughout the day Astragaloside IV: 250–500 mg daily Acetyl-L-carnitine: 2,000 mg or less daily	30 minutes exercise daily Dancing Adequate restorative sleep	Parasites and Lyme testing Dynamic Neural Retraining System
Recharge Your Heart	Essential fatty acids (EFAs) Antioxidant-rich foods Lower sodium intake Increase foods high in vitamin B 100 g protein daily Eat fiber-rich foods	Magnesium: 5 mg per lb of body weight Niacin: 250 mg at bedtime, then increase gradually to 1–2 g daily D-ribose: 5 g 3x daily UNI KEY's Super EPA fish oil: 1–2 g daily CoQ10: 100–300 mg daily L-carnitine: 2–3 g spread out through the day	Quit smoking Maintain a healthy weight Exercise daily Understand your emotions	Proper blood tests (see Chapter 12) Choose foods and cooking techniques that lower AGEs

TARGETED STRATEGIES	NUTRITION	SUPPLEMENTS	LIFESTYLE	OTHER
Repair Bones, Muscles, and Joints	Bone broth Great Lakes Collagen 4 prunes daily 100 g protein daily Foods rich in vitamin D; e.g., beef liver, cheese, egg yolks, fatty fish and fish oil, and mushrooms Foods rich in selenium; e.g., Brazil nuts, walnuts, and shiitake mushrooms	Vitamin D: 2,000–5,000 IU daily Selenium: 100–200 mcg daily Osteo-Key: 3 capsules 2x daily with meals UNI KEY's Advanced Daily Multivitamin: 3 capsules 2x daily with meals Turmeric: 200–500 mg daily Sea cucumber: 1,000 mg daily Bromelain: 2,000–6,000 mg on empty stomach	20–30 minutes sunshine daily Resistance or weight-bearing exercise Rebounding Super Slow training Balance training	Whole-body vibrational training Platelet-rich plasma (PRP)
Revitalize Your Skin	Phytonutrient-rich foods Omega-6 oils: 2 tablespoons daily of hemp, safflower, sesame, or Siberian pine nut oil	Black currant seed oil: 2 g daily Silica bamboo extract: 300 mg daily Vitamin C: up to 7 g daily Proline: 1–7 g daily Lysine: up to 3,000 mg daily Glycine: 3 g daily	Dry brushing Sweating Clay masks Regular sun exposure, but avoid toxic chemical sunscreens Avoid synthetic body products	Litmus test your creams, lotions, and serums
Reverse Hair Loss	Gluten-free diet Omega-3 fats: 1–2 g daily Aloe vera: 1–2 oz daily Increase biotin	Omega-3s: 1–2 g daily Biotin (vitamin B_7): 5 mg daily Pantothenic acid (vitamin B_5): 1–2 g daily Zinc: 45 mg daily Vitamin C: 1–7 g daily Methylsulfonylmethane (MSM): 500–3,000 mg daily UNI KEY Health's HCL+2: take as directed	Avoid chlorinated and fluoridated water Avoid prescription drugs Avoid chemical-laden hair products Ferritin level test: 50–70 ng/ml is optimal	Massage scalp with rosemary essential oil

TARGETED STRATEGIES	NUTRITION	SUPPLEMENTS	LIFESTYLE	OTHER
Reignite Your Sex Life	Warming foods; e.g., beans, green leafy vegetables, seeds, artichokes, mushrooms, oysters Longevity Blaster Cranberry Elixir Omega-6 Adrenal cocktail Go gluten free Fill up on fiber-rich foods	*Panax ginseng*: 300 mg daily Libido formula containing damiana, horny goat weed, yohimbe, *Mucuna pruriens*, *Tribulus terrestris* Vitamin A: 25,000 IU daily Magnesium: 5 mg per lb of body weight daily DHEA: 5 to 25 mg daily Niacin: 50–150 mg, 15 to 30 minutes prior to sexual activity ProgestaKey cream Vitamin D: 8,000 IU daily Zinc: 25–50 mg daily Saw palmetto oil: 320 mg daily Phosphatidyl serine: 300 to 400 mg daily	Get adequate restorative sleep Walk barefoot outside for 15 minutes daily Regular exercise; avoid overexercising Kegel exercises Avoid personal care products that contain endocrine disrupters Wash hands after handling gas, cash register, or ATM receipts	Salivary hormone test or blood test Serenity TMT ThermiVa radiofrequency treatment for women PRP "O-shot" solution for female sexual dysfunction PRP "P-shot" solution for male sexual dysfunction
Taking It to the Next Level	Bone broth made with rich bone marrow Dark, leafy greens Grass-fed dairy products Grass-fed meats Avoid foods containing synthetic folate	Astragaloside IV: 250–500 mg daily EGCG: 250–500 mg daily N-acetylcysteine (NAC): 1,800–2,400 mg daily Vitamin E: 400 IU daily Gamma tocotrienol: 20 mg daily L-carnosine: 1,000 mg daily	Regular exercise Short-term fasts Gentle daily detox through infrared sauna, deep breathing exercises, detox baths Colon cleanse	Stem cell activators Support methylation Platelet-rich plasma (PRP)

RECIPE LIST

BEVERAGES
Longevity Blaster

Live Longer Cocktail

Cranberry Elixir

Cranberry Water

SOUPS, SIDES, AND SNACKS
Radical Longevity Soup

Mediterranean Lentil Soup

White Bean and Spinach Soup
  (Slow Cooker)

Meatball Soup

Tofu Egg Drop Soup

Creamy Coconut Collard Greens

Bonus Recipes

Wild Mushroom Turkey Miso Soup

Spaghetti Squash Toss

Sautéed Escarole with Chickpeas

Flax or Chia "Eggs"

MAIN DISHES
Tempting Tempeh

Smoky Black Bean Burgers

Braised Coconut Milk Chicken

Red Wine and Rosemary Marinated
  Lamb Chops

Salmon en Papillote

Bonus Recipes

Tender Roast Beef

Poached White Fish with
  Mediterranean Herbed Sauce

Steamed Ginger Chicken with
  Sesame Garlic Sauce

DRESSINGS AND MARINADES
Cilantro Lime Dressing

Hemp Hemp Hooray Dressing

Zippy Ginger Miso Dressing

Tangy Tahini and Herb Vinaigrette

French Riviera Dressing

Bonus Recipes

Teresa's Longevity Marinade

Zesty Longevity Rosemary Marinade

Island Breezes Marinade

Long Life Mediterranean Marinade

Thai One On Marinade

Marvelous Marinade

TASTY TREATS

Macadamia Nut Crème
Mocha Chocolate Surprise Cake
Pomegranate Gelatin

Bonus Recipes

Red Wine Cranberry Poached Pears
Cashew Crème
Blueberry Crumble
Chocolate-Dipped Strawberries

GRATITUDE

I want to acknowledge all my personal health heroes who didn't have the opportunity to live into old age. I especially want to remember and honor Nathan Pritikin, Dr. Robert Atkins, Robert Crayhon; Shari Lieberman, PhD; Carol Simontacchi; Jack Challem; Marcia Zimmerman; Nan Kathryn Fuchs, PhD; Nathan Pritikin; Dr. Robert Atkins; Ann Boroch; Dr. Nicolas Gonzalez; Dr. Mitchell Gaynor; Andrew Cutler, PhD; Dr. James Bradstreet; Adelle Davis; Euell Gibbons; Jerome Irving Rodale; Jim Fixx; Michel Montignac; Dr. Abram Ber; Dr. Andreas Marx; Marty Zucker; Dr. Marcus Laux; Dr. Paul Eck; Susan Stockton; Dr. Theodore Baroody; Rachel Kranz; Alice Swanson; Rev. Dr. Roberta Herzog; Dr. Hanoch Talmor; Dr. Alan Pressman; and Ann Boroch. I also wish to acknowledge my dear friends who were not granted the privilege of living a long life including football legend Don Meredith, Gracie Aldworth, Ed Aldworth, Kathie Moe, Joan Lanning, and beloved cousins Gail Fannon, Dennis Hersh, David Hersh, Gary Lorber, Allen Gittleman, and Alan Kriwitzky.

I also must acknowledge my ever-tireless literary agent who was the editor of my very first book and has seen me through many nutritional tomes—Coleen O'Shea. My most sincere appreciation goes to my favorite editor, Renée Sedliar, who has been in my corner for decades, and the Radical Longevity team from Hachette Books, including Alison Dalafave, Michelle Aielli, Michael Barrs, Mary Ann Naples, LeeAnn Falciani, Cisca L. Schreefel, Iris Bass, and Amy Quinn.

And of course, I am absolutely thrilled to have been working with the legendary Nancy Hancock—whom I met back in the days of Dr. Atkins—who made my Fat Flush a household name.

Sincere thanks go to my team on the home front—Rhonda Burns, Anne Rhody, Tracy St. Peter, Liz Patton, Tricia Pearson, and Cheryl Edwards. Thank you, ladies, for offering all your assistance in the development and creation of the different generations of the manuscript. Many thanks also to Bernie Rosen for his "eagle eye."

I am deeply grateful to my moderators online who have been assisting and leading my Facebook groups. These wonderful people include Lynn Tapper, Amanda Troxell, Bernice Gannuscio Zampano, Denise Hanson, and Linda Davis. And also some of my very faithful fans who have been with me for many years, including Debi Clem, Leslie Halbower Barrett, Tara Gloor, Trina Grace, Rachel Samson, Hillary Tinsley, Diana Gongora, Brooke Shultz, Kristin Mismash, Julee Nall, Jeanne Petersen, Amy Taormina, Gina Moore, Gene Early, Judith Smith, Sharon Erb, Patricia Coburn, Lyle Milovina, Lori Bryan, Lisa Forbes, Samantha Cannon, and Diana Hitzelberg.

I would be very remiss if I didn't acknowledge my significant brother, Stuart Gittle-man, who handles all my day-to-day business and myriad of correspondence with finesse, humor, and lots of love.

Major kudos and thanks are extended to Ben Clark, Brian Clark, Brian Linehan, and Chris Mitlitsky. My appreciation also goes out to my staff at home—the wonderful nourishing food provided by Teresa Pfaff, and the home management skills wonderfully executed by Kathleen Sullivan, and my life partner for over thirty years, James William Templeton—my one and only.

SELECTED REFERENCES

INTRODUCTION

J. D. Beasley, "The Kellogg Report," Institute of Health Policy and Practice, Bard College Center, 1989, 171.

"Drugs in the Water," *Harvard Health*, accessed November 3 and 4, 2019, https://www .health.harvard.edu/newsletter_article/drugs-in-the-water.

"From Fat Flush to First Lady of Nutrition," *Mindful Mavericks*, no. 5, https://mindful mavericksmagazine.com/issue-5-ann-louise-gittleman-fat-flush-detox-diet/.

Nicholas Kristof, "Are You a Toxic Waste Disposal Site?" *New York Times*, February 13, 2016, accessed November 3, 2019, https://www.nytimes.com/2016/02/14/opinion/sunday/are -you-a-toxic-waste-disposal-site.html.

S. Ozen and S. Darcan, "Effects of Environmental Endocrine Disruptors on Pubertal Development," *Journal of Clinical Research in Pediatric Endocrinology* 3, no. 1 (2011): 1–6, https://doi.org/10.4274/jcrpe.v3i1.01, accessed November 3, 2019.

L. Tomljenovic, "Aluminum and Alzheimer's Disease: After a Century of Controversy, Is There a Plausible Link?" *Journal of Alzheimer's Disease* 23, no. 4 (2011): 567–598, https:// doi.org/10.3233/JAD-2010-101494, accessed November 4, 2019, https://www.ncbi.nlm.nih.gov /pubmed/21157018.

B. C. Wilding, K. Curtis, and K. Welker-Hood, "Hazardous Chemicals in Health Care," Physicians for Social Responsibility, http://www.psr.org/assets/pdfs/hazardous-chemicals -in-health-care.pdf.

CHAPTER 1: NEW RULE #1: IMMUNITY IS EVERYTHING

L. Alvarez-Rodriguez et al., "Age and Low Levels of Circulating Vitamin D Are Associated with Impaired Innate Immune Function," *Journal of Leukocyte Biology* 91 (May 2012), https://doi.org/10.1189/jlb.1011523.

Y. Longtin et al., "Hand Hygiene," *New England Journal of Medicine* 364 (2011): 324, https://doi.org/10.1056/NEJMvcm0903599.

L. L. Munasinghe et al., "The Prevalence and Determinants of Use of Vitamin D Supplements Among Children in Alberta, Canada: A Cross-Sectional Study," *BMC Public Health* 15 (2015): 1063, https://doi.org/10.1186/s12889-015-2404-z.

"Stem Cells and Sleep," *Stanford Medicine* (Spring 2016), accessed November 5, 2019, https://stanmed.stanford.edu/2016spring/upfront/stem-cells-and-sleep.html.

Stephanie Taylor and Walter Hugentobler, "Is Low Indoor Humidity a Driver for Healthcare-Associated Infections?" Harvard Medical School, Boston, MA, and Institut für

Hausarztmedizin, Universität und Universitätsspital Zürich, Switzerland, accessed August 12, 2020, https://www.isiaq.org/docs/Papers/Paper340.pdf.

Z. Zakay-Rones et al., "Randomized Study of the Efficacy and Safety of Oral Elderberry Extract in the Treatment of Influenza A and B Virus Infections," *Journal of International Medical Research* 32 (2002): 132–140.

CHAPTER 2: NEW RULE #2: TAKE ON TOXIC OVERLOAD

W. R. Adey, "Biological Effects of Electromagnetic Fields," *Journal of Cellular Biochemistry* 51, no. 4 (April 1993): 410–416.

W. R. Adey, "Cell Membranes: The Electromagnetic Environment and Cancer Promotion," *Neurochemical Research* 13, no. 7 (July 1988): 671–677.

P. Allain et al., "Bromine and Thyroid Hormone Activity," *Journal of Clinical Pathology* 46, no. 5 (May 1993): 456–458, accessed November 4, 2019, https://www.ncbi.nlm.nih.gov/pmc/articles/PMC501258/.

Norm Alster, "Captured Agency: How the Federal Communications Commission Is Dominated by the Industries It Presumably Regulates," Edmond J. Safra Center for Ethics, Harvard University, Cambridge, MA.

O. M. Amin, "Seasonal Prevalence of Intestinal Parasites in the United States During 2000," *American Journal of Tropical Medicine and Hygiene* 66, no. 6 (June 1, 2002): 799–803, accessed November 4, 2019, https://www.ajtmh.org/content/journals/10.4269/ajtmh.2002.66.799.

"Arsenic and Drinking Water from Private Wells," Centers for Disease Control and Prevention, accessed September 27, 2019, https://www.cdc.gov/healthywater/drinking/private/wells/disease/arsenic.html#targetText=Once%20on%20the%20ground%20or,or%20herbicides%20in%20the%20past.

S. M. Bawin and W. R. Adey, "Sensitivity of Calcium Binding in Cerebral Tissue to Weak Environmental Electric Fields Oscillating at Low Frequency," *Proceedings of the National Academy of Science USA* 73, no. 6 (June 1976): 1999–2003.

L. Bjorkman, G. Sandborgh-Englund, and J. Ekstrand, "Mercury in Saliva and Feces After Removal of Amalgam Fillings," *Toxicology and Applied Pharmacology* 144, no. 1 (May 1997): 156–162, accessed November 4, 2019, https://www.ncbi.nlm.nih.gov/pubmed/9169079.

"Body Burden: The Pollution in Newborns," Environmental Working Group (July 14, 2005), accessed November 3, 2019, https://www.ewg.org/research/body-burden-pollution-newborns.

Jerry Carlson, "The Purdue Professor Heard 'Round the World," *Renewable Farming* (January 2018), accessed November 7, 2019, https://www.renewablefarming.com/index.php/the-purdue-professor-heard-round-the-world.

Jill Carnahan, "Your Definitive Mold Clean Up Guide," Dr. Jill: Your Functional Medicine Expert, accessed November 4, 2019, https://www.jillcarnahan.com/2018/06/12/your-definitive-mold-clean-up-guide/.

Gaétan Chevallier et al., "Earthing: Health Implications of Reconnecting the Human Body to the Earth's Surface Electrons," *Journal of Environmental and Public Health*

(2012), Article ID 291541, accessed November 7, 2019, https://www.hindawi.com/journals/jeph/2012/291541/.

Y.-H. Chiou et al., "Nickel Accumulation in Lung Tissues Is Associated with Increased Risk of p53 Mutation in Lung Cancer Patients," *Environmental and Molecular Mutagenesis* 55 (2014): 624–632, https://doi.org/10.1002/em.21867, accessed November 4, 2019.

H. R. Chung, "Iodine and Thyroid Function," *Annals of Pediatric Endocrinology & Metabolism* 19, no. 1 (March 2014): 8–12, accessed November 4, 2019, https://www.ncbi.nlm.nih.gov/pmc/articles/PMC4049553/.

K. Daniel, "Chicken Soup with Lead? Looking into a Controversy," Dr. Kaayla Daniel: The Naughty Nutritionist, 2013, accessed November 4, 2019, http://drkaayladaniel.com/boning-up-is-broth-contaminated-with-lead/.

"Dentistry," Weston A. Price Foundation, accessed November 4, 2019, https://www.westonaprice.org/dentistry.

"Dirty Dozen Endocrine Disruptors," Environmental Working Group, accessed November 3, 2019, http://www.ewg.org/research/dirty-dozen-list-endocrine-disruptors.

D. Dominic, "10 Plants That Can Absorb Electromagnetic Radiation," EMF Advice, accessed November 4, 2019, https://emfadvice.com/plants-absorb-eliminate-radiation/.

C. Exley, "Aluminum Should Now Be Considered a Primary Etiological Factor in Alzheimer's Disease," *Journal of Alzheimer's Disease Reports* 1, no. 1 (June 8, 2017): 23–25, https://doi.org/10.3233/ADR-170010, accessed November 3, 2019.

K. E. Farsalinos, V. Voudris, and K. Poulas, "Are Metals Emitted from Electronic Cigarettes a Reason for Health Concern? A Risk-Assessment Analysis of Currently Available Literature," *International Journal of Environmental Research and Public Health* 12, no. 5 (2015): 5215–5232, accessed September 27, 2019, https://doi.org/10.3390/ijerph120505215.

Andrew Goldsworthy, "The Biological Effects of Weak Electromagnetic Fields" (unpublished research, 2007).

S. Guth et al., "Toxicity of Fluoride: Critical Evaluation of Evidence for Human Developmental Neurotoxicity in Epidemiological Studies, Animal Experiments and In Vitro Analyses," *Archives of Toxicology* 94 (2020): 1375–1415.

"Health Effects of Lead Exposure," Oregon Department of Human Services, http://www.oregon.gov/oha/ph/HealthyEnvironments/HealthyNeighborhoods/LeadPoisoning/MedicalProvidersLaboratories/Documents/introhealtheffectsmedicalprovider.pdf, accessed November 4, 2019.

C. A. Hess et al., "E-Cigarettes as a Source of Toxic and Potentially Carcinogenic Metals," *Environmental Research* 152 (January 2017): 221–225, accessed November 6, 2019, https://doi.org/10.1016/j.envres.2016.09.026, accessed November 6, 2019, https://www.ncbi.nlm.nih.gov/pmc/articles/PMC5135636/.

International Association of Fire Fighters, Division of Occupational Health, Safety and Medicine, "Position on the Health Effects from Radio Frequency/Microwave (RF/MW) Radiation in Fire Department Facilities from Base Stations for Antennas and Towers for the Conduction of Cell Phone Transmissions," https://ecfsapi.fcc.gov/file/109281319517547/20-Attachment%2020-%20Firefighters%20Inter%20Resolution%20Against%20Cell%20Towers.pdf.

"Leading Causes of Death," Centers for Disease Control and Prevention, accessed November 4, 2019, https://www.cdc.gov/nchs/fastats/leading-causes-of-death.htm.

"Lyme and Other Tickborne Diseases Increasing," Centers for Disease Control and Prevention, accessed November 4, 2019, https://www.cdc.gov/media/dpk/diseases-and-conditions /lyme-disease/index.html.

Douglas Main, "Glyphosate Now the Most-Used Agricultural Chemical Ever," *Newsweek*, February 2, 2016, accessed November 7, 2019, https://www.newsweek.com /glyphosate-now-most-used-agricultural-chemical-ever-422419.

R. Mehrandish, A. Rahimiam, and A. Shahriary, "Heavy Metals Detoxification: A Review of Herbal Compounds for Chelation Therapy in Heavy Metals Toxicity," *Journal of Herbmed Pharmacology* 8, no. 2 (2019): 69–77, https://doi.org/10.15171/jhp.2019.12, accessed November 4, 2019, http://www.herbmedpharmacol.com/PDF/jhp-9359.

Geoffrey Mohan, "California Jury Awards $289 Million to Man Who Claimed Monsanto's Roundup Pesticide Gave Him Cancer," *Los Angeles Times*, August 10, 2018, accessed November 4, 2019, https://www.latimes.com/business/la-fi-roundup-verdict-20180810-story.html.

Alan Mozes, "Toxic Metals Found in E-Cigarette Vapor," WebMD (February 26, 2018), accessed November 4, 2019, https://www.webmd.com/smoking-cessation/news/20180226 /toxic-metals-found-in-e-cigarette-vapor#1.

"NASA Clean Air Study," Wikipedia, accessed September 27, 2019, https://en.wikipedia .org/wiki/NASA_Clean_Air_Study.

Clinton Ober, Stephen T. Sinatra, and Martin Zucker, *Earthing: The Most Important Health Discovery Ever!* 2nd ed. (Laguna Beach, CA: Basic Health Publications, 2014).

S. Olson, "E-Cigs' Dangerous Duo: The Lowdown on Nickel and Chromium," *Medical Daily* (September 2, 2014), accessed November 4, 2019, http://www.medicaldaily.com /e-cigarettes-emit-levels-nickel-and-chromium-4-times-higher-tobacco-smoke-300704.

S. Ozen and S. Darcan, "Effects of Environmental Endocrine Disruptors on Pubertal Development," *Journal of Clinical Research in Pediatric Endocrinology* 3, no. 1 (2011): 1–6, https://doi.org/10.4274/jcrpe.v3i1.01.

Martin L. Pall, "Microwave Frequency Electromagnetic Fields (EMFs) Produce Widespread Neuropsychiatric Effects Including Depression," *Journal of Chemical Neuroanatomy* 75, Pt. B (September 2016): 43–51, https://doi.org/10.1016/j.jchemneu.2015.08.001.

Martin L. Pall, "Scientific Evidence Contradicts Findings and Assumptions of Canadian Safety Panel 6: Microwaves Act Through Voltage-Gated Calcium Channel Activation to Induce Biological Impacts at Non-Thermal Levels, Supporting a Paradigm Shift for Microwave/Lower Frequency Electromagnetic Field Action," *Reviews on Environmental Health* 30, no. (2015): 99–116, https://doi.org/10.1515/reveh-2015-0001.

"Public Health Statement for Formaldehyde," Agency for Toxic Substances & Disease Registry (September 2008), CAS# 50-00-0, accessed November 4, 2019, https://www.atsdr.cdc.gov /phs/phs.asp?id=218&tid=39.

Sara Shannon, *Diet for the Atomic Age* (New York: Avery Publishing Group, 1987).

R. L. Siblerud and E. Kienholz, "Evidence That Mercury from Dental Amalgam May Cause Hearing Loss in Multiple Sclerosis Patients," *Journal of Orthomolecular Medicine* 12 (4th

Quarter 1997), accessed November 4, 2019, http://www.orthomolecular.org/library/jom/1997/articles/1997-v12n04-p240.shtml.

O. Tarrago and Mary Jean Brown, "Lead Toxicity—What Is the Biological Fate of Lead in the Body?" *Case Studies in Environmental Medicine*, Agency for Toxic Substances & Disease Registry (June 12, 2017), accessed November 4, 2019, https://www.atsdr.cdc.gov/csem/csem.asp?csem=34&po=9.

"The BEST Article on Glyphosate with Comments from Jeffrey Smith," Institute for Responsible Technology (February 9, 2017), accessed November 4, 2019, http://responsibletechnology.org/best-article-glyphosate-comments-jeffrey-smith/.

L. Tomljenovic, "Aluminum and Alzheimer's Disease: After a Century of Controversy, Is There a Plausible Link?" *Journal of Alzheimer's Disease* 23, no. 4 (2011): 567–598, https://doi.org/10.3233/JAD-2010-101494.

T. M. Vance and O. K. Chun, "Zinc Intake Is Associated with Lower Cadmium Burden in US Adults," Department of Nutritional Sciences, University of Connecticut, Storrs, CT, *Journal of Nutrition* 145, no. 12 (December 2015): 2741–2748, https://doi.org/ 10.3945/jn.115.223099.

N. D. Vaziri, "Mechanisms of Lead-Induced Hypertension and Cardiovascular Disease," *American Journal of Physiology—Heart and Circulatory Physiology* 295, no. 2 (August 2008): H454–H465, https://doi.org/10.1152/ajpheart.00158.2008, accessed November 4, 2019.

R. S. Walker et al., "Galvanic Interaction Between Gold and Amalgam: Effect of Zinc, Time and Surface Treatments," *Journal of the American Dental Association* 134, no. 11 (November 2003): 1463–1467, accessed November 4, 2019, https://www.ncbi.nlm.nih.gov/pubmed/14664264.

R. Williamson, "Clinical Management of Galvanic Current Between Gold and Amalgam," *General Dentistry* 44, no. 1 (January–February 1996): 70–73, accessed November 4, 2019, https://www.ncbi.nlm.nih.gov/pubmed/8940574.

B. C. Wolverton and J. D. Wolverton, "Plants and Soil Microorganisms: Removal of Formaldehyde, Xylene, and Ammonia from the Indoor Environment," *Journal of the Mississippi Academy of Sciences* 38, no. 2 (1993): 11–15.

Q. Zhai, A. Narbad, and W. Chen, "Dietary Strategies for the Treatment of Cadmium and Lead Toxicity," *Nutrients* 7, no. 1 (January 2015): 552–571, accessed November 4, 2019, https://www.ncbi.nlm.nih.gov/pmc/articles/PMC4303853/.

CHAPTER 3: NEW RULE #3: STOP AGES (ADVANCED GLYCATION END PRODUCTS)

Michael Brownlee, "Advanced Protein Glycosylation in Diabetes and Aging," *Annual Reviews of Medicine* 36 (1995): 4223–4234.

K. E. Davis et al., "Advanced Glycation End Products, Inflammation, and Chronic Metabolic Diseases: Links in a Chain?" *Critical Reviews in Food Science and Nutrition* 56, no. 6 (2016): 989–998, https://doi.org/10.1080/10408398.2012.744738.

K. Hayes, "How Much Protein Do You Need After 50?" *AARP* (February 12, 2018), https://www.aarp.org/health/healthy-living/info-2018/protein-needs-fd.html.

H. Heyn et al., "Distinct DNA Methylomes of Newborns and Centenarians," *Proceedings of the National Academy of Sciences* 109, no. 26 (June 26, 2012): 10522–10527, https://doi.org/10.1073/pnas.1120658109.

N. J. Kellow and M. T. Coughlan, "Effect of Diet-Derived Advanced Glycation End Products on Inflammation," *Nutrition Reviews* 73, no. 11 (November 2015): 737–759, https://doi.org/10.1093/nutrit/nuv030.

C. Leung et al., "Dietary Glycotoxins Exacerbate Progression of Experimental Fatty Liver Disease," *Journal of Hepatology* 60, no. 4 (April 2014): 832–838, https://doi.org/10.1016/j.jhep.2013.11.033.

Anastacia Marx de Salcedo, "10 Food Favorites Invented by the U.S. Military," accessed September 19, 2019, https://www.military.com/undertheradar/2015/08/10-food-favorites-invented-by-the-u-s-military.

C. Neves et al., "Dietary Glycotoxins Impair Hepatic Lipidemic Profile in Diet-Induced Obese Rats Causing Hepatic Oxidative Stress and Insulin Resistance," *Oxidative Medicine and Cellular Longevity* 2019, Article ID 6362910, accessed November 1, 2019, https://doi.org/10.1155/2019/6362910.

K. Nowotny et al., "Advanced Glycation End Products and Oxidative Stress in Type 2 Diabetes Mellitus," *Biomolecules* 5, no. 1 (March 16, 2015): 194–222, https://doi.org/10.3390/biom5010194.

"Obesity and Overweight: Key Facts," World Health Organization (February 16, 2018), accessed September 19, 2019, https://www.who.int/news-room/fact-sheets/detail/obesity-and-overweight#targetText=Of%20these%20over%20650%20million,tripled%20between%201975%20and%202016.

R. Ramasamy at el., "Advanced Glycation End Products and RAGE: A Common Thread in Aging, Diabetes, Neurodegeneration, and Inflammation," *Glycobiology* 15, no. 7 (July 2005): 16R–28R.

J. Uribarri et al., "Elevated Serum Advanced Glycation End Products in Obese Indicate Risk for the Metabolic Syndrome: A Link Between Healthy and Unhealthy Obesity?" *Journal of Clinical Endocrinology and Metabolism* 100, no. 5 (2015): 1957–1966.

Dr. Helen Vlassara, *AGE-less Diet* (New York: Square One Publishers, 2017), 28–29.

H. Vlassara et al., "Cachectin/TNF and IL-1 Induced by Glucose-Modified Proteins: Role in Normal Tissue Remodeling," *Science* 240, no. 4858 (1988): 1546–1548.

H. Vlassara et al., "Protection Against Loss of Innate Defenses in Adulthood by Low Advanced Glycation End Products (AGE) Intake: Role of the Anti-Inflammatory AGE Receptor-1," *Journal of Clinical Endocrinology and Metabolism* 94, no. 11 (2009): 4483–4491.

W. Wang et al., "Phytochemicals from Berries and Grapes Inhibited the Formation of Advanced Glycation End-Products by Scavenging Reactive Carbonyls," *Food Research International* 44, no. 9 (November 2011): 2666–2673.

S. Zieman and D. Kass, "Advanced Glycation End Product Cross-Linking: Pathophysiologic Role and Therapeutic Target in Cardiovascular Disease," *Congestive Heart Failure* 10, no. 3 (May–June 2004): 144–149, https://doi.org/10.1111/j.1527-5299.2004.03223.x.

CHAPTER 4: NEW RULE #4: FREE UP FASCIA
FOR YOUTHFUL MOVEMENT

"About Us: Dr. Rath," Dr. Rath: Health Begins with Cells," accessed November 3, 2019, https://shop.drrath.com/pages/about-us.

B. Bordoni, D. Lintonbon, and B. Morabito, "Meaning of the Solid and Liquid Fascia to Reconsider the Model of Biotensegrity," *Cureus Journal of Medical Science* 10, no. 7 (July 2018): e2922.

R. Bridgett et al., "Effects of Cupping Therapy in Amateur and Professional Athletes: Systematic Review of Randomized Controlled Trials," *Journal of Alternative and Complementary Medicine* 24, no. 3 (March 2018): 208–219, https://doi.org/10.1089/acm.2017.0191.

L. Cugusi et al., "Effects of a Mini-Trampoline Rebounding Exercise Program on Functional Parameters, Body Composition and Quality of Life in Overweight Women," *Journal of Sports Medicine and Physical Fitness* 58, no. 3 (March 2018): 287–294, https://doi.org/10.23736 /S0022-4707.16.06588-9.

V. Ivanov et al., "Plant-Derived Micronutrients Suppress Monocyte Adhesion to Cultured Human Aortic Endothelial Cell Layer by Modulating Its Extracellular Matrix Composition," *Journal of Cardiovascular Pharmacology* 52, no. 1 (July 2008): 55–65, https://doi .org/10.1097/FJC.ob013e31817e692f, accessed November 3, 2019, https://www.ncbi.nlm.nih .gov/pubmed/18594473.

H. Lodish et al., "Section 22.3 Collagen: The Fibrous Proteins of the Matrix," *Molecular Cell Biology*, 4th ed., accessed November 3, 2019, https://www.ncbi.nlm.nih.gov/books /NBK21582/.

CHAPTER 5: NEW RULE #5: ACTIVATE
CELLULAR REJUVENATION

S. M. Aly, "Role of Intermittent Fasting on Improving Health and Reducing Diseases," *International Journal of Health Sciences* (Qassim) 8, no. 3 (July 2014): v–vi, www.ncbi.nlm.nih .gov/pmc/articles/PMC4257368/#b4-ijhs-8-3-v.

J. L. Barger et al., "A Low Dose of Dietary Resveratrol Partially Mimics Caloric Restriction and Retards Aging Parameters in Mice," *PLoS One* 3, no. 6 (June 4, 2008): e2264, https://doi .org/10.1371/journal.pone.0002264.

J. L. Barger et al., "Short-Term Consumption of a Resveratrol-Containing Nutraceutical Mixture Mimics Gene Expression of Long-Term Caloric Restriction in Mouse Heart," *Experimental Gerontology* 43, no. 9 (September 2008): 859–866, https://doi.org/10.1016/j .exger.2008.06.013.

C. A. Connor et al., "Changes in Tripeptides Produced by the LifeWave X39 Patch," *International Journal of Healing and Caring* 20, no. 2 (May 2020).

M. H. Connor et al., "LifeWave X39 Pilot Demonstrates Light Triggered Changes," *International Journal of Healing and Caring* 20, no. 2 (2020): 1–13.

A. Fujishiro et al., "Vitamin K2 Supports Hematopoiesis Through Acting on Bone Marrow Mesenchymal Stromal/Stem Cells," *Blood* 126, no. 23 (December 3, 2015): 1192, https://doi .org/10.1182/blood.V126.23.1192.1192.

M. M. Mihaylova et al., "Fasting Activates Fatty Acid Oxidation to Enhance Intestinal Stem Cell Function During Homeostasis and Aging," *Cell Stem Cell* 22, no. 5 (May 2018): 769–778, E4, https://doi.org/10.1016/j.stem.2018.04.001, accessed November 4, 2019.

P. Mukhopadhyay et al., "Restoration of Altered MicroRNA Expression in the Ischemic Heart with Resveratrol," *PLoS One* 5, no. 12 (December 23, 2010): e15705, https://doi.org/10.1371/journal.pone.0015705.

Homer Nazeran, "A Double-Blind Placebo-Controlled Heart Rate Variability Investigation to Evaluate the Quantitative Effects of the Organic Nanoscale Aeon Patch on the Autonomic Nervous System," *TANG Humanitas Medicine* 5, no. 1 (2015): e5.

"Redox Signaling Biochemistry," ASEA Frequently Asked Questions, ASEA, accessed November 4, 2019, https://www.redoxsignalingwater.com/Products/product-frequently-asked-questions.

Pierre Volckmann, "Osteoarthritis Double-Blind Placebo Controlled LifeWave Med Pain Relief Study," *PharmaScan* (June 2013).

Kenneth Ward, "Gene Expression Profile Changes Resulting from Ingestion of ASEA Redox Dietary Supplement: An Exploratory Study," Taueret Laboratories (September 18, 2017).

K. T. Won, "The Impact of Sleep and Circadian Disturbance on Hormones and Metabolism" *International Journal of Endocrinolology* (2015): 591729, https://doi.org/10.1155/2015/591729, www.ncbi.nlm.nih.gov/pmc/articles/PMC4377487/.

CHAPTER 6: NEW RULE #6: MIND YOUR MINERALS

A. M. Abdollahi et al., "Egg Consumption, Cholesterol Intake, and Risk of Incident Stroke in Men: The Kuopio Ischaemic Heart Disease Risk Factor Study," *American Journal of Clinical Nutrition* 110, no. 1 (2019): 169–176, https://doi.org/10.1093/ajcn/nqz066.

Erik R. Anderson and Yatrik M. Shah, "Iron Homeostasis in the Liver," *Comprehensive Physiology* 3, no. 1 (January 2013): 315–330, https://doi.org/10.1002/cphy.c120016.

B. Andriopoulos et al., "Sustained Hydrogen Peroxide Induces Iron Uptake by Transferrin Receptor-1 Independent of the Iron Regulatory Protein/Iron-Responsive Element Network," *Journal of Biological Chemistry* 282, no. 28 (July 13, 2007): 20301–20308.

S. Bagheri et al., "Role of Copper in the Onset of Alzheimer's Disease Compared to Other Metals," *Frontiers in Aging Neuroscience* 9 (January 23, 2018): 446, https://doi.org/10.3389/fnagi.2017.00446.

K. D. Barker et al., "Protein Binding and the Electronic Properties of Iron(II) Complexes: An Electrochemical and Optical Investigation of Outer Sphere Effects," *Bioconjugate Chemistry* 20, no. 10 (October 21, 2009): 1930–1939, https://doi.org/10.1021/bc900270a.

Max Bayard, Jim Holt, and Eileen Boroughs, "Nonalcoholic Fatty Liver Disease," *American Family Physician* 73, no. 11 (June 1, 2006): 1961–1968.

H. L. Bonkovsky et al., "Iron in Liver Diseases Other Than Hemochromatosis," *Seminars in Liver Disease* 16, no. 1 (February 1996): 65–82.

George J. Brewer, "How to Avoid Alzheimer's Disease," *Scientia*, Health and Medicine (November 21, 2018), accessed August 13, 2020, https://www.scientia.global/professor-george-brewer-how-to-avoid-alzheimers-disease/.

George J. Brewer, "Issues Raised Involving the Copper Hypotheses in the Causation of Alzheimer's Disease," *International Journal of Alzheimer's Disease* (2011): 537528.

U. T. Brunk and A. Terman, "Lipofuscin: Mechanisms of Age-Related Accumulation and Influence on Cell Function," *Free Radical Biology and Medicine* 33, no. 5 (September 2002): 611–619.

S. Cloonan et al., "The Iron-y of Iron Overload and Iron Deficiency in Chronic Obstructive Pulmonary Disease," *American Journal of Respiratory and Critical Care Medicine* 196, no. 9 (November 1, 2017): 1103–1112, https://doi.org/10.1164/rccm.201702-0311PP.

H. Brian Dunford, "Oxidations of Iron(II)/(III) by Hydrogen Peroxide: From Aquo to Enzyme," *Coordination Chemistry Reviews* 223–234 (November 2002): 311–318.

G. Forte et al., "Metals in Plasma of Nonagenarians and Centenarians Living in a Key Area of Longevity," *Experimental Gerontology* 60 (December 2014): 197–206.

H. Gerster, "High-Dose Vitamin C: A Risk for Persons with High Iron Stores?" *International Journal for Vitamin and Nutrition Research* 69, no. 2 (March 1999): 67–82.

E. Graf, K. L. Empson, and J. W. Eaton, "Phytic Acid. A Natural Antioxidant," *Journal of Biological Chemistry* 262, no. 24 (August 25, 1987): 11647–11650.

John M. C. Gutteridge and Barry Halliwell, *Antioxidants in Nutrition, Health, and Disease* (New York: Oxford University Press, 1994), 24–39.

"Iron Contributes to the Leading Causes of Vision Loss," Iron Disorders Institute, accessed November 1, 2019, http://www.irondisorders.org/iron-contributes-to-the-leading-causes-of-vision-loss.

Y. Jiao et al., "Iron Chelation in the Biological Activity of Curcumin," *Free Radical Biology and Medicine* 40, no. 7 (April 1, 2006): 1152–1160.

B. J. Lee and D. G. Hendricks, "Phytic Acid: New Doors Open for a Chelator," *Lancet* 2, no. 8560 (September 19, 1987): 664–666.

Luca Mascitelli, Mark R. Goldstein, and Leo R. Zacharski, "Iron, Oxidative Stress, and the Mediterranean Diet," *Journal of American Medicine* 127, no. 9 (September 2014): e49.

Z. K. Mathys and A. R. White, "Copper and Alzheimer's Disease," *Advances in Neurobiology* 18 (2017): 199–216, https://doi.org/10.1007/978-3-319-60189-2_10.

J. M. McCord, "Iron, Free Radicals, and Oxidative Injury," *Seminars in Hematology* 35, no. 1 (January 1998): 5–12.

Brandon J. Perumpail et al., "Clinical Epidemiology and Disease Burden of Nonalcoholic Fatty Liver Disease," *World Journal of Gastroenterology* 24, no. 47 (December 21, 2017): 8263–8276.

J. F. Quinn et al., "A Copper-Lowering Strategy Attenuates Amyloid Pathology in a Transgenic Mouse Model of Alzheimer's Disease," *Journal of Alzheimer's Disease* 21, no. 3 (January 2010): 903–914, https://doi.org/10.3233/JAD-2010-100408.

Maryam Rameshrad, Bibi Marjan Razavi, and Hossein Hosseinzadeh, "Protective Effects of Green Tea and Its Main Constituents Against Natural and Chemical Toxins: A Comprehensive Review," *Food and Chemical Toxicology* (2016): 100, https://doi.org/10.1016/j.fct.2016.11.035.

E. P. Raven et al., "Increased Iron Levels and Decreased Tissue Integrity in Hippocampus of Alzheimer's Disease Detected *in Vivo* with Magnetic Resonance Imaging," *Journal of Alzheimer's Disease* 37, no. 1 (2013): 127–136, https://doi.org/10.3233/JAD-130209.

S. Rehault-Godbert, N. Guyot, and Y. Nys, "The Golden Egg: Nutritional Value, Bioactivities, and Emerging Benefits for Human Health," *Nutrients* (March 22, 2019), https://doi.org/10.3390/nu11030684.

"Risk of Non-Alcoholic Fatty Liver Disease in Patients with Type-1 Diabetes," *Atlas of Science* (February 18, 2019).

V. Salomaa et al., "Decline of Coronary Heart Disease Mortality in Finland During 1983 to 1992: Roles of Incidence, Recurrence, and Case-Fatality," *Circulation* 94, no. 12 (December 15, 1996): 3130–3137, https://doi.org/10.1161/01.CIR.94.12.3130.

J. Salonen, "High Stored Iron Levels Are Associated with Excess Risk of Myocardial Infarction in Eastern Finnish Men," *Circulation* 86, no. 3 (September 1992): 803–811.

B. G. Schreurs, "Cholesterol and Copper Affect Learning and Memory in the Rabbit," *International Journal of Alzheimer's Disease* (2013): 518780, https://doi.org/10.1155/2013/518780.

Terrence Wong et al., "Prevalence of Alcoholic Fatty Liver Disease Among Adults in the United States, 2001–2016," *JAMA* 321, no. 7 (2019): 1723-1725, https://doi.org/10.1001/jama.2019.2276.

T. Wyss-Coray et al., "Prominent Neurodegeneration and Increased Plaque Formation in Complement-Inhibited Alzheimer's Mice," *Proceedings of the National Academy of Sciences of the United States of America* 99, no. 16 (August 6, 2002): 10837–10842.

I. M. Zijp, O. Korver, and L. B. Tijburg, "Effect of Tea and Other Dietary Factors on Iron Absorption," *Critical Reviews in Food Science and Nutrition* 40, no. 5 (September 2000): 371–398.

CHAPTER 7: NEW RULE #7: OPTIMIZE THE GUT-BRAIN CONNECTION

B. P. Chapman et al., "Emotion Suppression and Mortality Risk over a 12-Year Follow-Up," *Journal of Psychosomatic Research* 75, no. 4 (October 2013): 381–385, accessed November 4, 2019, https://www.ncbi.nlm.nih.gov/pmc/articles/PMC3939772/.

Louise L. Hay, *You Can Heal Your Life* (Carlsbad, CA: Hay House, Inc., 2007).

Gabor Maté, *When the Body Says No: Exploring the Stress-Disease Connection* (Hoboken, NJ: John Wiley & Sons, Inc., 2003).

A. Franco-Obregón and J. A. Gilbert, "The Microbiome-Mitochondrion Connection: Common Ancestries, Common Mechanisms, Common Goals," *Microbial Systems* (May 9, 2017), https://doi.org/10.1128/mSystems.00018-17, accessed November 4, 2019, https://www.ncbi.nlm.nih.gov/pmc/articles/PMC5425687/.

E. Mostofsky et al., "Risk of Acute Myocardial Infarction After the Death of a Significant Person in One's Life," *Circulation* 125, no. 3 (January 2012): 491–496, accessed November 5, 2019, https://www.ahajournals.org/doi/10.1161/CIRCULATIONAHA.111.061770.

Candace Pert, *Molecules of Emotion: The Science Behind Mind-Body Medicine* (New York: Scribner, 1997).

H. G. Prigerson et al., "Traumatic Grief as a Risk Factor for Mental and Physical Morbidity," *American Journal of Psychiatry* 154 (April 2006): 5, 616–623, accessed November 5, 2019, https://ajp.psychiatryonline.org/doi/abs/10.1176/ajp.154.5.616?url_ver=Z39.88-2003&rfr _id=ori%3Arid%3Acrossref.org&rfr_dat=cr_pub%3Dpubmed.

"Takotsubo Cardiomyopathy (Broken-Heart Syndrome)," *Harvard's Women's Health Watch*, Harvard Health Publishing (November 2010), accessed November 5, 2019, https://www.health.harvard.edu/heart-health/takotsubo-cardiomyopathy-broken-heart-syndrome.

CHAPTER 8: ENVIRONMENT, TESTING, NUTRIENT, AND LIFESTYLE STRATEGIES

S. Cloonan et al., "The Iron-y of Iron Overload and Iron Deficiency in Chronic Obstructive Pulmonary Disease," *American Journal of Respiratory and Critical Care Medicine* 196, no. 9 (November 1, 2017): 1103–1112, https://doi.org/10.1164/rccm.201702-0311PP.

Stephanie Taylor and Walter Hugentobler, "Is Low Indoor Humidity a Driver for Healthcare-Associated Infections?" Harvard Medical School, Boston, MA, and Institut für Hausarzt-medizin, Universität und Universitätsspital Zürich, Switzerland, accessed August 12, 2020, https://www.isiaq.org/docs/Papers/Paper340.pdf.

CHAPTER 9: STOCK YOUR KITCHEN

T. O. Ajiboye et al., "Antioxidant and Drug Detoxification Potentials of Hibiscus sabdariffa Anthocyanin Extract," *Drug and Chemical Toxicology* 34, no. 2 (April 2011): 109–115, https://doi.org/10.3109/01480545.2010.536767.

M. Aviram et al., "Pomegranate Juice Consumption Reduces Oxidative Stress, Atherogenic Modifications to LDL, and Platelet Aggregation: Studies in Humans and in Atherosclerotic Apolipoprotein E-Deficient Mice," *American Journal of Clinical Nutrition* 71 (May 2000): 1062–1076.

"Dark Chocolate," Harvard T. H. Chan School of Public Health, accessed November 4, 2019, https://www.hsph.harvard.edu/nutritionsource/food-features/dark-chocolate/.

R. Ferracane et al., "Effects of Different Cooking Methods on Antioxidant Profile, Antioxidant Capacity, and Physical Characteristics of Artichoke," *Journal of Agricultural Food Chemistry* 56, no. 18 (September 24, 2008): 8601–8608, http://doi/10.1021 /jf800408w.

Johns Hopkins Medicine, "Broccoli Sprout Compound May Restore Brain Chemistry Imbalance Linked to Schizophrenia," *ScienceDaily* (May 8, 2019), accessed November 4, 2019, www.sciencedaily.com/releases/2019/05/190508093733.htm.

Jon Johnson, "Hemp Oil Benefits List," *Medical News Today* (February 2019), accessed November 4, 2019, https://www.medicalnewstoday.com/articles/324450.php.

Marilyn Johnson-Kozlow et al., "Coffee Consumption and Cognitive Function Among Older Adults," *American Journal of Epidemiology* 156, no. 9 (November 1, 2002): 842–850, https://doi.org/10.1093/aje/kwf119.

A. Jundal et al., "Radioprotective Potential of *Rosemarinus officinalis* against Lethal Effects of Gamma Radiation: A Preliminary Study," *Journal of Environmental Pathology, Toxicology and Oncology* 25, no. 4 (2006): 633–634.

M. D. Kontogianni et al., "The Impact of Olive Oil Consumption Pattern on the Risk of Acute Coronary Syndromes: The CARDIO2000 Case-Control Study," *Clinical Cardiology* 30, no. 3 (March 2007): 125–129.

Tiffany La Forge, "The Ultimate Guide to Bitters," *Healthline*, accessed November 4, 2019, https://www.healthline.com/health/food-nutrition/how-to-use-bitters.

Alexandre Mendonca and Rodrigo Cunha, "Therapeutic Opportunities for Caffeine in Alzheimer's Disease and Other Neurodegenerative Disorders Preface," *Journal of Alzheimer's Disease* 20, suppl. 1 (2010): S1–2, https://doi.org/10.3233/JAD-2010-01420.

Nutrient Data Laboratory, Beltsville Human Nutrition Research Center (BHNRC), Agricultural Research Service (ARS), US Department of Agriculture (USDA), Little Rock, AR, "Oxygen Radical Absorbance Capacity (ORAC) of Selected Foods—2007" (November 2007).

E. Rusinek-Prystupa et al., "Content of Selected Minerals and Active Ingredients in Teas Containing Yerba Mate and Rooibos," *Biological Trace Element Research* 172, no. 1 (July 2016): 266–275, https://doi.org/10.1007/s12011-015-0588-9.

Ana Sandoiu, "Blueberries May Lower Cardiovascular Risk by Up to 20 Percent," *Medical News Today* (February 2019), accessed November 4, 2019, https://www.medicalnewstoday.com/articles/324526.php.

K. Seunghae et al., "Ginger Extract Ameliorates Obesity and Inflammation via Regulating MicroRNA-21/132 Expression and AMPK Activation in White Adipose Tissue," *Nutrients* 10, no. 11 (November 2018): 1567.

D. Soyal et al., "Modulation of Radiation-Induced Biochemical Alterations in Mice by Rosemary (*Rosemarinus officinalis*) Extract," *Phytomedicine* 14, no. 10 (October 2007): 701–705.

Carol Stockton, "Omega-7 Protects Against Metabolic Syndrome," *LifeExtension* (April 2014), accessed November 4, 2019, http://www.lifeextension.com/Magazine/2014/4/Omega-7-Protects-Against-Metabolic-Syndrome/Page-01.

Hiromitsu Watanabe, "Beneficial Biological Effects of Miso with Reference to Radiation Injury, Cancer and Hypertension," *Journal of Toxicologic Pathology* 26, no. 2 (June 2013): 91–103, accessed November 4, 2019, https://www.ncbi.nlm.nih.gov/pmc/articles/PMC3695331/.

CHAPTER 10: FUEL YOUR SYSTEM

Robert G. Carroll, "Endocrine System," *Elsevier's Integrated Physiology* (2007), accessed August 20, 2020, https://www.sciencedirect.com/topics/neuroscience/glucagon.

"No Need to Avoid Healthy Omega-6 Fats," *Harvard Heart Letter*, Harvard Medical School (May 2009; updated August 20, 2019), accessed August 20, 2020, https://www.health.harvard.edu/newsletter_article/No-need-to-avoid-healthy-omega-6-fats.

CHAPTER 11: RECLAIM YOUR BRAIN

M. S. Beeri et al., "Serum Concentration of an Inflammatory Glycotoxin, Methylglyoxal, Is Associated with Increased Cognitive Decline in Elderly Individuals," *Mechanisms of Ageing and Development* 132, no. 11–12 (November–December 2011): 583–587, https://doi .org/10.1016/ j.mad.2011.10.007.

S. Bengmark, "Advanced Glycation and Lipoxidation End Products—Amplifiers of Inflammation: The Role of Food," *Journal of Parenteral and Enteral Nutrition* 31, no. 5 (2007): 430–440.

"Brain Basics: Understanding Sleep," National Institute of Neurological Disorders and Stroke, accessed November 5, 2019, https://www.ninds.nih.gov/Disorders/Patient -Caregiver-Education/Understanding-Sleep.

R. Bucala et al., "Lipid Advanced Glycosylation: Pathway for Lipid Oxidation In Vivo," *Proceedings of the National Academy of Sciences USA* 90 (1993): 6434–6438.

W. Cai et al., "Oral Glycotoxins Are a Modifiable Cause of Dementia and the Metabolic Syndrome in Mice and Humans," *Proceedings of the National Academy of Sciences USA* 111, no. 13 (April 2014): 4940–4945, https://doi.org/10.1073/pnas.1316013111.

N. V. Chuyen et al., "Toxicity of the AGEs Generated from the Maillard Reaction: On the Relationship of Food-AGEs and Biological-AGEs," *Molecular Nutrition and Food Research* 50, no. 12 (2006): 1140–1149.

T. H. Crook et al., "Effects of Phosphatidylserine in Age-Associated Memory Impairment," *Neurology* 41, no. 5 (May 1, 1991): 644–649, https://doi.org/10.1212/wnl.41.5.644.

C. Liu, "ApoE4 Accelerates Early Seeding of Amyloid Pathology," *Neuron* 96, no. 5 (December 6, 2017): 1024–1032, e3, https://doi.org/10.1016/j.neuron.2017.11.013.

L. C. Maillard, "Action des acides aminés sur les sucres: Formation des melanoidines par voie méthodique," *Comptes rendus de l'Académie des Sciences* 154 (1912): 1653–1671.

Z. Makita et al., "Advanced Glycosylation Endproducts in Patients with Diabetic Nephropathy," *New England Journal of Medicine* 325 (1991): 836–842.

G. Malanga et al., "New Insights on DMAE Features as a Free Radical Scavenger," *Drug Metabolism Letters* 6, no. 1 (March 2012): 54–59.

J. O'Brien and P. A. Morrissey, "Nutritional and Toxicological Aspects of the Maillard Browning Reaction in Foods," *Critical Reviews in Food Science and Nutrition* 28, no. 3 (1989): 211–248.

X. Pan et al., "Long-Term Cognitive Improvement After Benfotiamine Administration in Patients with Alzheimer's Disease," *Neuroscience Bulletin* 32, no. 6 (2016): 591–596.

Monira Pervin et al., "Beneficial Effects of Green Tea Catechins on Neurodegenerative Disease," *Molecules* 23, no. 6 (June 2018): 1297.

S. Sang et al., "Thiamine Diphosphate Reduction Strongly Correlates with Brain Glucose Hypometabolism in Alzheimer's Disease, Whereas Amyloid Deposition Does Not," *Alzheimer's Research & Therapy* 10, no. 1 (March 1, 2018): 26, https://doi.org/10.1186 /s13195-018-0354-2, accessed November 5, 2019, https://www.ncbi.nlm.nih.gov/pubmed /29490669.

278   Selected References

S. H. Shim et al., "Ginkgo Biloba Extract and Bilberry Anthocyanins Improve Visual Function in Patients with Normal Tension Glaucoma," *Journal of Medicinal Food* 15, no. 9 (September 2012): 818–823.

A. Spilt et al., "Late-Onset Dementia: Structural Brain Damage and Total Cerebral Blood Flow," *Radiology* 236, no. 3 (September 2005): 990–995.

"Stem Cells and Sleep," *Stanford Medicine* (Spring 2016), accessed November 5, 2019, https://stanmed.stanford.edu/2016spring/upfront/stem-cells-and-sleep.html.

Joe Verghese et al., "Leisure Activities and the Risk of Dementia in the Elderly," *New England Journal of Medicine* 348 (June 19, 2003): 2508–2516, https://doi.org/10.1056/NEJMoa022252.

M. P. Vitek et al., "Advanced Glycosylation Endproducts Contribute to Amyloidosis in Alzheimer's Disease," *Proceedings of the National Academy of Sciences USA* 91 (1994): 4766–4770.

H. Vlassara and G. E. Striker, "AGE Restriction in Diabetes Mellitus: A Paradigm Shift," *Nature Reviews Endocrinology* 7, no. 9 (May 2011): 526–539, https://doi.org/10.1038/nrendo.2011.74, Review, MID: 21610689.

M. L. Volvert et al., "Benfotiamine, a Synthetic S-acyl Thiamine Derivative, Has Different Mechanisms of Action and a Different Pharmacological Profile Than Lipid-Soluble Thiamine Disulfide Derivatives," *BMC Pharmacology* 8 (June 2008): 10, https://doi.org/10.1186/1471-2210-8-10, accessed November 6, 2019, https://www.ncbi.nlm.nih.gov/pubmed/18549472.

"What Temperature Should Your Bedroom Be?" National Sleep Foundation, accessed November 5, 2019, https://www.sleepfoundation.org/bedroom-environment/touch/what-temperature-should-your-bedroom-be.

K. Wijarnpreecha et al., "Insomnia and Risk of Nonalcoholic Fatty Liver Disease: A Systematic Review and Meta-Analysis," *Journal of Postgraduate Medicine* 63, no. 4 (October–December 2017): 226–231, accessed November 5, 2019, https://www.ncbi.nlm.nih.gov/pmc/articles/PMC5664866/.

A. V. Witte et al., "Effects of Resveratrol on Memory Performance, Hippocampal Functional Connectivity, and Glucose Metabolism in Healthy Older Adults," *Journal of Neuroscience* 34, no. 23 (June 2014): 7862–7870, https://doi.org/10.1523/JNEUROSCI.0385-14.2014, accessed November 6, 2019, https://www.ncbi.nlm.nih.gov/pubmed/24899709.

J. D. Chris Zarafonetis, "Darkening of Gray Hair During Para-Amino-Benzoic Therapy," *Journal of Investigative Dermatology* 15, no. 6 (December 1950): 399–401.

C. Zhichun and C. Zhong, "Decoding Alzheimer's Disease from Perturbed Cerebral Glucose Metabolism: Implications for Diagnostic and Therapeutic Strategies," *Progress in Neurobiology* 108 (September 2013): 21–43, accessed November 6, 2019, https://www.sciencedirect.com/science/article/pii/S0301008213000531?via%3Dihub.

CHAPTER 12: RECHARGE YOUR HEART

P. L. da Luz et al., "High Ratio of Triglycerides to HDL-Cholesterol Predicts Extensive Coronary Disease," *Clinics* 63, no. 4 (August 2008): 427–432, accessed September 30, 2019, https://www.ncbi.nlm.nih.gov/pmc/articles/PMC2664115/?log$=activity.

L. Di Donna et al., "Statin-Like Principles of Bergamot Fruit (Citrus bergamia): Isolation of 3-Hydroxymethylglutaryl Flavonoid Glycosides," *Journal of Natural Products* 72, no. 7 (July 2, 2009): 1352–1354, https://doi.org/ 10.1021/np900096w.

J. DiNicolantonio et al., "L-Carnitine in the Secondary Prevention of Cardiovascular Disease: Systematic Review and Meta-Analysis," *Mayo Clinic Proceedings* (2013), accessed October 1, 2019, https://www.medpagetoday.com/upload/2013/4/12/jmcp_ft88_4_2.pdf.

"Grief's Effect on the Heart," *Edward-Elmhurst Health* (May 2, 2017), accessed September 30, 2019, https://www.eehealth.org/blog/2017/05/impact-of-grief-on-the-heart/.

D. Heber et al., "Cholesterol-Lowering Effects of a Proprietary Chinese Red-Yeast-Rice Dietary Supplement," *American Journal of Clinical Nutrition* 69, no. 2 (February 1999): 231–236, accessed October 5, 2019, https://www.ncbi.nlm.nih.gov/pubmed/9989685.

W. Herchi et al., "Phytosterols Accumulation in the Seeds of Linum usitatissimum L," *Plant Physiology and Biochemistry* 47 no. 10 (October 2009), accessed November 5, 2019, http://www.ncbi.nlm.nih.gov/pubmed/19616960.

"High Blood Pressure FAQ," Centers for Disease Control and Prevention (November 2016), accessed October 6, 2019, https://www.cdc.gov/bloodpressure/faqs.htm.

"Hugs Heartfelt in More Ways Than One," Harvard Health Publishing (March 2014), accessed October 14, 2019, https://www.health.harvard.edu/newsletter_article/In_brief_Hugs_heartfelt_in_more_ways_than_one.

S. K. Jain, J. L. Rains, and J. L. Croad, "Effect of Chromium Niacinate and Chromium Picolinate Supplementation on Lipid Peroxidation, TNF-α, IL-6, CRP, Glycated Hemoglobin, Triglycerides, and Cholesterol Levels in Blood of Streptozotocin-Treated Diabetic Rats," *Free Radical Biology and Medicine* 43, no. 8 (October 15, 2007): 1124–1131, accessed October 1, 2019, https://ncbi.nlm.nih.gov/pmc/articles/PMC3568689.

I. Konstantinov, N. Mejevoi, and N. Anichkov, "Nikolai N. Anichkov and His Theory of Atherosclerosis," *Texas Heart Institute Journal* 33, no. 4 (2006): 417–423, accessed October 3, 2019, https://www.ncbi.nlm.nih.gov/pmc/articles/PMC1764970/.

R. W. Kuncl, "Agents and Mechanisms of Toxic Myopathy," *Current Opinion in Neurology* 22 no. 5 (October 2009): 506–515, accessed November 5, 2019, http://www.ncbi.nlm.nih.gov/pubmed/19680127.

N. A. Lee and C. A. Reasner, "Beneficial Effect of Chromium Supplementation on Serum Triglyceride Levels in NIDDM," *Diabetes Care* 17, no. 12 (December 1994): 1449–1452, accessed October 10, 2019, https://www.ncbi.nlm.nih.gov/pubmed/7882815.

T. Nwankwo et al., "Hypertension Among Adults in the US: National Health and Nutrition Examination Survey," NCHS Data Brief, no. 133 (2011–2012); National Center for Health Statistics, Centers for Disease Control and Prevention (2013).

"Obesity and Cardiovascular Disease Risk," *Cardiology Magazine* (July 23, 2018), accessed October 6, 2019, https://www.acc.org/latest-in-cardiology/articles/2018/07/06/12/42/cover-story-obesity-and-cardiovascular-disease-risk#targetText=Obesity%20has%20consistently%20been%20associated,Harold%20Bays%2C%20MD%2C%20FACC.

Stephen Sinatra, "The Ideal Homocysteine Level for Cardiac Health," accessed October 6, 2019, https://www.drsinatra.com/the-ideal-homocysteine-level-for-cardiac-health.

C. P. Stanley, W. H. Hind, and S. E. O'Sullivan, "Is the Cardiovascular System a Therapeutic Target for Cannabidiol?" *British Journal of Clinical Pharmacology* 75, no. 2 (February 2013): 313–322, accessed October 10, 2019, https://www.ncbi.nlm.nih.gov/pmc/articles/PMC3579247/.

"Takotsubo Cardiomyopathy (Broken-Heart Syndrome)," *Harvard Women's Health Watch*, Harvard Health Publishing (April 2, 2018), accessed October 6, 2019, https://www.health.harvard.edu/heart-health/takotsubo-cardiomyopathy-broken-heart-syndrome.

C. B. Taylor et al., "Spontaneously occurring angiotoxic derivatives of cholesterol," *American Journal of Clinical Nutrition* 32, no. 1 (January 1979): 40–57, accessed November 6, 2019, https://www.ncbi.nlm.nih.gov/pubmed/367149.

"The American Heart Association Diet and Lifestyle Recommendations," accessed October 6, 2019, https://www.heart.org/en/healthy-living/healthy-eating/eat-smart/nutrition-basics/aha-diet-and-lifestyle-recommendations.

"The Health Consequences of Smoking: 50 Years of Progress. A Report of the Surgeon General," US Department of Health and Human Services, Centers for Disease Control and Prevention, National Center for Chronic Disease Prevention and Health Promotion, Office on Smoking and Health (2014), accessed November 7, 2019, https://www.ncbi.nlm.nih.gov/books/NBK179276/pdf/Bookshelf_NBK179276.pdf.

"The Surprising Truth About Pre-Diabetes," Centers for Disease Control and Prevention (January 2018), accessed October 6, 2019, https://www.cdc.gov/features/diabetesprevention/index.html#targetText=You%20can%20prevent%20or%20delay,t%20know%20they%20have%20it.

Elaine M. Urbina et al., "Triglyceride to HDL-C Ratio and Increased Arterial Stiffness in Children, Adolescents, and Young Adults," *Pediatrics* 131, no. 4 (April 2013): e1082–e1090.

V. Verhoeven et al., "Red Yeast Rice Lowers Cholesterol in Physicians—a Double Blind, Placebo Controlled Randomized Trial," *BMC Complementary and Alternative Medicine* 13 (July 18, 2013): 178, accessed October 5, 2019, https://www.ncbi.nlm.nih.gov/pubmed/23866314.

Z. H. Wei et al., "Time-and-Dose-Dependent Effect of Psyllium on Serum Lipids in Mild-to-Moderate Hypercholesterolemia: A Meta-Analysis of Controlled Clinical Trials," *European Journal of Clinical Nutrition* 63 no. 7 (July 2009): 821–827, accessed November 5, 2019, http://www.ncbi.nlm.nih.gov/pubmed/18985059.

"Your Guide to Lowering Your Cholesterol with TLC," National Institutes of Health, National Heart, Lung, and Blood Institute (December 2005): NIH Publication No. 06-5235, accessed October 1, 2019, https://www.nhlbi.nih.gov/files/docs/public/heart/chol_tlc.pdf.

CHAPTER 13: REPAIR BONES, MUSCLES, AND JOINTS

G. E. Abraham and G. Harinder, "A Total Dietary Program Emphasizing Bone in Postmenopausal Women on Hormonal Therapy," *Journal of Reproductive Medicine* 35, no. 5 (May 1990): 503–507.

Jeffrey Bland, "Building Stronger Bones," *Delicious* (July–August 1988): 12.

Edith M. Carlisle, "Silicon: An Essential Element for the Chick," *Science* 178, no. 4061 (November 10, 1972): 619–621, https://doi.org/10.1126/science.178.4061.619.

C. J. Carr and R. F. Shangraw, "Nutritional and Pharmaceutical Aspects of Calcium Supplementation," *American Pharmacy* NS27, no. 2 (February 1987): 49–50, 54–57, https://doi.org:10.1016/s0160-3450(15)32077-8.

J. W. Cha et al., "The Polyphenol Chlorogenic Acid Attenuates UVB-Mediated Oxidative Stress in Human HaCaT Keratinocytes," *Biomolecular Therapy (Seoul)* 22, no. 2 (March 2014): 136–142, https://doi.org/10.4062/biomolther.2014.006, accessed November 7, 2019, https://www.ncbi.nlm.nih.gov/pmc/articles/PMC3975475/.

R. Emmons et al., "Acute Exercise Mobilizes Hematopoietic Stem and Progenitor Cells and Alters the Mesenchymal Stromal Cell Secretome," *Journal of Applied Physiology* (March 2016), accessed November 4, 2019, https://www.ncbi.nlm.nih.gov/pubmed/26744505.

L. G. Glynn et al., "Platelet-Rich Plasma (PRP) Therapy for Knee Arthritis: A Feasibility Study in Primary Care," *Pilot and Feasibility Studies* (July 2018), accessed November 4, 2019, https://www.ncbi.nlm.nih.gov/pmc/articles/PMC6030745/.

Judith Graham, "For Older Adults, a Protein-Rich Diet Is Important for Health," *Washington Post*, January 19, 2019, accessed November 4, 2019, https://www.washington post.com/national/health-science/for-older-adults-a-protein-rich-diet-is-important-for-health/2019/01/18/886926ce-1a78-11e9-88fe-f9f77a3bcb6c_story.html.

Charlotte Hilton Anderson, "8 Benefits of High-Intensity Interval Training (HIIT)," *Shape*, accessed August 23, 2020, http://www.shape.com/fitness/workouts/8-benefits-high-intensityinterval-training-hiit.

A. Hruby et al., "Protein Intake and Functional Integrity in Aging: The Framingham Heart Study Offspring," *Journals of Gerontology Series A Biological Sciences and Medical Sciences* (September 2018): 1–8, https://doi.org/10.1093/gerona/gly201.

Ken Hutchins, *Super Slow: The Ultimate Exercise Protocol* (Ken Hutchins, 1992).

Morimasa Kato, "Effect of Chlorogenic Acid Intake on Cognitive Function in the Elderly: A Pilot Study," *Evidence-Based Complementary and Alternative Medicine* (March 7, 2018), accessed November 4, 2019, https://www.ncbi.nlm.nih.gov/pmc/articles/PMC5863 287/.

Hallie Levine, "Your Metabolism: A User's Manual," *Health* (November 2016): 109–112.

E. Loughrill et al., "Calcium to Phosphorus Ratio, Essential Elements and Vitamin D Content of Infant Foods in the UK: Possible Implications for Bone Health," *Maternal and Child Nutrition* 13, no. 3 (July 2017), https://doi.org/10.1111/mcn.12368, accessed November 6, 2019, https://www.ncbi.nlm.nih.gov/pubmed/27612307.

N. Mendonca et al., "Protein Intake and Disability Trajectories in Very Old Adults: The Newcastle 85+ Study," *Journal of the American Geriatrics Society* 67, no. 1 (January 2019): 50–56, https://doi.org/10.1111/jgs.15592.

L. Metcalfe et al., "Postmenopausal Women and Exercise for Prevention of Osteoporosis: The Bone, Estrogen, Strength Training (BEST) Study," ACSM's *Health & Fitness Journal* 5, (2001): 6–14.

L. L. Munasinghe et al., "The Prevalence and Determinants of Use of Vitamin D Supplements Among Children in Alberta, Canada: A Cross-Sectional Study," *BMC Public Health* 15 (2015): 1063, https://doi.org/10.1186/s12889-015-2404-z.

F. H. Neilson et al., "Effect of Dietary Boron on Mineral, Estrogen and Testosterone Metabolism in Postmenopoausal Women," *Applied Science of Experimental Biology* 1 (1987): 394–397.

Igho Onakpoya et al., "The Use of Green Coffee Extract as a Weight Loss Supplement: A Systematic Review and Meta-Analysis of Randomised Clinical Trials," *Gastroenterology Research and Practice* (2011), accessed November 4, 2019, https://www.ncbi.nlm.nih.gov/pmc/articles/PMC2943088/.

Robert R. Recker, "Calcium Absorption and Achlorhydria," *New England Journal of Medicine* 313 (1985): 70–73.

M. M. Robinson et al., "Enhanced Protein Translation Underlies Improved Metabolic and Physical Adaptations to Different Exercise Training Modes in Young and Old Humans," *Cell Metabolism* 25, no. 3 (March 7, 2017): 581–592.

Helen M. Shields, "Rapid Fall of Serum Phosphorus Secondary to Antacid Therapy," *Gastroenterology* 75, no. 6 (1978): 1137–1141.

A. R. Sousa-Santos and T. F. Amaral, "Differences in Handgrip Strength Protocols to Identify Sarcopenia and Frailty—a Systematic Review," *BMC Geriatrics* (October 2017), accessed November 4, 2019, https://www.ncbi.nlm.nih.gov/pmc/articles/PMC5644254/.

H. Spencer and L. Kramer, "Osteoporosis: Calcium, Fluoride, and Aluminum Interactions," *Journal of the American College of Nutrition* 4, no. 1 (1985): 121–128, accessed November 6, 2019, https://www.tandfonline.com/doi/abs/10.1080/07315724.1985.10720071.

Emily M. Stein and Shonni J. Silverberg, "Bone Loss After Bariatric Surgery: Causes, Consequences and Management," *Lancet Diabetes Endocrinology* 2, no. 2 (February 2014): 165–174, accessed November 6, 2019, https://www.ncbi.nlm.nih.gov/pmc/articles/PMC4467779/.

Evelyn Whitlock, *The Calcium Plus Workbook* (New Canaan, CT: Keats Publishing, 1988), 7, 15.

Sara Wykes, "Incredible Cartilage—Focusing on Gristle in the Effort to Improve Joint Replacements," *Stanford Medicine* (2014), accessed November 4, 2019, http://sm.stanford.edu/archive/stanmed/2014summer/incredible-cartilage.html.

CHAPTER 14: REVITALIZE YOUR SKIN

Joel Bamford et al., "Oral Evening Primrose Oil and Borage Oil for Eczema," Cochrane Database of Systematic Reviews (2013): CD004416, https://doi.org/10.1002/14651858.CD004416.pub2.

A. T. Dinkova-Kostova et al., "Protection Against UV-Light-Induced Skin Carcinogenesis in SKH-1 High-Risk Mice by Sulforaphane-Containing Broccoli Sprout Extracts," *Cancer Letters* 240, no. 2 (August 28, 2006): 243–252, accessed October 22, 2019, https://www.researchgate.net/publication/7497540_Protection_against_UV-light-induced_skin_carcinogenesis_in_SKH-1_high-risk_mice_by_sulforaphane-containing_broccoli_sprout_extracts.

C. A. Downs et al., "Toxicopathological Effects of the Sunscreen UV Filter, Oxybenzone (Benzophenone-3), on Coral Planulae and Cultured Primary Cells and Its Environmental Contamination in Hawaii and the U.S. Virgin Islands," *Archives of Environmental Contamination and Toxicology* 70, no. 2 (February 2016): 265–288.

Y. Duan et al., "Toxicological Characteristics of Nanoparticulate Anatase Titanium Dioxide in Mice," *Biomaterials* 31, no. 5 (February 2010): 894–899, https://doi.org/10.1016/j.biomaterials.2009.10.003.

Elizabeth Plourde, *Sunscreens—Biohazard: Treat as Hazardous Waste* (Irvine, CA: New Voice Publications, 2011).

L. E. Rhodes et al., "Recommended Summer Sunlight Exposure Levels Can Produce Sufficient (> or =20 ng ml(–1)) but Not the Proposed Optimal (> or =32 ng ml(–1)) 25(OH)D Levels at UK Latitudes," *Journal of Investigative Dermatology* 130, no. 5 (May 2010): 1411–1418, https://doi.org/10.1038/jid.2009.417.

M. C. Rhodes et al., "Carcinogenesis Studies of Benzophenone in Rats and Mice," *Food and Chemical Toxicology* 45, no. 5 (2007): 843–851, https://doi.org/10.1016/j.fct.2006.11.003.

M. Skocaj et al., "Titanium Dioxide in Our Everyday Life: Is It Safe?" *Radiology and Oncology* 45, no. 4 (December 2011): 227–247, https://doi.org/10.2478/v10019-011-0037-0.

CHAPTER 15: REVERSE HAIR LOSS

J. Caba, "Baldness Myths: 5 Things That May or May Not Be Causing Hair Loss," *Medical Daily* (July 2014).

A. A. Cerman et al., "Vitamin D Deficiency in Alopecia Areata," *British Journal Dermatology* 170, no. 6 (June 2014): 1299–1304, PMID: 24655364, https://doi.org/10.1111/bjd.12980.

M. G. Davis et al., "A Novel Cosmetic Approach to Treat Thinning Hair," *British Journal of Dermatolology* 165, suppl. 3 (December 2011): 24–30, PMID: 22171682, https://doi.org/10.1111/j.1365-2133.2011.10633.x.

Q. Q. Dinh and R. Sinclair, "Female Pattern Hair Loss: Current Treatment Concepts," *Clinical Interventions in Aging* 2, no. 2 (June 2007): 189–199, PMCID: PMC2684510.

N. Gedgaudas, "Don't Fall for This New Study About the New 'Key to Burning Fat' (Please)," *Primal Body Primal Mind* (June 2016), https://www.primalbody-primalmind.com/dont-fall-new-study-new-key-burning-fat/.

A. Glynis, "A Double-Blind, Placebo-Controlled Study Evaluating the Efficacy of an Oral Supplement in Women with Self-Perceived Thinning Hair," *Journal of Clinical Aesthetic Dermatology* 5, no. 11 (November 2012): 28–34, PMCID: PMC3509882.

V. R. Gottumukkala et al., "Phytochemical Investigation and Hair Growth Studies on the Rhizomes of *Nardostachys jatamansi* DC," *Pharmacognosy Magazine* 7, no. 26 (April–June 2011): 146–150, https://doi.org/10.4103/0973-1296.80674.

E. D. Harris et al., "Copper and the Synthesis of Elastin and Collagen," *Ciba Foundation Symposium* 79 (1980): 163–182, PMID:6110524.

D. H. Kim et al., "Successful Treatment of Alopecia Areata with Topical Calcipotriol," *Annals of Dermatology* 24, no. 3 (August 2012): 341–344, https://doi.org/10.5021/ad.2012.24.3.341.

C. Le Floc'h et al., "Effect of a Nutritional Supplement on Hair Loss in Women," *Journal of Cosmetic Dermatology* 14, no. 1 (March 2015): 76–82, PMID: 25573272, https://doi.org/10.1111/jocd.12127.

M. Moeinvaziri et al., "Iron Status in Diffuse Telogen Hair Loss Among Women," *Acta Dermatovenerologica Croatica* 17, no. 4 (2009): 279–284, PMID: 20021982.

S. Murugusundram, "Serenoa Repens: Does It Have Any Role in the Management of Androgenetic Alopecia?" *Journal of Cutaneous and Aesthetic Surgery* 2, no. 1 (January–June 2009): 31–32, https://doi.org/10.4103/0974-2077.53097.

Y. Pahahi et al., "Rosemary Oil vs Minoxidil 2% for the Treatment of Androgenetic Alopecia: A Randomized Comparative Trial," *Skinmed* 13, no. 1 (January–February 2015): 15–21, PMID: 25842469.

H. Park et al., "The Therapeutic Effect and the Changed Serum Zinc Level After Zinc Supplementation in Alopecia Areata Patients Who Had a Low Serum Zinc Level," *Annals of Dermatology* 21, no. 2 (May 2009): 142–146, https://doi.org/10.5021/ad.2009.21.2.142.

C. A. Perry et al., "Pregnancy and Lactation Alter Biomarkers of Biotin Metabolism in Women Consuming a Controlled Diet," *Journal of Nutrition* 144, no. 12 (December 2014): 1977–1984, https://doi.org/10.3945/jn.114.194472.

L. I. Smith-Mungo and H. M. Kagan, "Lysyl Oxidase: Properties, Regulation and Multiple Functions in Biology," *Matrix Biology* 16, no. 7 (February 1998): 387–398, PMID: 9524359.

M. Tarameshloo et al., "Aloe Vera Gel and Thyroid Hormone Cream May Improve Wound Healing in Wistar Rats," *Anatomy and Cell Biology* 45, no. 3 (September 2012): 170–177, https://doi.org/10.5115/acb.2012.45.3.170.

L. B. Trost et al., "The Diagnosis and Treatment of Iron Deficiency and Its Potential Relationship to Hair Loss," *Journal of the American Academy of Dermatology* 54, no. 5 (May 2006): 824–844, PMID: 16635664, https://doi.org/10.1016/j.jaad.2005.11.1104.

R. M. Trueb, "Oxidative Stress in Ageing of Hair," *International Journal of Trichology* 1, no. 1 (January–June 2009): 6–14, https://doi.org/10.4103/0974-7753.51923.

Nina van Beek et al., "Thyroid Hormones Directly Alter Human Hair Follicle Functions: Anagen Prolongation and Stimulation of Both Hair Matrix Kerantinocyte Proliferation and Hair Pigmentation," *Journal of Clinical Endocrinology and Metabolism* 93, no. 11 (November 2008): 4381–4388.

CHAPTER 16: REIGNITE YOUR SEX LIFE

G. Benedek et al., "Estrogen Protection Against EAE Modulates the Microbiota and Mucosal-Associated Regulatory Cells," *Journal of Neuroimmunology* 15, no. 310 (September 2017): 51–59, https://doi.org/10.1016/j.jneuroim.2017.06.007. www.ncbi.nlm.nih.gov/pubmed/28778445.

R. H. Boger et al., "Restoring Vascular Nitric Oxide Formation by L-Arginine Improves the Symptoms of Intermittent Claudication in Patients with Peripheral Arterial Occlusive Disease," *Journal of the American College of Cardiology* 32, no. 5 (November 1998): 1336–1144.

S. Bolour and G. Braunstein, "Testosterone Therapy in Women: A Review," *International Journal of Impotence Research* 17, no. 5 (September–October 2005): 399–408, www.ncbi.nlm.nih.gov/pubmed/15889125.

Gaétan Chevallier et al., "Earthing: Health Implications of Reconnecting the Human Body to the Earth's Surface Electrons," *Journal of Environmental and Public Health* (2012), Article ID 291541, accessed November 7, 2019, https://www.hindawi.com/journals/jeph/2012/291541/.

L. Cormio et al., "Oral L-Citrulline Supplementation Improves Erection Hardness in Men with Mild Erectile Dysfunction," *Urology* 77, no. 1 (January 2011): 119–122.

J. Dabbs Jr., "Salivary Testosterone Measurements: Collecting, Storing, and Mailing Saliva Samples," *Physiology & Behavior* 49, no. 4 (1991): 815–817.

C. Dees et al., "Dietary Estrogens Stimulate Human Breast Cells to Enter the Cell Cycle," *Environmental Health Perspectives* 105, no. 3 (1997): 633–636.

Endocrine Society, "Overweight Men Can Boost Low Testosterone Levels by Losing Weight," *ScienceDaily*, accessed October 10, 2019, www.sciencedaily.com/releases/2012/06/120625124914.htm.

M. Euan, "Balancing Your Hormones Through Diet and Lifestyle," *Price-Pottenger Journal* 39 no. 4 (2016): 14.

Y. Y. Fan, K. S. Ramos, and R. S. Chapkin, "Dietary Gamma-Linolenic Acid Enhances Mouse Macrophage-Derived Prostaglandin E1 Which Inhibits Vascular Smooth Muscle Cell Proliferation," *Journal of Nutrition* 127, no. 9 (1997): 1765–1771.

C. J. Fuller, "Effects of Antioxidants and Fatty Acids on Low Density Lipoprotein Oxidation," *American Journal of Clinical Nutrition* 60, no. 6 (supplement) (December 1994): 1010F–1013F.

Ronald Hoffman, "Estrogen Dominance Syndrome," Ronald L. Hoffman, MD, website (October 4, 2013), accessed November 6, 2019, https://drhoffman.com/article/estrogen-dominance-syndrome-2/.

Stephen Holt, "Phytoestrogens for a Healthier Menopause," *Alternative and Complementary Therapies* 3, no. 3 (2009): 187–193.

C. Lauritzen, "Results of a 5 Year Prospective Study of Estriol Succinate Treatment in Patients with Climacteric Complaints," *Hormone and Metabolic Research* 19, no. 11 (November 1987): 579–584, www.ncbi.nlm.nih.gov/pubmed/3428874.

D. M. Lee et al., "Sexual Health and Well-Being Among Older Men and Women in England: Findings from the English Longitudinal Study of Ageing," *Archives of Sexual Behavior* (January 27, 2015), https://doi.org/10.1007/s10508-014-0465-1.

C.-S. Lin, "Advances in Stem Cell Therapy for Erectile Dysfunction," *Advances in Andrology* (2014), Article ID 140618.

E. Marcuccio et al., "A Survey of Attitudes and Experiences of Women with Heart Disease," *Women's Health Issues* 13 (2003): 23.

Vakkat Muraleedharan and T. Hugh Jones, "Testosterone and Mortality," *Clinical Endocrinology* 81 (May 2014): 477–487.

K. P. Nunes, H. Labazi, and R. C. Webb, "New Insights into Hypertension-Associated Erectile Dysfunction," *Current Opinion in Nephrology and Hypertension* 21, no. 2 (2012): 163–170.

Claes Ohlsson et al., "High Serum Testosterone Is Associated with Reduced Risk of Cardiovascular Events in Elderly Men—the MrOS (Osteoporotic Fractures in Men) Study in Sweden," *Journal of the American College of Cardiology* 58 no. 16 (October 11, 2011): 1674–1681.

S. Sandhaus and C. Schuler, "DHEA Restoration Therapy," Life Extension Foundation, www.lifeextension.com/Protocols/Metabolic-Health/Dhea-Restoration/Page-03.

J. B. Schmidt et al., "Treatment of Skin Aging with Topical Estrogens," *International Journal of Dermatology* 35, no. 9 (September 1996): 669–674.

E. Steels et al., "Physiological Aspects of Male Libido Enhanced by Standardized Trigonella foenum-graecum Extract and Mineral Formulation," *Phototherapy Research* 25, no. 9 (September 2011): 1294–1300.

CHAPTER 17: TAKING IT TO THE NEXT LEVEL

J. L. Barger et al., "Short-Term Consumption of a Resveratrol-Containing Nutraceutical Mixture Mimics Gene Expression of Long-Term Caloric Restriction in Mouse Heart," *Experimental Gerontology* 43, no. 9 (September 2008): 859–866, https://doi.org/10.1016/j.exger.2008.06.013, accessed October 12, 2019, https://www.ncbi.nlm.nih.gov/pubmed/18657603.

M. A. Blasco et al., "Telomere Shortening and Tumor Formation by Mouse Cells Lacking Telomerase RNA," *Cell* 91, no. 1 (October 1997): 25–34, accessed November 7, 2019, https://www.ncbi.nlm.nih.gov/pubmed/9335332.

Catherine de Lange, "Golfer Jack Nicklaus Says Stem Cell Therapy Cured His Back Pain," *New Scientist* (April 27, 2018), accessed November 5, 2019, https://www.newscientist.com/article/2167552-golfer-jack-nicklaus-says-stem-cell-therapy-cured-his-back-pain/.

"EPA Releases First Major Update to Chemicals List in 40 Years," US Environmental Protection Agency Press Office (February 19, 2019), accessed August 17, 2020, https://www.epa.gov/newsreleases/epa-releases-first-major-update-chemicals-list-40-years.

Michael Fossel, Greta Blackburn, and Dave Woynarowski, *The Immortality Edge* (Hoboken, NJ: John Wiley & Sons, 2011).

A. Fujishiro et al., "Vitamin K2 Supports Hematopoiesis Through Acting on Bone Marrow Mesenchymal Stromal/Stem Cells," *Blood* 126, no. 23 (December 3, 2015): 1192, accessed November 5, 2019, http://www.bloodjournal.org/content/126/23/1192.

H. Jiang et al., "Proteins Induced by Telomere Dysfunction and DNA Damage Represent Biomarkers of Human Aging and Disease," *PNAS* 105, no. 32 (August 2008): 11299–11304, accessed November 7, 2019, https://www.pnas.org/content/pnas/105/32/11299.full.pdf.

N. W. Kim et al., "Specific Association of Human Telomerase Activity with Immortal Cells and Cancer," *Science* 266, no. 5193 (December 1994): 2011–2015.

M. M. Mihaylova et al., "Fasting Activates Fatty Acid Oxidation to Enhance Intestinal Stem Cell Function During Homeostasis and Aging," *Cell Stem Cell* 22, no. 5 (May 2018): 769–778, E4, https://doi.org/10.1016/j stem.2018.04.001, accessed November 4, 2019, https://www.ncbi.nlm.nih.gov/pubmed/29727683.

Stephen Moll and Elizabeth A. Varga, "Homocysteine and *MTHFR* Mutations," *Circulation* 132 (July 7, 2015): e6–e9, https://doi.org/10.1161/CIRCULATIONAHA.114.013311.

A. J. Montpetit et al., "Telomere Length: A Review of Methods for Measurement," *Nursing Research* 63, no. 4 (July–August 2014): 289–299, accessed November 4, 2019, https://www.ncbi.nlm.nih.gov/pmc/articles/PMC4292845/.

A. Satyanarayana, M. P. Manns, and K. L. Rudolph, "Telomeres and Telomerase: A Dual Role in Hepatocarcinogenesis," *Hepatology* 40, no. 2 (August 2004): 276–283, accessed November 7, 2019, https://www.ncbi.nlm.nih.gov/pubmed/15368430.

RESOURCES

1. SUPPORT

My team and I are here to support you on your Radical Longevity journey. Visitors to my website and subscribers to my email list never miss my latest blogs and are the first to know about news and upcoming events. Plus, you can stay up to date with my latest online summits, interviews, podcasts, and television appearances.

Visit me at www.annlouise.com.

I also invite you to join my communities on Facebook or any of my other private Facebook groups for a 24/7 connection. I'll be there along with other team leaders and members to lend our support, advice, knowledge, and guidance!

Ann Louise Gittleman
www.facebook.com/
annlouisegittleman
Radical Longevity www.facebook
.com/groups/radicallongevity

Radical Metabolism www.facebook
.com/groups/radicalmetabolism
Fat Flush www.facebook.com
/groups/fatflushcommunity
Inner Circle www.facebook.com
/inner-circle

2. LONGEVITY SUPPLEMENTS AND PRODUCTS
CORE SUPPLEMENTS

The following supplements may be found at www.annlouise.com. As brand ambassador, I've proudly partnered with UNI KEY Health for over twenty-five years to provide these custom-developed formulas. They are the highest quality, combining cutting-edge science with ancient healing wisdom, and are formulated to deliver gentle yet deeply effective supplementation.

Advanced Daily Multivitamin

This iron-Free and copper-free specially designed multivitamin supplement for adults of all ages and stages of life features more than thirty key vitamins, minerals, enzymes, and antioxidants. It also contains methylated B vitamins and is uniquely designed to support optimized metabolism and weight maintenance.

Dosage: Take three (3) capsules twice daily with meals.

Mag-Key

This is a full-spectrum magnesium supplement with four highly absorbable forms plus vitamin B_6.

Dosage: Take two (2) capsules up to four times daily.

Ultra H-3 Plus

Ultra H-3 Plus, the upgraded Ultra H-3, is designed to help soothe aching joints, increase energy, help with sleep, improve mood and sense of well-being, and reawaken the brain for more mental vibrancy.

Dosage: For adults, take one (1) capsule three (3) times daily, between meals.

Daily Greens Formula

The Daily Greens Formula contains heavy metal chelating chlorella in a blend of eleven organic, non-GMO greens that can be easily mixed into the daily Live Longer Cocktail (page 132) and/or other smoothies. This combination was specifically designed to provide a variety of chlorophyll cleansing greens without the radioactive contamination typically found in seaweed and algae.

Dosage: Mix one (1) scoop (included) into smoothie, water, or beverage of your choice.

HCL+2

HCL+2 is a hydrochloric acid with bile supplement. Heartburn and GERD can often be misinterpreted as too much stomach acid when in essence, in many cases, it is too little. Optimizing the body's HCl levels can help restore comfortable digestion.

Dosage: Take one to two (1–2) caplets three (3) times daily.

Digesta-Key

Digesta-Key provides a diverse combination of pancreatic enzymes and anti-inflammatory enzymes with antioxidants and metabolic cofactors that include pancreatin, papain, rutin, bromelain, trypsin, chymotrypsin, and serrapeptase. These digestive enzymes reportedly aid the small intestine's role in digesting proteins, fats, and carbohydrates.

Dosage: Take at least two (2) with meals and two to three (2–3) between meals.

Bile Builder

Essential for those with a sluggish metabolism, poor detox genetics, and/or missing gallbladder, Bile Builder's key lipotropic ingredients (including choline, taurine, pancreatic lipase, ox bile, collinsonia root, and beet root) help thin the bile and increase bile flow. It also helps break down fats and decreases fat deposition in the liver.

Dosage: Take one to two (1–2) capsules with each meal. For those without a gallbladder, the suggested dosage is two (2) capsules per meal.

Fat Flush Body Protein

Body Protein is made from non-GMO pea and rice. It provides a complete source of essential amino acids and packs 20 g of protein per serving. Each batch is third-party tested for heavy metals, including lead, arsenic, cadmium, and mercury, and is free of sugar, gluten, dairy, and soy.

Dosage: Use one (1) scoop per smoothie (scoop included).

Fat Flush Whey Protein

This nondenatured whey protein concentrate comes from A2 grass-fed cows. It provides natural CLA as well as building blocks of glutathione It is also GMO-free, soy-free, and sugar-free.

Dosage: Use one (1) scoop per smoothie (scoop included).

Vitality C

This is the most highly bio available, buffered, neutral pH vitamin C powder on the market. It provides a whopping 4 grams of vitamin C per scoop.

Dosage: Adults can take one (1) to four (4) scoops daily.

ProgestaKey

ProgestaKey is an all-natural progesterone creme sourced from wild yam to help balance estrogen for optimal health.

Dosage: Dosage: Apply one (1) pump on days 12–25 of the calendar month.

Thyro-Key

Thyro-Key is a nonherbal combination of glandular extracts including bovine thyroid, parotid gland, pituitary gland, hypothalamus, adrenal, and liver tissue that are designed to support optimal thyroid function.

Dosage: Take one (1) tablet two to three (2–3) times daily.

Osteo-Key

As an all-inclusive bone-building formula, Osteo-Key contains a complete vitamin K complex (vitamin K_1 and two forms of vitamin K) as well as a 1:1 ratio of calcium to magnesium with the highly absorbable form of calcium microcrystalline hydroxyapatite. It also contains phosphorus, vitamin D, zinc, and boron, all balanced for maximum bone-strengthening support.

Dosage: Take three (3) capsules twice daily with meals as a dietary supplement.

Adrenal Formula

Adrenal Formula provides the building blocks to promote optimal adrenal function with whole adrenal gland and raw bovine adrenal cortex; important revitalizing nutrients include vitamin C, pantothenic acid, zinc, vitamins A and B_6, and tyrosine (a thyroid-supportive amino acid).

Dosage: Take three (3) times per day, ideally at the adrenal "times" of seven a.m., eleven a.m., and three p.m. It is recommended that individuals begin with one (1) caplet at each of these times and increase gradually until two (2) caplets are taken at the allotted times.

Y-C Cleanse

Y-C Cleanse is a homeopathic yeast and candida cleanse that contains ingredients to help neutralize the candida and enhance immunity with additional homeopathic ingredients, including echinacea.

Dosage: Adults take four (4) droppers or one (1) teaspoon in two (2) ounces of water.

My Colon Cleansing Kit (for parasites)

My Colon Cleansing Kit provides an advanced yet gentle intestinal parasite cleanse for microorganism detoxification support. As an effective natural colon cleanse to target hidden invaders, it also targets accumulated waste and toxins to promote a balanced GI tract for optimum nutrient absorption, and overall intestinal health. The addition of probiotics promotes a balanced microbiome inhospitable to all types of uninvited guests.

Dosage: Para-Key—Take two (2) capsules three (3) times daily, twenty to thirty minutes before meals. For children 40 to 80 pounds, take half the adult dosage.

Dosage: Verma-Plus—Take one-quarter (¼) teaspoon in four (4) ounces of water three (3) times daily: twice between meals on an empty stomach and once at bedtime or as directed by a health-care professional.

Immune Formula

This immune formula is unique because it contains the RNA, DNA blueprint of the two organs that play major roles in the immune systems: the thymus and the spleen. It also features "astragalus," the longevity herb that has been known for thousands of years in traditional Chinese medicine. It is further supported by the top immune-boosting nutrients vitamins A, C, D, and zinc in their most absorbable forms.

ADDITIONAL LONGEVITY SUPPLEMENTS AND PRODUCTS

ASEA

I am a proud brand ambassador for ASEA. As the only certified redox signaling supplement on the market, its unique signaling technology enables critical communication and connection between the body's cells, which ensure optimal revitalization and renewal.

Dosage: Take four (4) ounces twice daily.

888-438-5971

www.aseaglobal.com

Longevinex

Longevinex is a micronized and bioavailable form of resveratrol combined with a synergistic array of molecules designed to maximize and intensify healing benefits on the cellular level.

Dosage: Take one or two (1 or 2) tablets daily.

https://longevinex.com

LifeWave X39 Patches

As an advanced form of phytotherapy, LifeWave nano patches contain organic crystals that, when stimulated by body heat, reflect low levels of light in the infrared invisible band. The X39 stem cell patch has been clinically shown to reset four thousand genes to a younger state and help with pain relief, collagen production, and wound healing.

https://supernaturalmom.com/cellularhealth

Medix4Life Stem Cell Activators

Medix4Life offers a variety of stem cell activators to target specific body systems and organs. Medix4Life's powerful healing serums contain natural bio-regulatory peptides obtained from natural sources. You can register for an account at www.biolightstore.com/medix.html or call 770-302-6900 ext. 1 for assistance.

Biome Medic

Biome Medic is an anti-GMO supplement that helps protect your gut from glyphosate, as well as other herbicides and pesticides; its fulvic and humic acid minerals can help offset glyphosate toxicity. *Use as directed.*

Available on Amazon.

Restore

Restore promotes gut-brain health. Its ingredients are comprised of purified water and a unique soil-based mineral supplement, Terrahydrite (aqueous humic substances, mineral amino acid complexes). Environmental factors that impact the gut—GMOs, gluten, herbicides, and antibiotics—can also impact the blood-brain barrier, another critical tight junction system in the body, which is why Restore users report enhanced mental clarity. Use as directed.

Available on Amazon.

Kannaway CBD Oil

Kannaway is a "company of firsts" in CBD. Its founder, Dr. Stuart Titus, was the first person to legally bring nonpsychoactive hemp CBD to the United States in 2012. Kannaway offers the most efficacious, triple-lab-tested, natural choice when it comes to hemp CBD. As a proud member of the US Hemp Authority, Kannaway sets the standard for safety and quality. I personally recommend Kannaway's Green Oral Applicator (1,500 mg of full-spectrum CBD), Pure Gold (oil and capsules—broad spectrum), and the Salve (500 mg of CBD).

https://cbd4longlife.com

Perfect Amino

Perfect amino tablets or powder contains the eight essential fatty acids the body needs to support and maintain its skeletal, muscular, hormonal, and enzymatic systems that can be weakened with age.

800-791-3395

advancedbionutritionals.com

Telomere Benefits

Telomere Benefits is a product that features a standardized extract of Astragaloside IV (AG-IV). AG-IV supports the expression of the telomerase enzyme, which supports healthy DNA and telomere length, resulting in aging support at the genetic level.

800-325-1776

www.davincilabs.com

Gotu Kola Complex

Gotu Kola Complex is a combination of gotu kola, grape seed, and ginkgo biloba that support the normal tissue repair process and can soften scar tissue.

www.standardprocess.com

3. LIFESTYLE UPGRADES
SAFE COOKWARE

VitaClay

VitaClay is quite possibly the world's very best slow cooker with no dangerous coatings. Winner of the Good Housekeeping Best Slow Cooker Award and Top Kitchen Pick by Weight Watchers. Use coupon code "ALG+10" when ordering.

www.vitaclaychef.com

Römertopf Clay Cookers

Clay pot cooking is a centuries-old method that produces outstanding results! The Römertopf Clay Cooking Pot, glazed with a glass finish, is a healthy and natural way to cook by steaming food and allowing it to braise in its own juices.

https://www.romertopfdirect.com/USA

Xtrema Pure Ceramic Cookware

Whereas nonstick and metal cookware can leach metals and toxic chemicals into foods, Xtrema 100% ceramic cookware was developed to give home cooks a healthier alternative.

www.xtrema.com

FOOD AND BEVERAGE

Bone Broth

Kettle & Fire's bone broth provides all the health benefits of traditional bone broth without the hassle. Every batch is made with bones from 100% grass-fed, pasture-raised cattle that are hormone- and antibiotic-free.

https://www.kettleandfire.com/ann

Purity Coffee

This coffee is lab tested to be two to ten times higher in antioxidants and free of molds, pesticides, and mycotoxins. Save 10 percent off your first order with code "Detox10."

https://puritycoffee.com/

Pique Tea

Pique Tea Crystals are hot and cold water–soluble and deliver up to twelve times the antioxidant polyphenols of regular tea. Organic and triple-screened for pesticides, mycotoxins, and heavy metals as well as fluoride.

www.piquetea.com

Traditional Medicinals

Hibiscus Tea from Traditional Medicinals is one of the finest organic red hibiscus teas, known for its rich source of antioxidants and great cardiovascular benefits.

www.traditionalmedicinals.com

HEALTHY RESTAURANT GUIDE

The Templeton List

The Templeton List is your guide to the healthiest restaurants in America. This free service, provided by the Templeton Wellness Foundation, gives us an option to eat healthy when away from home. In this work in progress and labor of love, hundreds of restaurants have been contacted and interviewed to find the ones that offer healthy food options and adhere to strict ingredient, preparation, and environmental standards for smart options when eating out.

http://templetonlist.com

SAFE SKIN PRODUCTS

EssentiaClenz

EssentiaClenz is a pure and waterless natural soap whose ingredients include coconut oil, geranium, pine needle extract, chamomile, nutmeg, lemon, thyme, passionflower, apple cinnamon, eucalyptus, raspberries, sea salt, and mycelized oil of oregano. Absorbs immediately into the skin, no rinsing or washing necessary.

www.northamericanherbandspice.com

BeauCle Skin Care

With nature's purest healing herbs, beautifying botanicals, and a unique probiotic complex, BeauCle products contain the safest ingredients to restore your skin's health and youthful appearance from the outside in. The BeauCle Ultra Hydrating Moisturizer is unusual because it fades brown spots while supporting immediate hydration and sun damage repair.

800-888-4353

http://www.unikeyhealth.com/beaucle-ultra-hydrating-moisture

3rd Rock Essentials

3rd Rock Essentials offers 3rd Rock SunBlock and other chemical-free skin and body products. Let the company know I sent you by using the code "CLEANSUN."

757-486-2088

www.3rdrockessentials.com

Moremo

Moremo hair and skin care products are derived from natural ingredients, such as lemongrass, orange peel, jojoba, and avocado. Their innovative formulations treat, repair, and luxuriously moisturize your hair and skin.

www.moremo.com

PAIN RELIEF

The MELT Method

Sue Hitzmann, MS, CST, NMT, is the creator of the MELT Method, a simple self-treatment technique to relieve chronic pain. Hitzmann has developed specialty products, such as a uniquely designed foam roller and a hand and foot treatment kit that have been proven to be successful in joint and muscle pain relief.

www.meltmethod.com

Cupping Therapy

The Health Community and Health Conscience Consumers have developed a renewed interest in one of the most ancient of therapeutic healing practices: "cupping," the application of suction to the body. This traditional, time-honored treatment remains favored by millions of people worldwide because it is safe, comfortable, and remarkably effective for many health disorders. To find a qualified cupping therapist in your area, check out their website.

www.cuppingtherapy.org

Clear Passage

The Clear Passage Approach is a revolutionary hands-on technique designed to break up adhesions, scar tissue, and other blockages that prevent the muscles, organs, and systems of your body from working properly. Their technique is a natural, nonsurgical, drug-free solution that treats the core problem, not just the symptoms.

USA and Canada: 1-866-222-9437

UK: 0-808-145-3738

www.clearpassage.com

John F. Barnes Myofascial Release Approach

John F. Barnes, PT, LMT, NCTMB, is an internationally recognized physical therapist, lecturer, author, and the leading authority on myofascial release. Through his fifty years of experience and creative insight, he has developed an innovative and highly effective whole-body approach for the evaluation and treatment of pain and dysfunction. Myofascial release has exploded on the therapeutic scene with an unprecedented impact and is recognized as the most effective form of health-care therapy.

www.myofascialrelease.com/

Restoration Healthcare

The center specializes in radical antiaging and pain relief through the use of Wharton's jelly stem cells, amnion injections, ozone and UV infusions, vitamin and chelation treatments, NAD, shockwave, and so much more. Mention that Ann Louise sent you and receive 10 percent off any procedure. Ask about their Rest and Renew Package that includes a stay at the beautiful Coeur d'Alene Resort during your treatment.

208-231-1018

www.restoration-healthcare.com/

Active Release Technique (ART)

Active release technique focuses on relieving tissue tension via the removal of adhesions that can develop in tissues as a result of repetitive use and overload stress. These disorders may lead to muscular weakness, numbness, aching, tingling, and burning sensations. For more information and to find a practitioner in your area, check out

www.activerelease.com

NEURO-COGNITIVE
ImPACT Test

ImPACT test professionals are experts in concussion care and management. Because concussions normally do not show up on a CT scan or MRI, a concussion specialist can use several other tools to diagnose a concussion and recommend a tailored treatment. These include balance screening, neurocognitive testing, a physical examination, and vestibular ocular examination. They can also assist you in finding a concussion specialist in your area.

www.impacttest.com

NEURAL RETRAINING

The Dynamic Neural Retraining System

The Dynamic Neural Retraining System offers a natural, drug-free healing program that can help you recover from many disorders, including chronic fatigue syndrome, multiple chemical sensitivity, fibromyalgia, chronic Lyme disease, food sensitivities, anxiety, chronic pain, postural orthostatic tachycardia syndrome, and more.

800-947-9389

https://retrainingthebrain.com

DENTAL HEALTH

Huggins Applied Healing

Dr. Huggins addresses the issue of dental toxicity due to mercury in amalgam fillings as the cause of many unexplained diseases and health issues. Other services include standard dental practices, such as root canals, also shown to contribute to many health issues for which the medical community often has no explanation.

866-948-4638

www.HugginsAppliedHealing.com

Directory of Biological Dentists, Doctors, and Allied Professionals

https://iabdm.org/location

The International Academy of Oral Medicine and Toxicology

https://iaomt.org

FITNESS TRAINING

Super Slow

Super Slow is a slow-motion strength training program popularized by Ken Hutchins during his research on osteoporosis. It requires less workout time than traditional weight training. Check for a location near you.

Power Plate

Whole-body vibration was first used by the cosmonauts to combat muscle and bone loss caused by extended stays in zero gravity. Today, Power Plate (known as advanced acceleration training) has continued developing the technology to create products and training programs that deliver legendary performance for professional sports teams, medical facilities, health clubs, studios, and individuals around the globe.

877-877-5283

http://powerplate.com

WOMEN'S HEALTH

MoisturePom

MoisturePom is an all-natural vaginal ointment for tissue renewal and provides ongoing relief from the burning, irritation, and itching due to vaginal dryness.

800-661-5176

www.pomhealth.com

Serenity TMT—Pelvic Floor Massage Tool

The curved design of the Serenity pelvic floor massage tool is ideal for intravaginal use. The smooth tapered end allows for easy insertion, while the longer handle allows for more controlled maneuverability.

800-382-5879

https://www.cmtmedical.com/ or amazon.com

ThermiVa

ThermiVa is a quick, noninvasive, nonablative treatment delivering physician-controlled radiofrequency energy using a thoughtfully designed handpiece to gently heat tissue.

www.thermiva.com

FOR YOUR HOME

Water and Air Filtration

Highly recommended filtration systems are the under-counter or countertop water filters with Metalgon that remove chlorine, parasites, and lead for safe drinking water straight out of the tap.

800-888-4353

http://www.unikeyhealth.com/under-counter-ultra-ceramic-water-filter

Clean Water Revival (CWR)

CWR specializes in custom-designed water filtration equipment, including its Ultra-Ceramic Water Filter, under-counter or countertop, as well as showerhead filter. CWR also has air purifiers and survival and personal protection equipment. For a free consultation to determine the exact type of water filtration for your home, based on your geographical locale, see contact info below:

800-444-3563

www.cwrenviro.com

Environmental Protection Agency Safe Drinking Water Hotline

800-426-4791

National Testing Laboratories, Inc.

800-458-3330

www.ntllabs.com

Suburban Water Testing

800-433-6595

www.suburbantestinglabs.com

HOME REMEDIATION

International Institute for Bau-Biology & Ecology

The International Institute for Bau-Biology & Ecology is a nonprofit North American organization that combines building biology, ecological principles, and technical expertise to support healthy living and a more sustainable environment, according to the precautionary principle. Certified building biology professionals can check for mold, volatile organic compounds (VOCs), electromagnetic fields (EMFs), and radon.

http://hbelc.org

ELECTROPOLLUTION

Aulterra Global

Aulterra's products for the office, car, and home provide powerful protection from the harmful effects of EMF radiation, including a whole-house plug, cell phone neutralizers, and protective pillows. Aulterra's EMF neutralizing products are scientifically proven to neutralize EMF exposure, including 5G.

208-635-5034

https://aulterra.com

Less EMF

Less EMF provides a wide range of products designed for identifying and protecting against electromagnetic pollution. The Less EMF Air Tube Headset is especially a must-have, since no radiation can travel up the wire to the earpiece.

518-608-6479

www.lessemf.com

Smart Meter Guard

Smart Meter Guard safely shields over 98 percent of the EMF, radio frequency, and radiation emitting from smart meters. No drilling or grounding wires needed. Portable, so you can take it with you if you move.

info@smartmeterguard.com

https://smartmeterguard.com/

Faraday Bag

Faraday bags block GPS, radio frequency, wireless, cell phone, and Bluetooth signals from both being sent and received to an electronic device, such as a mobile phone, car key, or laptop. They come in a range of sizes to shield different devices and can stop cyberattacks to your important digital device.

https://faradaybag.com/

Greenwave

Greenwave provides a meter and filters that measure and reduce dirty electricity present on electrical wiring in homes, schools, businesses, and more.

800-506-6098

https://greenwavefilters.com

Shungite Queen—EMF Protective Shungite Jewelry and Home Goods

This nearly metal-free jewelry is handmade from natural stones and crystals with natural electromagnetic field (EMF) protective qualities, such as genuine Russian shungite. Customizable and special orders are welcome.

www.shungitequeen.com

The Earthing Institute

All the latest scientific studies proving the efficacy of earthing can be found at this site as well as earthing technologies for your lifestyle.

info@earthinginstitute.net

www.earthinginstitute.net

SAUNA

Influence

Influence Sauna provides the most advanced Infrared Therapy available with unprecedented temperatures of 170 degrees (which is crucial for optimized detoxification), and the lowest

EMF-ELF on the market. There are no toxins used in manufacturing, no off-gassing, and the Canadian cedar smells like heaven and will not mold. And the price is much better than any other high-quality units by other brands.

866-626-6532

www.influencesauna.com/bestsauna

Relax FAR Infrared Sauna

This portable sauna uses patented ceramic semiconductor chips that filter out all nonhealing energies. The FDA has verified that the invisible light rays produced by the Relax Sauna radiators are between 4 and 14 microns, which means that these rays are 100 percent absorbable for infrared light.

614-262-7087

www.relaxsaunas.com

4. DIAGNOSTIC TESTS
MINERALS AND HEAVY METAL TESTING
Tissue Mineral Analysis (Hair)

The analysis includes a full report, up to twenty pages, which graphically shows the levels of thirty-two major minerals and six toxic metals in the body. Each mineral is fully evaluated in terms of its relationship with other minerals, which is a key to glandular function and metabolism rate. This report provides information on the effect of vitamin deficiency and excesses. There is also a complete discussion regarding environmental influences and disease tendencies, based upon mineral levels and ratios. A list of recommended food choices and supplements, based upon the individual findings, is included at the end of the report. UNI KEY uses Trace Elements, an independent testing laboratory specializing in hair tissue mineral analysis for health-care professionals worldwide.

800-888-4353

www.unikeyhealth.com/tissue-mineral-analysis

OTHER HEAVY METAL TESTING LABS
Analytical Research Laboratories (ARL)

Based on the work of Dr. Paul C. Eck, ARL provides a quality line of dietary supplements specifically formulated to balance body chemistry based on hair tissue mineral analysis.

602-995-1580

https://arltma.com

Doctor's Data

Doctor's Data is a specialist and forerunner in essential and toxic elemental testing, as well as other innovative specialty tests including tissue mineral analysis.

800-323-2784

www.doctorsdata.com

Cyrex Labs

Cyrex Labs is an advanced clinical laboratory that tests for antibody response to heavy metals, mold, and chemicals.

877-772-9739

www.cyrexlabs.com

LEAD TESTING

If you want to test your antique china pattern for possible lead contamination, you can order a lead-testing kit available at

https://www.epa.gov/lead/lead-test-kits

MERCURY TESTING

Quicksilver Scientific

The Tri-Test measures methylmercury and inorganic mercury, allowing analysis of exposure sources, body burden, and the ability to excrete each form of mercury.

303-531-0861

https://www.quicksilverscientific.com/testing/mercury-tri-test

Ferritin Blood Test

Ferritin testing is crucial; whereas a high level of ferritin is associated with iron overload, low ferritin levels can indicate that one may be at risk of being iron deficient. A ferritin test can be ordered online without a doctor's prescription from the following:

https://requestatest.com

https://www.lifeextension.com

RBC Zinc Test

Request A Test lab offers affordable consumer direct testing, including Zinc RBC.

888-732-2348

www.requestatest.com

PARASITES AND GASTROINTESTINAL TESTING

Expanded GI Panel (for parasite treatment)

The Expanded GI Panel done through DiagnosTechs can detect parasites and find possible causes for digestive problems, gluten intolerance and other food sensitivities, hyperactivity, leaky gut syndrome, inflammatory bowel disease (IBD), chronic fatigue, constipation, and fibromyalgia. The Expanded GI Panel tests for

1. *H. pylori*, *C. difficile*, *Candida albicans*, and fungus

2. Protozoa and worms, including giardia, *Blastocystis hominis*, roundworm, toxoplasma, *Trichinella spiralis* (from swine), and tapeworm

3. Allergies to gluten, cow's milk, eggs, and soy

4. Intestinal function markers including GI immunity-SIgA, pancreatic enzyme output, colon inflammation, blood in stool, and stool pH

800-888-4353

www.unikeyhealth.com/expanded-gi-panel

OTHER GUT AND STOOL TESTING

Genova Diagnostics

Genova Diagnostics is a provider of comprehensive and innovative clinical laboratory services for the prevention, diagnosis, and treatment of complex chronic disease. Its GI Effects Comprehensive Stool Profile is an advanced stool test that provides immediate clinical information for the management of gastrointestinal health. The company also offers a genetic detoxification profile called DetoxiGenomic Profile.

800-522-4762

www.gdx.net

Viome

Viome offers gut microbiome testing with the ability to analyze all the organisms in the gut and offer personalized nutrition and diet recommendations intended to optimize your gut ecosystem. It is the first company to offer an at-home test to measure RNA for improving individual health.

www.viome.com

LYME

IGeneX, Inc.

This team of talented scientists utilize cutting-edge technology to find new solutions that challenge the status quo of testing for Lyme and associated tick-borne diseases. It was the first to introduce Relapsing Fever Western Blot testing and the first to introduce comprehensive Lyme ImmunoBlot and TBRF ImmunoBlot testing.

800-832-3200

https://igenex.com

CHEMICAL TOXICITY

The Great Plains Laboratory, Inc.

The Great Plains Laboratory is the provider for glyphosate testing. Glyphosate is the world's most widely produced herbicide and is the primary toxic chemical in Roundup, as well as in many other herbicides. This lab also offers the MycoTOX Profile for mold exposure and a GPL-TOX Profile—a toxic nonmetal chemical profile—that screens for the presence of 173 different toxic chemicals.

800-288-0383

https://www.greatplainslaboratory.com

MOLD

Mycometrics

Founded in 2005, Mycometrics is a microbiology laboratory specializing in the identification of fungi (e.g., molds) and bacteria from the environments. Its EPA-approved test called the ERMI (Environmental Relative Moldiness Index) Analysis can identify the molds, bacteria, toxins, and viruses that may be negatively affecting your health.

732-355-9018

www.mycometrics.com

Visual Contrast Sensitivity

Visual contrast sensitivity testing measures your ability to see details at low contrast levels and is often used as a nonspecific test of neurological function. It can be used to identify mold sensitivity or toxicity.

www.vcstest.com

Mycotoxin Urine Test from Realtime Labs

The RealTime Labs mycotoxin test detects fifteen different mycotoxins. Testing is done using competitive ELISA, a very sensitive detection method using antibodies prepared against mycotoxins.

Patients: 972-521-9975

Doctors: 972-492-0419

https://realtimelab.com/mycotoxin-testing

ALLERGY TESTING
Immuno Laboratories

Immuno Laboratories in Fort Lauderdale, Florida, is widely recognized as one of the leading food and environmental allergy testing facilities in the world. Since its inception, the company has conducted over thirty-three million food sensitivity tests, with 97 percent of its physicians continuing testing for ten years or more—a clear indication of physician and patient satisfaction.

800-231-9197

www.immunolabs.com

HORMONES
Salivary Hormone Test

A feature of this test is that your result and a personal letter of recommendation from my office are mailed directly to you using the DiagnosTechs lab, a pioneer and leader in offering salivary hormone testing. Unlike blood tests, which do not measure bioavailable hormone activity, saliva testing is considered to be the most accurate measure of free, bioavailable hormonal activity. This personal hormone evaluation can be used to profile up to six hormones: estradiol, estriol, progesterone, testosterone, DHEA, and cortisol.

800-888-4353

www.unikeyhealth.com/salivary-hormone-test

OTHER HORMONE LABS AND TESTS
Precision Analytical Inc.

This lab uses a unique and comprehensive new dried urine testing method that measures hormones and how estrogen is being secreted.

https://dutchtest.com

ZRT's Urine Metabolites Profile

ZRT offers a blood spot hormone test kit with results equivalent to conventional blood tests.

www.zrtlab.com

Meridian Valley Lab

Meridian Valley Lab offers the CompletePLUS hormone profile. This is a comprehensive twenty-four-hour urine hormone and metabolite test that helps doctors use bioidentical hormone replacement therapy safely and effectively. The lab also offers dried urine hormone testing as well as tests for food sensitivities and allergies.

206-209-4200

http://meridianvalleylab.com

GENOMIC (DNA)
23andMe

Perhaps the best-known personal genetics company, 23andMe helps you begin your gene exploration using a saliva sample. Upon receiving your results, you can use 23andMe's relative finder in addition to learning about your disease risks based on your unique profile and can determine common genetic mutations that can impair detoxification. You can then upload the data to a genome tool like geneticgenie.org to analyze the information.

800-239-5230

www.23andme.com

LivingDNA

Using a saliva sample, you can uncover your DNA story, optimize your well-being, improve the quality of your life, and discover your family ancestry.

www.livingdna.com

METHYLATION AND DETOX ANALYSIS
Genetic Genie

This website works in conjunction with your 23andMe results to provide a methylation and/ or detoxification profile. Your 23andMe results grant full access to view your methylation and detox profiles.

http://geneticgenie.org

TELOMERE
SpectraCell Laboratories

Telomere testing is the best marker in quantifying biological age and it serves as a useful biomarker for risk assessment.

800-227-5227

www.spectracell.com/patients/patient-telomere-testing

5. NEWSLETTERS, MAGAZINES, BOOKS, AND WEBSITES
NEWSLETTERS
The Health Sciences Institute (HSI) Newsletter

HSI is an independent organization dedicated to uncovering and researching the most urgent advances in modern underground medicine. As a member of the professional advisory panel, I can verify that this cutting-edge newsletter is devoted to presenting extraordinary products to its members before the products hit the marketplace. HSI provides private access to hidden cures, powerful discoveries, breakthrough treatments, and advances in modern medicine.

888-213-0764

http://hsionline.com

MAGAZINES

First for Women Magazine

First for Women delivers helpful tips and credible information you can't get anywhere else, with numerous motivational articles on living a well-rounded life, nurturing family, owning a pet, preparing healthy menus, and just having fun! I am proud to be a regular contributor.

201-569-6699

www.firstforwomen.com

Total Health Online Magazine

The mission of *Total Health Online* magazine is to advocate self-managed natural health, emphasize the importance of becoming the cocaptain of your own health-care team, and address the imperatives to wellness. The magazine provides readers with the information and resources needed to establish and maintain optimum health. I am an associate editor for this outstanding publication.

http://totalhealthmagazine.com

Taste for Life

Taste for Life in-store magazines can be found in health food stores, natural product chains, food co-ops, and supermarkets nationwide. The publication provides excellent articles on pertinent health issues and serves as an informative educational source on a variety of levels. I am proud to sit on *Taste for Life*'s editorial board. The online website also provides a one-stop natural health resource.

www.tasteforlife.com

Woman's World Magazine

A magazine with information and inspiration on topics ranging from food to decor to beauty to nutrition, it boasts a circulation of approximately 1.6 million readers. It has held the title of the most popular newsstand women's magazine for many years. My "Radical Health Tips" column can be found in each weekly edition.

www.womansworld.com

BOOKS
BOOKS BY ANN LOUISE GITTLEMAN, PHD, CNS

Here are a list and brief descriptions of my books that are noteworthy companions for your Radical Longevity journey.

Radical Metabolism: A Powerful New Plan to Blast Fat and Reignite Your Energy in Just 21 Days

ISBN: 0738234702

In my national bestselling book, I give you menu plans, fifty sumptuous recipes, an extensive resource section, and everything you need to supercharge your metabolism and transform your body into a fat-burning dynamo in just twenty-one days.

www.radicalmetabolism.com

The NEW Fat Flush Plan

ISBN: 9781259861130

A fully updated edition of my *New York Times* bestseller. Like its pioneering predecessor, *The NEW Fat Flush Plan* offers evidence-based detox and diet strategies that are simple, safe, and effective, with a heightened emphasis on the role of liver health and the metabolic impact of foods.

HERE ARE SOME OF MY PERSONAL FAVORITES

I Used to Have Cancer: How I Found My Own Way Back to Health

James Templeton, founder of UNI KEY Health Systems, Inc., and the Templeton Wellness Foundation, ISBN 0757004784

James Templeton's memoir is an inspiring look back at his unique journey in overcoming Stage IV melanoma and remaining cancer free for over three decades and counting. James takes you with him on a trip crisscrossing America, during which he shares the various natural approaches he followed to battle his cancer—from diet and supplements to meditation and lifestyle adjustments.

www.iusedtohavecancer.com

Harmonic Healing: Restore Your Vital Force for Lifelong Wellness

Linda Lancaster

ISBN-13: 9781635653175

From "a pioneer in integrative medicine" comes a comprehensive program anchored in Ayurveda, yoga, energy medicine, homeopathy, and nutrition.

PROFESSIONAL ORGANIZATIONS FOR BETTER HEALTH

Academy for Comprehensive Integrative Medicine (ACIM)

ACIM's mission is to bring the best in integrative medical education, research, and professional referrals regarding all aspects of human health to the broadest segment of global society. Exceptional online courses are available with professors from all over the world.

800-958-0703

www.acimconnect.com

Academy of Integrative Health & Medicine (AIHM)

AIHM is a global organization that educates and trains clinicians in integrative health and medicine. Its focus is on individualized health care backed by evidence-based research.

858-240-9033

www.aihm.org/

American Academy of Anti-Aging (A4M)

The A4M is dedicated to the advancement of technology to detect, prevent, and treat aging-related disease and educating physicians, scientists, and members of the public about biomedical sciences, breaking technologies, and antiaging issues.

561-997-0112

www.a4m.com

American Academy of Craniofacial Pain (AACP)

AACP specializes in the relief of craniofacial pain, temporomandibular disorders, and dental sleep-related disorders. It also supports the advancement of education, research, and skills in these areas.

800-322-8651

www.aacfp.org

American Academy of Environmental Medicine

The American Academy of Environmental Medicine is an international association of physicians and other professionals who study the effects of our complex environment and our physical health. Topics studied include air pollution, mold, mycotoxins, and more. The academy also provides a physician referral for various conditions.

316-684-5500

www.aaemonline.org

American Academy of Stem Cell Physicians (AASCP)

AASCP is an organization created to advance research and the development of therapeutics in regenerative medicine. It is also an excellent educational resource for physicians, scientists, and the public in this new field of stem cell therapy.

305-891-4686

www.aascp.net

American College for Advancement in Medicine (ACAM)

ACAM enables the public to connect with integrative physicians and learn about integrative medicine treatment options in their area.

800-532-3688

www.acam.org

Best Answer for Cancer Foundation (BAFC)

BAFC's mission is to improve the quality of life and treatment of cancer patients with a holistic platform, targeted cancer therapies, and a patient-centered approach.

512-342-8181

https://bestanswerforcancer.org

International Academy of Oral Medicine and Toxicology (IAOMT)

The IAOMT is an organization that supports the effort to inform consumers about health risks from amalgam mercury, water fluoridation, and safe ways to eliminate these risks.

863-420-6373

http://iaomt.org

International Association for Colon Hydrotherapy (I-ACT)

This association strives to ensure continuing and progressive education in the field of colon hydrotherapy.

210-366-2888

www.i-act.org

International College of Craniomandibular Orthopedics (ICCMO)

For over thirty-five years, ICCMO has specialized in the scientific advancement and education in occlusion, neuromuscular dentistry, and TMJ/TMD diagnosis and treatment.

866-379-3656

http://iccmo.org

National Association of Nutrition Professionals (NANP)

If you are interested in pursuing a nutrition consultant or natural chef certification, the NANP has developed two rigorous sets of educational standards for both. Every school that appears on its Recommended Educational Programs page has been approved by NANP's thorough review process, ensuring a comprehensive and well-rounded curriculum.

800-342-8037

www.nanp.org

NeuroLipid Research Foundation

The NeuroLipid Research Foundation pursues the core cause of the patient's disease/disorder and recommends addressing membrane fatty acid disturbances and epigenetic (toxic exposure) factors as a means of healing and health.

856-431-5505

www.neurolipid.store

Templeton Wellness Foundation

James Templeton created the Templeton Wellness Foundation to help you fight and win your battle against cancer. After staring death in the face over thirty years ago and beating cancer using a natural, radical approach to healing, James is living his best life now. It is his personal mission to inspire HOPE and to provide the latest resources and information for anyone facing a similar battle or seeking cancer prevention. The foundation has compiled an extensive collection of first-hand interviews with late-stage cancer survivors as well as many of the foremost cancer experts from across the world today.

https://templetonwellness.com

INDEX